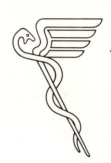

1981
YEAR BOOK OF

**SPORTS
MEDICINE**

THE 1981 YEAR BOOKS

The YEAR BOOK series provides in condensed form the essence of the best of the recent international medical literature. The material is selected by distinguished editors who critically review more than 500,000 journal articles each year.

Anesthesia: *Drs. Eckenhoff, Bart, Brunner, Cane and Linde.*

Cancer: *Drs. Clark, Cumley and Hickey.*

Cardiology: *Drs. Harvey, Kirkendall, Kirklin, Nadas, Resnekov and Sonnenblick.*

Clinical Pharmacy: *Dr. Woolley.*

Dentistry: *Drs. Hale, Hazen, Moyers, Redig, Robinson and Silverman.*

Dermatology: *Drs. Dobson and Thiers.*

Diagnostic Radiology: *Drs. Whitehouse, Adams, Bookstein, Gabrielsen, Holt, Martel, Silver and Thornbury.*

Drug Therapy: *Drs. Hollister and Lasagna.*

Emergency Medicine: *Dr. Wagner.*

Endocrinology: *Drs. Schwartz and Ryan.*

Family Practice: *Dr. Rakel.*

Medicine: *Drs. Rogers, Des Prez, Cline, Braunwald, Greenberger, Bondy and Epstein.*

Neurology and Neurosurgery: *Drs. De Jong and Sugar.*

Nuclear Medicine: *Drs. Hoffer, Gottschalk and Zaret.*

Obstetrics and Gynecology: *Drs. Pitkin and Zlatnik.*

Ophthalmology: *Dr. Hughes.*

Orthopedics: *Dr. Coventry.*

Otolaryngology: *Drs. Paparella and Strong.*

Pathology and Clinical Pathology: *Dr. Brinkhous.*

Pediatrics: *Drs. Oski and Stockman.*

Plastic and Reconstructive Surgery: *Drs. McCoy, Brauer, Haynes, Hoehn, Miller and Whitaker.*

Psychiatry and Applied Mental Health: *Drs. Freedman, Friedhoff, Kolb, Lourie, Nemiah and Romano.*

Sports Medicine: *Col. Anderson, Mr. George, Drs. Krakauer, Shephard and Torg.*

Surgery: *Drs. Schwartz, Najarian, Peacock, Shires, Silen and Spencer.*

Urology: *Drs. Gillenwater and Howards.*

The YEAR BOOK of

Sports Medicine

1981

Editors

Col. JAMES L. ANDERSON, PE.D.
Director of Physical Education
United States Military Academy

FRANK GEORGE, A.T., C., R.P.T.
Head Athletic Trainer
Brown University

LEWIS J. KRAKAUER, M.D., F.A.C.P.
Adjunct Professor of Health, Oregon State University
Assistant Clinical Professor of Medicine,
University of Oregon Medical School

ROY J. SHEPHARD, M.D., Ph.D.
Director, School of Physical and Health
Education and Professor of Applied Physiology,
Department of Preventive Medicine and Biostatistics,
University of Toronto

JOSEPH S. TORG, M.D.
Professor of Orthopedic Surgery and Director,
Sports Medicine Center, University of Pennsylvania
School of Medicine

YEAR BOOK MEDICAL PUBLISHERS, INC.
CHICAGO • LONDON

22, 62, 117-9, 321 347.
121-2.

Table of Contents

The material covered in this volume represents literature reviewed up to February 1981.

Acknowledgments

We sincerely thank Hiroyuki Nakajima, M.D., for his efforts again this year in surveying Japanese-language articles and providing English abstracts and expert commentary. The illustrations appearing in this YEAR BOOK were obtained from the authors of the original papers, and we thank them for their cooperation.

Journals Represented

Acta Chirurgica Scandinavica
Acta Endocrinologica
Acta Odontologica Scandinavica
Acta Orthopaedica Scandinavica
Acta Paediatrica Scandinavica
Acta Radiologica: Diagnosis
Alaska Medicine
American Corrective Therapy Journal
American Heart Journal
American Journal of Cardiology
American Journal of Clinical Nutrition
American Journal of Diseases of Children
American Journal of Physical Medicine
American Journal of Physiology
American Journal of Roentgenology
American Journal of Sports Medicine
American Review of Respiratory Disease
American Surgeon
Angiology
Annals of Emergency Medicine
Annals of Internal Medicine
Archives of Internal Medicine
Archives of Pathology and Laboratory Medicine
Archives of Physical Medicine and Rehabilitation
Athletic Training
Aviation Space and Environmental Medicine
British Heart Journal
British Journal of Diseases of the Chest
British Journal of Radiology
British Medical Journal
Canadian Family Physician
Canadian Medical Association Journal
Chest
Circulation
Consultant
Contemporary Orthopedics
Deutsche Medizinische Wochenschrift
Diabetologia
European Journal of Applied Physiology and Occupational Physiology
Foot and Ankle
Hawaii Medical Journal
Injury
Journal of Allergy and Clinical Immunology
Journal of the American Medical Association
Journal of Applied Physiology
Journal of Bone and Joint Surgery: American Volume

Journal of Bone and Joint Surgery: British Volume
Journal of Cardiovascular Surgery
Journal of Clinical Endocrinology and Metabolism
Journal of Clinical Investigation
Journal of Laboratory and Clinical Medicine
Journal of Nuclear Medicine
Journal of Orthopaedics and Sports Physical Therapy
Journal of Pediatrics
Journal de Radiologie
Journal of Sports Medicine and Physical Fitness
Journal of Thoracic and Cardiovascular Surgery
Journal of Trauma
Lancet
Medical Journal of Australia
Medicine and Science in Sports
Metabolism
New England Journal of Medicine
New York State Journal of Medicine
Nouvelle Presse Medicale
Ophthalmic Surgery
Orthopedics
Pain
Pediatrics
Physical Therapy
Physician and Sports Medicine
Postgraduate Medicine
Quintessence International
Radiology
Research Quarterly for Exercise and Sports
Respiration Physiology
Revue de Chirurgie Orthopedique
Runner's World
Scandinavian Journal of Clinical and Laboratory Investigation
Schweizerische Medizinische Wochenschrift
South African Medical Journal
Southern Medical Journal
Spine
Surgery, Gynecology and Obstetrics
Thorax
Thrombosis and Haemostasis
Topics in Emergency Medicine
Undersea Biomedical Research
Undersea Medical Society, Bethesda, Md.
Urology
Western Journal of Medicine
Yale Journal of Biology and Medicine

1. Exercise Physiology

1–1 **Regional Distribution of Cerebral Blood Flow During Exercise in Dogs.** Paul M. Gross, Melvin L. Marcus, and Donald D. Heistad (Univ. of Iowa) sought to determine whether exercise produces vasodilatation in regions of the brain associated with motor functions despite the associated vasoconstrictor effect of hypocapnia. Nine dogs were trained to run on a treadmill before catheterization. Total and regional cerebral blood flow (CBF) were measured with microspheres during moderate treadmill exercise. Exercise was at averages of 7 mph and 3% grade and 10 mph and 9% grade. Cerebral vascular responses at rest were studied by stimulation of ventilation with doxapram. This stimulus produced arterial hypertension and hypocapnia similar in magnitude to those during exercise.

During moderate exercise, the dogs experienced substantial tachycardia and hypertension. Exercise redistributed CBF. Total blood flow to the brain was not significantly changed at either level of exercise, but flow to the motor-sensory cerebral cortex, spinal cord, and cerebellum was significantly increased during the higher level of exercise. The increase in blood flow to the cerebellum occurred primarily in the cortical layers. Vascular resistance increased in all regions of the brain except the cerebral and cerebellar cortex and spinal cord, in which resistance was unchanged (table). Injection of doxapram in resting, restrained dogs increased arterial pressure and produced arterial hypocapnia. Doxapram produced hyperventilation but did not appear to produce discomfort. Total and regional CBFs were de-

EFFECT OF EXERCISE ON REGIONAL CEREBRAL VASCULAR RESISTANCE

	Rest	Exercise 1	Exercise 2
Regional cerebral vascular resistance, $Torr \cdot ml^{-1} \cdot min^{-1} \cdot 100\ g^{-1}$			
Total brain	1.9 ± 0.3	$2.4 \pm 0.4^*$	$2.2 \pm 0.4^*$
Motor-sensory cortex	1.4 ± 0.2	1.8 ± 0.3	1.2 ± 0.2
Cerebral white matter	4.4 ± 0.1	$5.4 \pm 0.2^*$	$5.7 \pm 0.2^*$
Brain stem	2.4 ± 0.3	$3.4 \pm 0.5^*$	$3.0 \pm 0.5^*$
Cerebellar cortex	1.6 ± 0.2	1.7 ± 0.3	1.4 ± 0.3
Spinal cord	5.7 ± 0.1	6.0 ± 0.3	5.8 ± 0.3

*Significantly different from rest at $P < .05$. All values are means $\pm$ SE for 9 dogs.

(1–1) J. Appl. Physiol. 48:213–217, February 1980.

creased significantly during resting arterial hypocapnia. In contrast to exercise, which also was associated with hypocapnia, there was a fairly uniform reduction in blood flow to all regions of the brain after doxapram.

Exercise in conscious dogs increases blood flow in regions of the brain associated with movement despite the associated vasoconstrictor stimulus of arterial hypocapnia. Thus, during exercise, local dilator influences that presumably result from increases in metabolism predominate over a potent constrictor stimulus in regulation of cerebral vascular resistance.

▶ [Exercise in man has generally been thought to have little effect on cerebral blood flow. However, technical factors have permitted examination only of the total cerebral blood flow. The present study of dogs is interesting in showing that regions of the brain involved in the control of physical activity have an increased regional perfusion during exercise.—R.J.S.] ◀

1–2 **Alteration by Hyperoxia of Ventilatory Dynamics During Sinusoidal Work.** Richard Casaburi, Richard W. Stremel, Brian J. Whipp, William L. Beaver, and Karlman Wasserman (Torrance, Calif.) studied the responses of normal subjects to sinusoidal variations of work rate and rate of pedaling. They sought to determine whether the carotid chemoreceptors contribute to ventilatory dynamics during sinusoidal exercise and to quantitate the effects of acute decreases in the sensitivity of carotid chemoreceptors on the kinetics of ventilatory control during exercise.

Subjects were studied while breathing oxygen and while breathing air so that each might serve as his own control. Ventilatory and gas exchange responses were analyzed so that changes in ventilatory kinetics could be related to any concomitant changes in carbon dioxide-related variables. Five subjects exercised on 14 occasions on a cycle ergometer for 30 minutes with a sinusoidally varying work load. Tests were performed at seven frequencies of work load during air or 100% oxygen inspiration. From the breath-by-breath responses to the tests, dynamic characteristics were analyzed.

The responses to normoxic and hyperoxic exercise showed no appreciable variation of the mean of the sinusoidal fluctuation with the period of the fluctuation for any of the variables examined for either inhalate. Figure 1–1 presents the average amplitude of the end-tidal oxygen tension (PET_{CO_2}) fluctuation for the subjects studied as a function of the period of the work rate sinusoid during normoxic and hyperoxic exercise. The fluctuation amplitude increased from its steady-state level and then dropped off sharply at the higher forcing frequencies for both inhalates. The PET_{CO_2} fluctuated more during hyperoxia than during normoxia, suggesting that arterial carbon dioxide tension was less tightly regulated.

The increased amplitude of the PET_{CO_2} fluctuations seen during hyperoxia probably reflects increased arterial carbon dioxide tension fluctuation. Hyperoxia apparently "loosens" the link between carbon dioxide output and ventilation; the kinetics of ventilation are slowed

(1–2) J. Appl. Physiol. 48:1083–1091, June 1980.

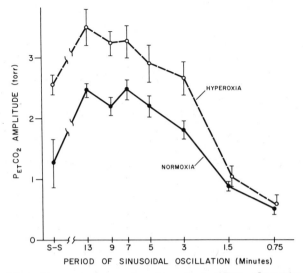

Fig 1–1.—Effect of hyperoxia on mean-to-peak amplitude of Pet_{CO_2} fluctuation at each sinusoidal work rate period and in steady state *(S-S)*. Points are mean response (±SE) of five subjects. (Courtesy of Casaburi, R., et al.: J. Appl. Physiol. 48:1083–1091, June 1980.)

relative to those of carbon dioxide output, and, consequently, arterial carbon dioxide tension is less tightly controlled. The carotid bodies play a role in respiratory control during exercise, tracking changes in metabolically produced carbon dioxide and thus minimizing potential changes in arterial carbon dioxide tension.

▶ [Breathlessness is probably the most common clinical reason for halting vigorous exercise. Nevertheless, argument continues over mechanisms of ventilatory control during physical activity. Ventilation seems closely related to carbon dioxide output, but there has been no very convincing demonstration of the pulmonary venous carbon dioxide receptors that such a relationship might imply. The present authors have developed an interesting technique for application of a sinusoidally varying work load; this enables them to explore phase relationships among work output, ventilation, and arterial carbon dioxide tension. The experiments described in this report show a larger fluctuation of end-tidal (and, by implication, arterial) carbon dioxide tension during hyperoxia than during normoxia. Because the carbon dioxide sensitivity of the carotid bodies is depressed by hyperoxia, the authors conclude that these structures contribute to ventilation during exercise. This is probably true of sinusoidally varying activity, but may not necessarily apply to steady-state work.—R.J.S.] ◀

1–3 **Energy Expended During Oxygen Deficit Period of Submaximal Exercise in Man.** It is known that the rate of creatine phosphate (CP) hydrolysis is greater than the CP production rate during the oxygen deficit of the early phase of exercise. Thus, the total energy released during oxygen deficit exercise can be expected to be less than during steady-state exercise. P. Pahud, E. Ravussin, and E. Jequier (Univ. of Lausanne) investigated this hypothesis by studying aerobic and anaerobic metabolic rates during the transition from mild (50 W external work) to more strenuous exercise (50% $\dot{V}O_2$max) in 6

(1–3) J. Appl. Physiol. 48:770–775, May 1980.

healthy male volunteers. Overall exercise efficiency on a cycle ergometer was calculated during oxygen deficit exercise and steady-state exercise. Aerobic metabolism (MR) was determined by indirect calorimetry, while anaerobic metabolism (M_{an}) was obtained by solving the heat balance equation: $MR + M_{an} - S = (R + C + E) + W$, where radiant (R), convective (C), and evaporative (E) heat losses were measured by direct calorimetry; work output (W) was measured by cycle ergometry; and heat storage (S) was measured by thermometry.

During oxygen deficit exercise, $MR + M_{an}$ was lower than MR during steady-state exercise. The mean mixed work efficiency (aerobic and anaerobic) was 33% during the first minute of exercise, compared with 26.6% aerobic efficiency during steady-state exercise, while the anerobic efficiency of oxygen deficit exercise was 41%. The difference in efficiencies indicates that the energy released by splitting of preformed high-energy bonds, such as CP, is less than the energy released when high-energy bonds, expended for the mechanical work performed, are continuously regenerated through oxidative phosphorylation.

The results indicate that almost two thirds of the energy liberated by the oxidation of foods are captured in the form of high-energy bonds.

▶ [Anaerobic exercise is generally held to be only about half as efficient as aerobic activity (see Shephard, R. J.: *Textbook of Exercise Physiology and Biochemistry,* Praeger, New York, 1981). However, traditional calculations assume resynthesis of creatine phosphate (CP). In the early phases of activity, breakdown of CP exceeds resynthesis. The authors show, by a nice application of heat balance equations, that this phase of effort has an efficiency of about 41%. Aerobic resynthesis has an efficiency of 64%, so that the combined efficiency of CP breakdown and reformation is $\left(\dfrac{41 \times 64}{100}\right)\% =$ 26.2% Their estimate for steady-state exercise of 26.6% $\pm$ 0.5% is close to this figure when work is done on a cycle ergometer. However, in the early phase of oxygen deficit the contribution from CP breakdown boosts the apparent efficiency to 33%.—R.J.S.] ◀

1-4 **Ventilatory Response to Carbon Dioxide in Hyperoxic Exercise.** J. Duffin, R. R. Bechbache, R. C. Goode, and S. A. Chung (Univ. of Toronto) measured the sensitivity of the ventilatory response to carbon dioxide in hyperoxia during light exercise in 14 healthy volunteers (13 men), aged 21 to 31 years. The rebreathing method of Read was used to measure the respiratory response. During all of the experimental runs, the volunteers wore earphones playing music devoid of strong rhythmic content. They breathed through a wide-bore, three-way Y valve. One side of the valve was connected to a T piece and tubing so that controlled gas compositions from a set of rotameters could be breathed without rebreathing. The other side of the Y valve was connected directly to a rebreathing bag. At rest, the bag was filled with 6 L of a mixture of 50% oxygen, 43% nitrogen, and 7% carbon dioxide. The subjects were studied at rest while they sat on the cycle ergometer in the same posture as in the exercise runs. After 5 minutes of breathing a hyperoxic mixture containing 50% oxygen-50% nitrogen and when stable end-tidal carbon dioxide and ox-

(1–4) Respir. Physiol. 40:93–105, April 1980.

ygen readings were obtained, the subjects were switched from the T piece to the rebreathing bag. They rebreathed for 4 minutes or until discomfort was felt. The carbon dioxide concentration was then gradually decreased to zero to prevent possible headaches. The same procedure was followed during exercise, except that the carbon dioxide concentration in the rebreathing bag was increased to 9.5% during 25-W exercise. The occurrence of a proper plateau in end-tidal carbon dioxide was essential for continuance of the rebreathing test. Two volunteers underwent steady-state measurements of the ventilatory response to carbon dioxide at rest and during exercise (25 W) as a check on the results obtained from the rebreathing tests.

Two factors produced artifactual changes in the slope of the response during exercise. (1) Breath-by-breath response lines showed that the maximum limit of ventilation was reached in 3 volunteers before the end of rebreathing, despite the low exercise load. The inclusion of such breaths in the calculation of the slope of the response could produce an artifactual decrease in slope. (2) Most of the response lines showed an increase in their slopes during exercise. However, a model of rebreathing in exercise showed that an increase in sensitivity could be the result of variation in the difference between end-tidal and central chemoreceptor carbon dioxide values during exercise. A criterion derived from the model, proportional to the variation in this difference, was found to be correlated with the increase in sensitivity from rest to exercise.

The sensitivity of the ventilatory response to carbon dioxide during light exercise is unchanged from that at rest.

▶ [Many studies of respiratory control during exercise have used the slope of the ventilation versus end-tidal carbon dioxide pressure as an index of responsiveness. This article makes a useful contribution by pointing out two errors in this basic index: (1) Some subjects may reach the limit of ventilation, depressing the slope (this would be a major difficulty in older patients with chest disease). (2) Discrepancies between end-tidal and central chemoreceptor carbon dioxide pressures tend to increase the slope (again, such differences would likely be augmented in respiratory disease).—R.J.S.] ◀

1–5 **Strength Training Effects on Aerobic Power and Short-Term Endurance.** R. C. Hickson, M. A. Rosenkoetter, and M. M. Brown (Univ. of Illinois, Chicago) assessed a training regimen developed to strengthen the quadriceps muscles to determine if differences in maximum oxygen uptake during bicycle and treadmill exercise are due to inadequate muscle strength. Circuit training results in little or no improvement in work capacity and maximal oxygen uptake, but it is possible that strenuous heavy resistance training involving few repetitions can increase strength to levels at which work capacity or maximal oxygen uptake are improved. Nine healthy men aged 18–27 years participated in the study. Weight training was carried out 5 days a week for 10 weeks. Parallel squats, knee flexions and extensions, leg presses, and calf raises were carried out.

Endurance time to exhaustion on cycling increased significantly after training with a 47% change. Endurance time while running in-

(1–5) Med. Sci. Sports Exerc. 12:336–339, 1980.

EFFECTS OF STRENGTH TRAINING ON MAXIMUM OXYGEN UPTAKE AND ENDURANCE DURING BICYCLE AND TREADMILL EXERCISE

	$\dot{V}O_2{}_{max}$ (Liters · min⁻¹)		$\dot{V}O_2{}_{max}$ ml·kg⁻¹·min⁻¹		Endurance (sec.)	
	Bicycle	Treadmill	Bicycle	Treadmill	Bicycle	Treadmill
Pre-training	3.40 ±0.22	3.70 ±0.16	44.0 ±2.3	47.8 ±1.5	278 ±27	291 ±14
Post-training	3.54[a] ±0.22	3.85 ±0.20	44.6 ±2.4	48.8 ±2.0	407[b] ±32	325[b] ±12

Values are means ± SE for 9 persons.
[a]Pretraining vs. posttraining ($P<.05$).
[b]Pretraining vs. posttraining ($P<.01$) (paired t test).

creased 12% when the men exercised at their pretraining maximal oxygen uptake. A small increase in maximal oxygen uptake was noted during bicycle exercise after training (table). Training had no effect on maximal oxygen uptake during treadmill exercise. Absolute differences between bicycle and treadmill oxygen uptake values were about the same after and before training. Blood lactate levels on endurance testing were not elevated more after training. Thigh girth increased significantly, and muscle strength increased by 40% with training.

Heavy resistance training can dramatically increase short-term endurance when the muscles involved are used almost exclusively during testing without an accompanying increase in maximal oxygen uptake. Differences in maximal oxygen uptake between bicycle and treadmill exercise appear not to result from inadequate muscle strength.

▶ [Further data are provided here that endurance is not a function of aerobic exercise alone, but can be significantly influenced by heavy resistance training. Predictably, this does not influence Vo_2 max, and Vo_2 max therefore is not the only indicator of endurance. This is a further argument for the complementary use of heavy resistance training coupled with aerobic exercise.—L.J.K.] ◀

1–6   **Blood Pyruvate Recovery Curves After Short Heavy Submaximal Exercise in Man.** H. Freund, J. Marbach, C. Ott, J. Lonsdorfer, A. Heitz, P. Zouloumian, and P. Kehayoff (Strasbourg, France) studied the evolution of the arterial blood pyruvate concentrations after short heavy submaximal exercise. They also set up an equation representing its evolution as a function of time and determined the relationship between the arterial blood lactate and pyruvate recovery curves.

TECHNIQUE.—Six male subjects began the experiment in the morning after an overnight fast of 12 hours. For 5 subjects, the tests involved, in order, a 10-minute rest, a 10-minute moderate exercise, a 30-minute recovery, a 3-minute heavy exercise, and a 60- to 70-minute recovery. For the sixth subject, there was an initial 15-minute rest, four 1-minute strenuous exercises, each interspaced with a 4-minute rest, followed by a 90-minute recovery period after the last bout. Exercise consisted of pedaling a cycle ergometer in the sitting position at a rate of 60 rpm. Arterial and venous blood were withdrawn from the humeral artery and brachiocephalic vein, respectively, and analyzed continuously for lactate and pyruvate levels (Fig 1–2).

All of the subjects' recovery curves showed a similar pattern: when work stops, the pyruvate level decreases for about 1 minute. Subsequently, it increases and reaches its maximum value between the fifth and ninth minute of recovery. It then decreases with time.

The velocity constant of the final arterial blood pyruvate decrease was similar to that of the simultaneously measured lactate value, indicating that the rate of lactate removal is closely related to that of pyruvate. This is consistent with the fact that pyruvate is a necessary intermediate in the lactate metabolism.

▶ [Exercise physiologists often discuss when to collect "grab" samples of arterial

(1–6)   Eur. J. Appl. Physiol. 43:83–91, February 1980.

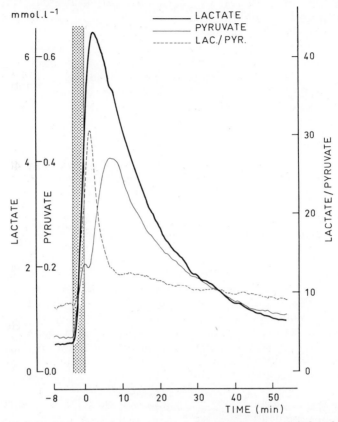

Fig 1–2.—Arterial blood lactate and pyruvate, and lactate-pyruvate ratio before, during, and after 3 minutes of heavy submaximal exercise on a bicycle ergometer (average values, $\eta = 5$). The shaded portion between the vertical lines locates the working period. (Courtesy of Freund, H., et al.: Eur. J. Appl. Physiol. 43:83–91, February 1980; Berlin-Heidelberg-New York: Springer.)

blood for lactate measurements. This article provides a rather pretty continuous curve of arterial lactate levels during and after exercise producing a heart rate of 170 beats per minute. The arterial lactate level starts to rise concurrently with the onset of exercise, but there is some phase lag, a peak being reached 1 to 2 minutes after the end of exercise. A curve of the blood pyruvate level is more complex, peaking about 5 to 9 minutes after exercise.—R.J.S.] ◄

1–7 **Transcutaneous Oxygen Monitoring During Exercise Stress Testing.** Tommy Schonfeld, Charles W. Sargent, Daisy Bautista, Marla A. Walters, Margaret H. O'Neal, Arnold C. G. Platzker, and Thomas G. Keens (Univ. of Southern California) measured arterial oxygen tension (Pa_{O_2}) and transcutaneous oxygen tension ($tcPo_2$) in 4 children with chronic lung disease and in 3 normal young adult volunteers at rest and during exercise. The aim was to evaluate the usefulness of these measurements in monitoring the patients during

(1–7) Am. Rev. Respir. Dis. 121:457–462, March 1980.

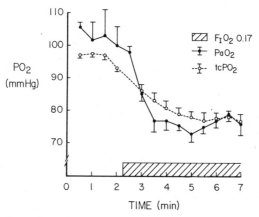

Fig 1–3.—This figure shows the Pa_{O_2} and $tcPo_2$ response after a step change in $F_{I_{O_2}}$ during exercise. Closed circles represent Pa_{O_2}; open circles represent $tcPo_2$. (Courtesy of Schonfeld, T., et al.: Am. Rev. Respir. Dis. 121:457–462, March 1980.)

exercise testing. The same graded exercise stress test on an electronically braked cycle ergometer was performed on all subjects.

A total of 358 sets of simultaneous Pa_{O_2} and $tcPo_2$ values were obtained on all subjects. Figure 1–3 shows the correlation between Pa_{O_2} and $tcPo_2$ at rest and during exercise. At rest, the regression coefficient for $tcPo_2$ on Pa_{O_2} was 0.78 ± 0.03 (SE) ($r = 0.924$; $P < .0005$)

Fig 1–4.—This figure shows the correlation between Pa_{O_2} and $tcPo_2$ at rest and during exercise. Individual data points are shown. Crosses represent values at rest, and closed circles represent those during exercise. Linear regressions are shown for rest *(dashed line)* and exercise *(solid line)*. (Courtesy of Schonfeld, T., et al.:Am. Rev. Respir. Dis. 121:457–462, March 1980.)

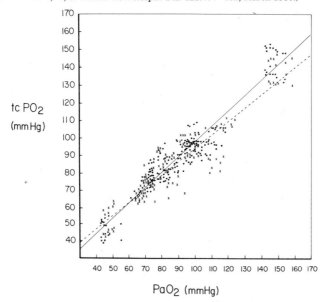

compared with 0.88 ± 0.02 ($r = 0.958$; $P < .0005$) during exercise. Both regression coefficients were significantly different from each other ($P < .01$) and from unity ($P < .001$). The correlation coefficient during exercise was significantly greater than the correlation coefficient at rest ($P < .005$). These results suggest that $tcPO_2$ may approximate Pa_{O_2} more closely during exercise than at rest. The response of Pa_{O_2} and $tcPO_2$ to a step change in inspired oxygen concentration (FI_{O_2}) from 0.21 to 0.17 is shown during exercise in Figure 1–4. The Pa_{O_2} and $tcPO_2$ changes after each change in FI_{O_2} were similar at rest and during exercise by analysis of variance ($P = .20$). The time constants for $tcPO_2$ at rest and during exercise were not significantly different ($P = .30$). These results indicate that $tcPO_2$ followed the change in Pa_{O_2} after a step change in FI_{O_2}.

Measurements of transcutaneous oxygen tension are affected by skin perfusion, skin oxygen consumption, and skin thickness. Skin perfusion and oxygen consumption change during exercise, and adult skin is thicker than that of the neonate. Results of evaluation of the clinical usefulness of transcutaneous oxygen monitoring during exercise stress testing in this study indicate a tendency for correlation between Pa_{O_2} and $tcPO_2$ to be better during exercise than at rest. This may be explained by the increase in skin blood flow during exercise.

▶ [There are many clinical situations, particularly during exercise, when it would be a great asset to have a simple noninvasive indicator of arterial oxygen pressure. Over the past few years, the transcutaneous oxygen electrode has been gaining in popularity. It was used initially for the monitoring of neonates and worked particularly well in this situation because skin was thin. During exercise, an increase of skin blood flow facilitates the use of transcutaneous data in adults. The present data illustrate a reasonable matching of transcutaneous and arterial results under both steady-state and step-change conditions. At rest, discrepancies amount to 3 torr for normal subjects and 13 torr for patients with chest disease; however, the corresponding figures for vigorous exercise are only 1 and 3 torr, respectively.—R.J.S.] ◀

1–8 **Mixed Venous CO_2 Tension During Exercise.** The determination of exercise cardiac output using carbon dioxide (CO_2) as the test gas requires estimation of mixed venous CO_2 tension. J. Howland Auchincloss, Robert Gilbert, Mitchell Kuppinger, and David Peppi (SUNY, Upstate Med. Center) conducted a series of experiments in 95 adults, 25 of whom had coronary artery disease, to evaluate the reproducibility of the extrapolation (Defares) CO_2 rebreathing method and the equilibrium (Collier) method for estimating mixed venous CO_2 tension. The Collier method was modified slightly by using a fixed 3-L bag rather than a variable bag volume. Values for the Collier method were corrected for the downstream effect, whereas the Defares values were uncorrected. Both methods were validated by comparison with the results of other studies.

The subjects were tested on a walking treadmill at 82 or 123 W. Both methods gave similar mean values for normal subjects walking at 123 W for 3 minutes. However, the coefficient of variation for the Collier values in duplicate determinations was 2.5%, whereas the Defares values had a coefficient of variation of 4.5%. In paired compari-

(1–8) J. Appl. Physiol. 48:933–938, June 1980.

sons, Defares values usually were either higher or lower than the Collier values; the differences were related to variations in technique and to the analysis of Defares tracings. The duration of the rebreathing period (10 seconds and 15 seconds) did not markedly affect the Collier values.

Although the Collier procedure was noticeably more uncomfortable for the subjects than the Defares technique, there was little difficulty in completing the tests in subjects with coronary artery disease. The results confirm other findings favorable to the Collier method and enhance its superiority by proposing simplifications that minimize trial and error. The findings also demonstrate difficulties with the Defares technique that are not readily apparent.

▶ [Some authors who estimate cardiac output by CO_2 rebreathing fail to specify the method they have used. There are several available procedures, with differing reproducibility and results. Two of the better known are those of Collier and Defares. The former apparently leads to very erroneous values of mixed venous CO_2 tension during exercise, and it is necessary to apply a horrendous 10–15 mm Hg "downstream" correction to the apparent plateau values of CO_2 tension. The Defares data are not usually "corrected" in this way, and perhaps because the bag CO_2 tension is lower, it does not seem to need the drastic "fudge-factor."

The Defares method also causes less discomfort, making it potentially more suitable for vigorous exercise. However, the present authors find it less reproducible than the Collier approach. The other difficulty is that the Defares technique needs a reasonable number of data points after lung-bag mixing, but before recirculation; there is some discussion as to how far this can be accomplished in vigorous exercise.—R.J.S.] ◀

1–9 **Effect of Work Intensity and Duration on Recovery O$_2$.** The slow component of the two-component recovery of O_2 (O_2 debt) after exercise has been attributed to the effects of lactate metabolism. Recently, it has been suggested that the greater part of the slow component of recovery O_2 can be explained by the effect of temperature on metabolism. J. M. Hagberg, J. P. Mullin, and F. J. Nagle (Univ. of Wisconsin, Madison) assessed the involvement of rectal temperature and blood lactate levels in the slow component of recovery O_2 in 18 young men exercised at work intensities of 50%, 65%, and 80% of maximal O_2 consumption ($\dot{V}O_2$ max) for 5 and 20 minutes. Baseline $\dot{V}O_2$ was established by cycling at 150 kpm·minute^{-1} before and after each exercise period.

The magnitude of the rapid component of recovery O_2 was proportional to the relative work load, but was not affected by the duration of exercise. The duration or intensity of exercise did not markedly alter the magnitude of the slow component of recovery O_2 at work intensities of 50% and 65% of $\dot{V}O_2$ max. However, 20 minutes of exercise at 80% $\dot{V}O_2$ max resulted in an almost fivefold increase in the magnitude of the slow component of recovery O_2 ($P < .01$). Rectal temperature was significantly ($P < .01$) increased after 20 minutes of exercise compared with the increase after 5 minutes of exercise at all three work intensities, and was proportional to increased exercise intensity. The only significant difference between the end-exercise blood lactate levels after 5 and 20 minutes of exercise was found at

(1–9) J. Appl. Physiol. 48:540–544, March 1980.

the 80% $\dot{V}O_2$ max level. Lactate metabolism could account for only 30%, at most, of the changes in magnitude of the slow components of recovery O_2 after 5 and 20 minutes of exercise at 80% intensity, while the Q_{10} effect of temperature accounted for 60%–70% of the slow component increase at all work rates and durations.

The study demonstrated that the time course of the slow component of recovery O_2 is independent of work load and duration of exercise unless the exercise is greater than 64% of $\dot{V}O_2$ max and the duration of exercise is longer than 5 minutes. The greater part of the slow component of recovery O_2 can be accounted for by the effect of temperature on metabolism.

▶ [The classic views of Margaria and his colleagues are built around a two-component oxygen recovery curve, the first representing "alactate" (adenosine triphosphate, creatine phosphate, and tissue oxygen stores) and the second representing lactic acid. However, recent authors have recognized that unless an arbitrary time is set for completion of the second phase, this can be overshadowed by effects due to an increase of tissue temperature and secretion of hormones that augment resting metabolism. This article by Hagberg et al. shows that the temperature effect is four times greater after 20 than after 5 minutes of work, and the change (0.8 C) is said to be large enough to account for 60%–70% of the second component if the exercise bout lasts 20 minutes. Plainly, if lactate is to be assessed from oxygen recovery curves, it is prudent to keep the exercise bout short.—R.J.S.] ◀

1–10   **Subcutaneous Interstitial Pressure in Man and Dogs Exposed to Heat and Exercise Stress.** H. A. Davis and P. L. Jooste assessed the validity of interstitial fluid pressure (IFP) as a measure of the balance between outward and inward filtration through capillary endothelium and lymphatic fluid removal. They compared their measurements of IFP with reports of others on changes in filtration occurring during heat exposure and anesthesia.

TECHNIQUE.—Six healthy male volunteers from the gold mining industry were studied. Their ages ranged from 19 to 29 years and their treadmill maximum oxygen uptake (VO_2 max) ranged from 3.03 to 3.57 L · minute^{-1}. The subjects were randomly allocated to three groups of 2 subjects each. Measurements were taken while the first 2 subjects (unacclimatized to heat) ran on a treadmill at approximately 75% VO_2 max. The second group of subjects, also unacclimatized, and the third group of highly heat-acclimatized subjects performed block-stepping at about 50% VO_2 max for 30 minutes. Heat acclimatization was carried out over 8 days according to the method of Wyndham and Strydom (1969). Before entry into the climatic chamber, a cotton wick was inserted into the dorsum of the hand for IFP measurements. Three dogs were also used in the study. The IFP was recorded in the dogs during exposure to heat to 20–22 C and after they were killed.

Results showed that, with the onset of exercise in heat, the IFP of highly heat acclimatized men changed rapidly from 1 mm Hg to +1 mm Hg (relative to atmospheric) (Fig 1–5). Thereafter, the IFP steadily decreased until cessation of exercise. In contrast, changes in IFP of unacclimatized men with onset of exercise was always negative and gradually became more negative as exercise in heat continued (Fig 1–6). After exercise ended, the IFP remained reasonably stable for approximately 10 minutes. The IFP of anesthetized dogs gradually

(1–10)   Eur. J. Appl. Physiol. 44:117–122, August 1980.

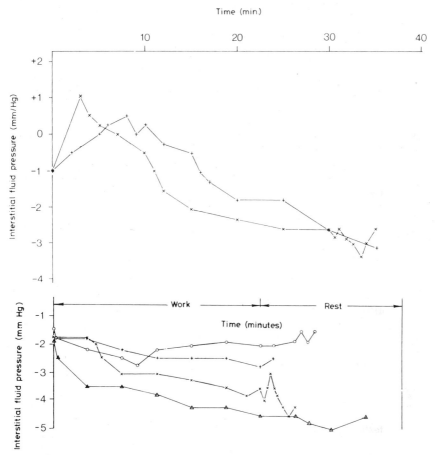

Fig 1–5 (top).—Interstitial pressure in acclimatized man during exercise and heat exposure: *plus*, subject 1; *x*, subject 2.

Fig 1–6 (bottom).—Interstitial pressure in unacclimatized man during exercise and heat exposure: *plus*, subject 1; *circle*, subject 2; *triangle*, subject 3; *x*, subject 4.

(Courtesy of Davis, H. A., and Jooste, P. L.: Eur. J. Appl. Physiol. 44:117–122, August 1980; Berlin-Heidelberg-New York: Springer.

became more negative during heat exposure. In contrast, the IFP of the same dogs tended toward atmospheric when the dogs were exposed to room temperatures (20–22 C).

The authors conclude that there are changes in heat-acclimatized men in forces operating across the capillary wall, and transient formation of free fluid occurs in the cutaneous interstitial space during the initial 10 minutes of exercise. Further research is needed to confirm and clarify this interpretation.

▶ [It is believed that considerable movement of both fluid and low molecular weight protein occurs between the capillaries and the extracellular space during the first few minutes of exercise; among other indications, there is a 5%–10% increase of hematocrit. This article concerns the possibility of using small wicks to measure the interstitial fluid pressure directly. Because the pressure falls during exercise, this technique suggests that extravascular fluid is diminishing during exercise. The explanation may lie in the relatively mild exercise used (50% of Vo_2 max). Under such conditions, muscle contraction may favor return of fluid via the lymphatic system.—R.J.S.] ◄

1–11   **Coronary Artery Status of Apparently Healthy Subjects With Frequent and Complex Ventricular Ectopy.** Although ventricular ectopy itself does not indicate coronary artery disease, many clinicians believe that most persons with frequent and complex ventricular ectopy have covert coronary disease. Harold L. Kennedy, Janet E. Pescarmona, Richard J. Bouchard, and Robert J. Goldberg (Johns Hopkins Univ.) performed cardiac catheterization and coronary angiography in 25 apparently healthy subjects with frequent and complex ventricular ectopy. Ectopy was most often found during routine resting ECG study or physical examination. Six patients developed symptoms once ectopy was known. Four patients were thought to have psychoneurologic stressful traits. Most subjects were men with a history of hypertension, cigarette smoking, or hyperlipemia.

Six subjects had coronary luminal narrowing of 50% or more, and 5 had lesser narrowing. Seven of the 14 subjects with normal coronary arteries had an elevated left ventricular end-systolic volume index, and 9 had an elevated left ventricular end-diastolic volume index. Those with coronary narrowing had normal volumes. Two subjects with significant coronary stenosis had abnormal wall motion on left ventricular angiography, as did 2 without coronary stenosis. No ischemic S-T segment change was found in any subject on exercise testing. All ectopy ceased at maximal exercise in 17 of 24 subjects, including 5 of 6 with significant coronary stenosis. Holter recordings did not distinguish subjects with from those without coronary artery disease. Complex ventricular ectopy was identified in 18 subjects. Most foci in subjects with significant coronary disease had ectopic beat patterns of right ventricular origin, although two- and three-vessel coronary disease was present.

The definitive long-term prognosis of apparently healthy subjects with frequent and complex ventricular ectopy remains to be defined, but the present findings indicate that most such subjects do not have covert coronary artery disease, and the findings support a conservative approach to these subjects.

► [Twenty-five subjects in apparent good health but who presented with significant ventricular ectopic beats as frequent or complex ventricular patterns were studied with cardiac catheterization and coronary angiography. Of this group, only 6 had significant coronary artery disease, defined as greater than 50% of luminal narrowing. Maximal exercise testing and 24-hour Holter ambulatory monitoring did not differentiate those subjects with coronary artery disease from those with normal coronary arteries, and this has obvious clinical significance for the practical management of this group of people in a medical or cardiologic practice. It would document further that a minority of the apparently healthy subjects with ventricular arrhythmia have significant coronary artery disease, and it certainly supports the conservative approach to the management of such patients.

The problem could be turned around. If approximately 25% of this subject group had significant coronary artery disease, is it worth putting such potential subjects through cardiac catheterization and coronary angiography? Is this justified especially

(1–11)   Ann. Intern. Med. 92(Pt. 1):179–185, February 1980.

if the aforementioned testing of maximal exercise stress test or Holter ECG monitoring was not definitive? This position would have some obvious appeal, especially as the safety of angiography has improved so greatly. This will be an ongoing debate.— L.J.K.] ◄

1–12 **The Acute Cardiac Risk of Strenuous Exercise.** There is some evidence, though not conclusive, that regular vigorous exercise helps to protect against coronary heart disease. Larry W. Gibbons, Kenneth H. Cooper, Betty M. Meyer, and R. Curtis Ellison (Inst. for Aerobic Res., Dallas) reviewed the computer logs of the amount and intensity of exercise performed by 2,935 adults (mean age, 37 years) over a 65-month period to estimate the acute cardiac risk of strenuous exercise. The computer logs represented 374,798 person-hours of exercise, which included 2,726,272 km of running and walking.

During the study period, there were two cardiovascular complications; both subjects survived and resumed regular exercise. Based on age-specific categories, maximum risk estimates (MREs) consistent with the upper 95% confidence limits for the data range from 0.3 to 2.7 cardiac events per 10,000 person-hours of exercise for men and 0.6 to 6.0 events per 10,000 person-hours for women. The higher MRE for women is attributable to the relatively low number of women in the study. It is calculated that if exercise were performed three times a week for 30 minutes per session for 52 weeks, the MRE would be 0.002 to 0.027 events per person-year for men and 0.005 to 0.05 events for women. However, actual risks are likely to be lower.

It appears that the combination of exercise and preexistent coronary disease together, rather than exercise alone, poses the major risk factor. Factors such as competition and smoking may also modify the risk of cardiac episodes occurring as a result of exercise.

► [The philosophic debate as to whether vigorous exercise can protect the heart against coronary disease continues. The weight of the evidence would suggest that there is some protective benefit from exercise. The ongoing concern remains that strenuous exercise may be associated with arrhythmia, myocardial infarction, and sudden death. Several attempts have been made to assess this risk directly. This article is one such attempt at quantitation of the risk factors. No deaths occurred in this rather extensive series involving 2,935 adults and about 375,000 person-hours of exercise. Nevertheless, sudden death and acute cardiac catastrophe are ongoing risks that we must accept. It is reasonable to recognize that sudden death rarely, if ever, will occur from the simple combination of exercise with a "healthy" heart. The unhealthy heart is not always recognized. Coexistent or preexistent coronary artery disease is certainly a predisposing factor to a cardiac episode. The data would also suggest that the factors of pressure and excitement of the competitive environment via sympathetic pathways are other contributory elements. A third factor to be faced squarely is that those subjects who smoke, and particularly who smoke heavily, are further predisposed to the risks of such activity. It is only fair to recognize that vigorous physical activity is not a guarantee of immortality and that it must be weighed against its own substrate of risks. The factor of common sense is the most difficult to quantitate in participants and in enthusiasts.—L.J.K.] ◄

1–13 **Chronobiology of Cardiac Sudden Death in Men.** Sudden cardiac death is a frequent mode of premature death from ischemic heart disease. Simon W. Rabkin, Francis A. L. Mathewson, and Robert B.

(1–12) J.A.M.A. 244:1799–1801, Oct. 17, 1980.
(1–13) J.A.M.A. 244:1357–1358, Sept. 19, 1980.

Tate (Univ. of Manitoba) examined daily variation in the occurrence of sudden deaths in a cohort study of cardiovascular disease in 3,983 men found fit for pilot training in World War II and observed since 1948. In 1948, the subjects had no clinical evidence of ischemic heart disease. Over two-thirds were aged 25 to 34 years. A total of 152 sudden cardiac deaths occurred in the next 29 years. Sixty-three patients had no clinical evidence of ischemic heart disease before death.

Among men without clinically evident ischemic heart disease, sudden cardiac deaths occurred most often on Mondays. Among those with clinical evidence of ischemic heart disease, sudden cardiac deaths occurred more uniformly throughout the week. There was no significant daily variation in total myocardial infarctions either in survivors or in patients who died within a week of infarction. Among men who had no previous evidence of ischemic heart disease, 75% of deaths known to occur at work and 46.7% of those occurring at home were on Mondays.

A significant excess of sudden cardiac deaths on Mondays was found among subjects without previous evidence of ischemic heart disease. Reintroduction to occupational stress, activity, or pollutants after a weekend may precipitate arrhythmias. Psychologic stress has been related to sudden cardiac death, and return to work may be a stressor. It also is possible that weekly oscillations in neurophysiologic function may be responsible. In men with known ischemic heart disease, factors related to myocardial disease may predominate over factors that influence daily variation in sudden deaths.

▶ [A further intriguing factor in the equation of sudden death is discussed by this article offering data that Monday is the day of greatest threat in terms of sudden cardiac death. The data appear to be solid, but the reasons are not clear. Possibilities raised are the sum of various stress factors, psychologic factors, and perhaps an internal biologic time clock. This statement is not made in jest, and the point that this warrants further research would appear to have merit in terms of this syndrome of sudden death.—L.J.K.] ◀

1–14 **Mural Left Anterior Descending Coronary Artery, Strenuous Exercise, and Sudden Death.** Azorides R. Morales, Renzo Romanelli, and Robert J. Boucek (Miami, Fla.) present the reports of 2 ostensibly healthy men, aged 54 and 34 years, respectively, who died suddenly while jogging, and of a girl, aged 17 years, who died after swimming. Postmortem studies showed an unobstructed but mural left anterior descending artery (LAD), diminished vascularity to the posterior left ventricle and ventricular septum, and morphological evidence of patchy, ischemic necrosis of the ventricular septum in different stages of healing.

These morphological findings, coupled with reports that cyclic compression of a mural LAD produces ischemia, strongly suggest that, in selected subjects, such an artery may be critically constricted during systole and produce myocardial ischemia and fibrosis. This intramyocardial location of the LAD may represent a potentially lethal anatomical variant.

(1–14) Circulation 62:230–237, August 1980.

The incidence of mural LAD in autopsy series varies widely. In various series it was found in 449 of 1,652 cases (27%). In one series of more than 5,000 patients with coronary arteriograms, there was a 0.51% incidence of LAD overbridging producing systolic compression. Recently, an incidence of 1.6% was reported in an arteriographic evaluation of 313 patients. Perhaps mural LAD might be suspected in young patients with angina-like pain, the ECG syndrome of septal fibrosis, and a positive exercise stress ECG response. These patients may warrant coronary arteriographic and myocardial scintigraphic examinations to document systolic compression of the LAD and reduced perfusion of the posterior septum and left ventricle. The study should include atrial pacing and coronary sinus lactate measurements. Recognition of a mural LAD with associated myocardial ischemia and fibrosis as a potentially lethal variant should direct attention to possible left ventricular myotomies.

▶ [Atherosclerotic coronary artery obstruction is recognized as a major cause of myocardial ischemia and infarction, but myocardial changes and death may occur without advanced obstructive coronary artery disease. This can be due to coronary spasm, inappropriate α-adrenergic receptor activity, or compression of a major epicardial artery by contraction of an overbridging left ventricular muscle. It is this last category that these cases relate to. The very real practical implication is that if this subgroup can be identified in young patients with anginal pain and the ECG syndrome of septal fibrosis and positive stress ECG responses, these patients may then properly undergo coronary arteriography and myocardial scintigraphy to document the systolic compression of the left anterior descending artery with reduced perfusion of the septum and left ventricle. The recognition of this syndrome as a potentially lethal variant would direct attention to left ventricular myotomy.—L.J.K.] ◀

1–15 **Effects of Exercise Training on Left Ventricular Function in Normal Subjects: Longitudinal Study by Radionuclide Angiography.** Although intensive exercise training can lead to extraordinary levels of cardiac performance in trained athletes, no unified concept of the effect of exercise conditioning on the heart has been formulated. Stephen K. Rerych, Peter M. Scholz, David C. Sabiston, Jr., and Robert H. Jones (Duke Univ.) used nuclide angiocardiography to examine the effects of physical training on ventricular function in 12 male and 6 female normal athletes (mean age 19 years), studied before and after a 6-month period of intensive training for competitive swimming. Jogging and weight lifting were also performed. Radionuclide studies were done at rest and during bicycle exercise with the use of ^{99m}Tc-labeled human albumin.

Although the direction of hemodynamic change during exercise was the same before and after exercise conditioning, the magnitude of change in several variables was influenced by conditioning (table). Ejection fraction increased by 19% during exercise before training and by 28% after training. Training did not alter the peak heart rate at maximal exercise. Exercise cardiac output increased by 21% after training, but resting output was not altered significantly. Pulmonary blood volume increased both at rest and during exercise after training. Total body blood volume at rest increased 31% after training.

(1–15) Am. J. Cardiol. 45:244–252, February 1980.

Measurements of Cardiac Function at Rest and During
Maximal Exercise

	Heart Rate (beats/ min)	Ejection Fraction (%)	End-Dia-stolic Volume (ml)	Cardiac Output (liters/ min)	Total Body Blood Volume (liter)
Rest					
BT	74 ± 11	73 ± 6	133 ± 35	6.9 ± 1.1	8.7 ± 0.8
AT	61 ± 7	67 ± 7	167 ± 40	6.7 ± 1.0	11.4 ± 2.2
Exercise					
BT	185 ± 10	87 ± 4	166 ± 34	25.5 ± 5.7	8.0 ± 0.9
AT	181 ± 14	86 ± 5	204 ± 39	32.0 ± 8.7	10.8 ± 2.3

There was no significant change in stroke work at rest or on exercise in the posttraining state.

These findings emphasize the hemodynamic importance of an increase in end-diastolic volume at rest after training. The acute increase in end-diastolic volume in response to exercise stress appears to be important for increased cardiac output. Increased output on maximal exercise after intensive training is due chiefly to the ability of the left ventricle to dilate from rest to exercise and to eject fully the increased end-diastolic volume at about the same or a lower heart rate. Cardiac output at rest is maintained at the same level after training, although increased vagal tone decreases the heart rate. This is achieved through an increase in stroke volume which appears to depend on an increase in left ventricular preload, reflected by increased end-diastolic volume.

▶ [The hemodynamic importance of the increase in end-diastolic volume at rest after training is emphasized. This training increases the capacity of the heart to utilize the Frank-Starling mechanism, increasing its effectiveness at rest and during the periods of maximal cardiac output. The study further suggests that increased left ventricular volume after training is accompanied by increases in pulmonary blood volume and total body blood volume.—L.J.K.] ◀

1–16 **Effects of Oral Propranolol on Left Ventricular Size and Performance During Exercise and Acute Pressure Loading.** Michael H. Crawford, JoAnn Lindenfeld, and Robert A. O'Rourke (Univ. of Texas, San Antonio), with the technical assistance of K. Wray Amon, used M-made echocardiography to examine the effects of chronic oral propranolol administration on left ventricular performance in 19 normal persons aged 19–36 years. The study group took 160 mg propranolol daily for 2 weeks. Serum propranolol levels at the time of study ranged from 23 to 151 ng/ml (mean, 70 ng/ml). Studies were done at rest, during supine bicycle exercise, and in conjunction with acute pressure loading with phenylephrine after atropine administration.

Resting heart rate was significantly reduced with propranolol administration. The systolic blood pressure also was lower than baseline after propranolol was taken. The left ventricular end-diastolic dimen-

(1–16) Circulation 61:549–554, March 1980.

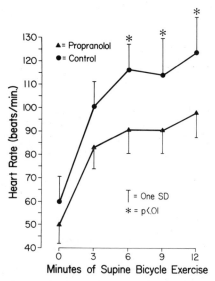

Fig 1–7.—Average values for heart rate during exercise in 10 persons prior to and during propranolol treatment. (Courtesy of Crawford, M. H., et al.: Circulation 61:549–554, March 1980; by permission of the American Heart Association, Inc.)

sion was greater with propranolol treatment, but percent left ventricular dimensional shortening was unchanged. Heart rate during exercise was lower with propranolol usage (Fig 1–7). The left ventricular end-diastolic dimension was larger when propranolol was taken, and the percent left ventricular dimensional shortening was lower at each stage of exercise. With acute pressure loading, there were no significant differences between the propranolol and control states in heart rate, systolic blood pressure, or echographic measures of left ventricular size or performance.

Oral propranolol administration reduces resting heart rate and blood pressure in normal persons, but the drug does not alter left ventricular performance significantly. Left ventricular size is greater and the percent dimensional shortening is reduced during exercise, but no significant effects are noted during acute pressure loading. Propranolol appears to have little if any intrinsic depressant effect on the myocardium. Its major action on the heart seems to be β-blockade, which is most manifest during periods of intense sympathetic stimulation, e.g., exercise. Patients having a history of overt congestive heart failure who are dependent on sympathetic tone for maintenance of resting ventricular performance would be expected to be affected adversely by orally administered propranolol. Patients with more subtle left ventricular dysfunction may benefit from concomitant digoxin therapy.

▶ [The conclusions of this study are consistent with those of others who studied the effects of intravenous β-blockade with the use of varying techniques in animals and man. The point should be stressed that patients with a history of overt congestive failure and dependent on sympathetic tone for maintenance of resting ventricular performance are a subgroup adversely affected by β-blockers, and this is a pretty absolute contraindication.

Frisk-Holmberg et al. (1980 YEAR BOOK, p. 48) in an article discussing metabolic changes in muscle during long-term administration of alprenolol, state that this drug appears to prevent lactase translocation from muscle cell to blood and limit lactate release. Thus, there is a peripheral effect on local circulation, with an impaired adaptation of the microcirculation that may be common both to myocardium and skeletal muscle.—L.J.K.] ◀

METABOLISM, NUTRITION, AND DRUGS

1-17 **Blood Lipid and ECG Responses to Carbohydrate Loading.** Many long-distance runners use carbohydrate loading before a race to increase muscle glycogen stores, as this is believed to enhance endurance. Steven Blair, Roger Sargent, Dennis Davidson, and Richard Krejci monitored changes in the ECG and blood lipid concentrations before and after competition in 10 runners who loaded carbohydrate (loaders) and 4 runners who maintained their normal diets (nonloaders) to determine whether carbohydrate loading had adverse effects.

Blood lipid analyses were carried out at baseline, after the depletion phase of carbohydrate loading, after carbohydrate loading, and after the race. The only statistically significant change in blood lipid concentrations was an increase in after-marathon triglyceride values over baseline in loaders. The only pronounced change in the ECG study was a marked decrease in R wave height after carbohydrate loading; this change was not significant by Fisher's exact test. The ECG voltage criteria for left ventricular hypertrophy were observed in 5 of 10 loaders and 3 of 4 nonloaders.

Although some of the changes observed were statistically significant, the values remained within normal limits, and therefore the changes were considered to be clinically trivial. There were no significant changes in T wave amplitude, S-T segment deviation, or heart rate before and after carbohydrate loading. It is concluded that carbohydrate loading had no adverse effects on blood lipid concentrations or ECGs in these runners.

▶ [In theory, carbohydrate loading could be bad for athletes who have had a coronary thrombosis, because the loading process may distort serum potassium levels while unloading may again affect serum potassium levels and reduce the amount of fat burned during a distance run. Although some trends of this type were observed with loading, the effects do not seem of major importance in practice.—R.J.S.] ◀

1-18 **High-Density Lipoprotein Cholesterol, Total Cholesterol and Triglycerides in Serum After a Single Exposure to Prolonged Heavy Exercise.** Sven Chr. Enger, Sigmund B. Strømme, and Harald E. Refsum (Univ. of Oslo) studied the effect of a single exposure to exercise on the levels of high-density lipoproteins (HDL).

TECHNIQUE.—Two groups of well-trained men (10 subjects each) participated in a 70-km ski race. During the race, the subjects had free access to warm and cold beverages at six places along the track. The beverages contained known amounts of sugar, but no salts, proteins, or fat. Blood sampling

(1–17) Physician Sportsmed. 8:68–75, July 1980.
(1–18) Scand. J. Clin. Lab. Invest. 40:341–345, June 1980.

SERUM LIPID AND TOTAL PROTEIN LEVELS IN 20 MEN BEFORE AND AFTER 70-KM
CROSS-COUNTRY SKI RACE

		Day before	Race day	Day after	2 days after	4 days after
Total cholesterol (mmol/l)	mean	5.35	5.37	4.93**	5.08**	5.28
	range	3.7–7.8	3.2–8.5	3.2–7.8	3.2–7.6	3.3–7.7
HDL cholesterol (mmol/l)	mean	1.46	1.64**	1.71**	1.62**	1.52**
	range	0.9–2.3	1.1–2.6	1.1–2.6	1.1–2.5	1.1–2.3
LDL+VLDL cholesterol	mean	3.89	3.73	3.22**	3.46**	3.76
(mmol/l)	range	2.4–6.1	1.6–5.9	1.5–5.2	1.7–5.1	1.9–6.0
Triglycerides (mmol/l)	mean	1.16	0.81**	0.82*	1.10	1.30
	range	0.1–1.9	0.1–1.8	0.1–2.1	0.5–2.3	0.5–2.4
Total proteins (g/l)	mean	73.1	76.2**	·70.6**	69.2**	71·9
	range	67–81	70–82	63–77	64–77	65–81

Note: Level of statistical significance between observations before and after exercise: $*P<.05; **P<.01$.

was performed on the day before the race, immediately after the race, and on the first second, and fourth day after the race.

The results show that total protein levels increased immediately after the exercise, fell to below the initial level on the following 2 days, but were essentially back to the pre-race level 4 days after the exercise (table). The total serum cholesterol level was unchanged immediately after exercise, was reduced by 8% and 5% of the pre-race level on the 2 following days, but was back at the initial level 4 days after the exercise. The HDL cholesterol level was definitely increased immediately after the race, rose to 17% above the pre-race level on the following day, and was still elevated on the fourth day after the exercise, whereas mean levels of low-density and very low-density lipoprotein (VLDL) cholesterol were correspondingly reduced. Triglyceride levels were reduced by 30% of the initial level immediately after the race, were still low on the following day, but were restored to the pre-race level 2 days after the race. The pre-race total serum cholesterol and HDL cholesterol levels were higher in the subjects in the 50- to 60-year-old group than in the 20- to 30-year-old group.

In accordance with previous observations after similar exercise, the variations in serum total protein level most probably indicate that the subjects were slightly dehydrated at the end of exercise and slightly overhydrated during the following days. The authors believe that the present report confirms previous studies showing that prolonged heavy exercise is accompanied by major changes in fat metabolism of several days' duration. The lipid changes suggest an increased catabolism of triglyceride-rich lipoproteins (chylomicrons and VLDL) during the race. It is concluded that a single exposure to prolonged heavy exercise induces changes in the HDL metabolism, showing that the physical exercise per se plays an important role in the increased HDL level seen in well-trained athletes.

▶ [It has been unclear whether the high levels of high-density lipoproteins of the well-trained athlete are due directly to physical activity or whether there is some less immediate explanation. This article shows that a single, long-sustained bout of vigorous exercise is sufficient to change the ratio of high-density lipoproteins to low-density lipoproteins for several days. Thus, physical activity has a causal role, rather than acting through possible changes in body mass, smoking, drinking, and dietary habits. In extrapolating these results to the average "keep-fit" class for the middle-aged man, we must recognize that exercise was prolonged to the point of glycogen depletion, with a need to burn fat. It is less certain that 15–30 minutes of moderate calisthenics or jogging will produce parallel changes.—R.J.S.] ◄

1–19 **Elevated High-Density Lipoprotein Levels in Marathon Runners.** Many reports have strongly suggested an inverse relationship between the amount of physical activity and the incidence of coronary artery disease, but a causal relationship has not been established. Marvin M. Adner and William P. Castelli (Framingham, Mass.) conducted a long-term, prospective study of 50 distance runners and 43 controls matched as closely as possible with the runners. There was 1 woman in each group. The runners ran over 500 miles a year; the controls were not long-distance runners. There was no significant group difference in family history of coronary disease.

Blood pressures were comparable in the two groups, but the runners had significantly slower resting pulse rates. There was no evidence of cardiovascular disease in the running group. The runners as a group had significantly lower relative weight than the control group, who participated actively in a variety of exercises for an average of 2 to 3 hours a week. The mean high-density lipoprotein (HDL) cholesterol concentrations were 54 mg/dl in the runners and 45 mg/dl in the controls, a highly significant difference. Values did not correlate significantly with relative weight in either group. There were no significant group differences in total cholesterol, low-density lipoprotein cholesterol, or triglyceride concentrations. Carbohydrate loading by runners did not result in a substantial elevation of triglyceride concentration.

Runners in this study had elevated HDL cholesterol concentrations compared with matched controls. Distance running may somehow result in HDL cholesterol elevation. If HDL cholesterol concentration and development of coronary artery disease are inversely correlated, distance runners should be at a lower risk of developing coronary disease than nonrunners. This hypothesis is undoubtedly an important motivating factor for many persons who take up distance running, but it is unproved.

1–20 **Alcohol Consumption and High-Density Lipoprotein Cholesterol in Marathon Runners.** Both alcohol consumption and physical activity are related inversely to coronary heart disease, and both are associated positively with increased levels of high-density lipoprotein cholesterol (HDL-C), presumably protective against coronary heart disease. Walter Willett, Charles H. Hennekens, Arthur J. Siegel, Marvin M. Adner, and William P. Castelli examined relationships of alcohol consumption and physical activity to HDL-C in 90 male physicians aged 27–68 years (median age, 42) who participated in the 1979 Doctors' Marathon.

The overall mean HDL-C level was 55.6 mg/dl. Levels correlated

(1–19)   J.A.M.A. 243:534–536, Feb. 8, 1980.
(1–20)   N. Engl. J. Med. 303:1159–1161, Nov. 13, 1980.

closely with alcohol consumption, increasing with the weekly alcohol intake. The relationship was not altered by consideration of weight or height. Intensity of exercise, based on miles run per week and the best marathon time, was not related to HDL-C levels or alcohol use. Only 1 runner reported smoking cigarettes. Alcohol intake was positively associated with total cholesterol level, but even the heavier drinkers had no elevation of triglyceride concentration, and there was no meaningful association between weight, height, or Quetelet's index and any lipid component.

These findings indicate a strongly positive association between alcohol consumption and HDL-C levels which is not explained by the effect of vigorous physical exercise. This association may help to explain why rates of myocardial infarction are lower in moderate drinkers than in nondrinkers, but the findings do not provide a sufficient basis for recommending that nondrinkers adopt a habit of moderate alcohol consumption. Additional epidemiologic studies are needed to examine further the relationships among alcohol consumption, blood lipid levels, myocardial infarction, and nutritional factors.

▶ [The preceding article reaches no conclusion other than to set the data base for a future prospective study, noting that there appears to be an inverse relationship between vigorous physical activity and the incidence of coronary artery disease and that there appears to be a relationship between vigorous physical activity and the presence of high-density lipoprotein cholesterol. This study goes one step further and suggests that in that subgroup characterized by vigorous physical activity, there is a positive association with alcohol consumption and the high-density lipoprotein cholesterol level. Vice may have its rewards.—L.J.K.] ◀

1–21 **Zinc Lowers High-Density Lipoprotein Cholesterol Levels.** The administration of zinc to rats has been found to increase serum cholesterol levels. Philip L. Hooper, Laurent Visconti, Philip J. Garry, and Gregory E. Johnson (Albuquerque, N.M.) studied the effect of zinc administration on serum lipoprotein levels in 20 healthy, nonobese men with normal serum cholesterol levels. Twelve subjects received a capsule containing 220 mg of zinc sulfate (80 mg of elemental zinc) twice a day with meals for 5 weeks. Fasting lipid levels were measured on a weekly basis. Eight men served as controls.

High-density lipoprotein cholesterol (HDL cholesterol) levels showed a marked decrease after 4 weeks of zinc administration. Two weeks after zinc supplementation was discontinued, serum HDL cholesterol levels had decreased 25% from baseline values (40.5 to 30.1 mg/dl) (Fig 1–8). Serum cholesterol, triglyceride, and low-density lipoprotein cholesterol levels did not show any significant changes during the study. Plasma zinc concentrations became elevated during the study, but did not correlate with the decrease in HDL cholesterol levels.

Because epidemiologic studies have shown a negative correlation between HDL and the risk of coronary heart disease, it is suggested that the sustained decrease in HDL concentration associated with zinc administration may increase the risk of coronary artery disease.

(1–21) J.A.M.A. 244:1960–1961, Oct. 24/31, 1980.

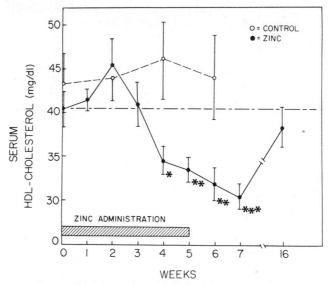

Fig 1–8.—High-density lipoprotein cholesterol levels of patients receiving zinc supplementation *(solid circles)* compared with baseline and control group *(open circles)*. *Single asterisk, P* = .002; *double asterisks, P* = .001; and *triple asterisks, P* = .0001 (paired Student's t test). (Courtesy of Hooper, P. L., et al.: J.A.M.A. 244:1960–1961, Oct. 24/31, 1980; copyright 1980, American Medical Association.)

Since the effect of zinc on serum lipoprotein values was without benefit, it is recommended that zinc supplementation be reserved for clinically indicated disease states.

▶ [The use of vitamin supplementation and megavitamin therapy often includes multivitamins with trace metal supplements, especially urged by some for individuals engaged in vigorous activity. Examples of such "high-powered" vitamins are Z-Bec, Surbex-750, and Berocca-Plus. If these data are corroborated, a strong case can be made for *not* taking zinc supplements in the absence of deficiency disease. This assumes replication of this study and further documents that HDL lipids are possibly correlated with a decreased incidence of coronary heart disease.—L.J.K.] ◀

1–22 **Hypozincemia in Runners.** Zinc, the most abundant trace mineral in tissues other than blood, must be eaten almost daily to prevent deficiency because it is lost from the body in feces, sweat, and urine. The recommended daily allowance of zinc for adults is 15 mg. Rudolph H. Dressendorfer and Ronald Sockolov (Univ. of California, Davis) investigated whether endurance training such as distance running might increase zinc loss and thus raise the dietary requirement for it.

Of 98 apparently healthy men (mean age, 38 years) who volunteered for blood sampling, 77 had run 6–84 miles (average, 22 miles) per week for longer than 1 year, and 21 did not run. Although dietary studies were not performed, each of 14 men who ran in marathons attempted to eat the high-carbohydrate, low-animal-protein diets popular among endurance athletes. Blood samples were drawn after a

(1–22) Physician Sportsmed. 8:97–100, April 1980.

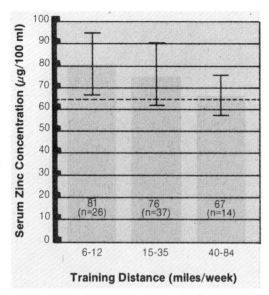

Fig 1–9.—Serum zinc concentrations in three groups of male runners classified according to their training distance. Values are mean ± standard deviation. Differences between groups are not statistically significant. Dashed line shows extreme lower limit of normal zinc concentration (65 µg/100 ml). (Courtesy of Dressendorfer, R. H., and Sockolov, R.: Physician Sportsmed. 8:97–100, April 1980.)

12-hour fast and before exercise for analysis of zinc and copper levels.

The mean serum zinc level was 76 µg/100 ml in runners and 94 µg/100 ml in nonrunners (P<0.05). Copper levels were similar in the 2 groups (96 and 93 µg/100 ml, respectively). The zinc level of 76 µg/100 ml is about 20% below normal, and 18 of the runners (23%) had zinc levels below normal, and 18 of the runners (23%) had zinc levels below 65 µg/100 ml, the extreme lower limit of normal. Serum zinc levels tended to decrease with greater training distance (Fig 1–9).

Experienced runners may be hypozincemic without showing signs or symptoms of zinc deficiency. Oral zinc supplementation is probably not necessary, but endurance athletes should be counseled to eat more protein foods, the major source of dietary zinc, to prevent zinc deficiency.

▶ [The question raised by this article as to whether endurance activity results in a lower zinc level remains to be further studied in other groups. The basis of zinc loss via sweat is discussed. That the high-carbohydrate and low-protein diet could contribute further to zinc deficiency is a theoretical possibility. The argument surely would be for a balanced diet. It has long been argued that there may be a place for multivitamins and increments of trace metals for high-endurance sports. The case could be made that it does no harm if taken in a reasonable single tablet multiple vitamin and mineral replacement. I should like to see more data before I am convinced that zinc should be obligatorily replaced. (See comments on zinc and high-density lipoprotein in the preceding article.)—L.J.K.] ◀

1–23 **Evidence That Body Size Does Not Determine Voluntary Food Intake in the Rat.** Lawrence B. Oscai (Univ. of Illinois, Chi-

(1–23)   Am. J. Physiol. 238:E318–E321, April 1980.

cago) studied the effect of body weight and size of adipocytes on voluntary food intake in rats. The size of the litters was controlled by redistribution of pups at birth. At about age $5^{1}/_{2}$ weeks, one group of rats was put on a food-restricted diet for 30 days; a comparable group was allowed to feed ad libitum.

Rats raised in litters of 13 had a slightly higher ratio of weight gain to food consumption than rats raised in litters of 4 ($P<.01$) and in litters of 22 ($P<.05$). These differences were not evident after the fifth week of life. Rats that were food restricted for 30 days were a mean of 142 gm lighter than unrestricted rats ($P<.001$). The mean diameter of adipocytes in epididymal fat pads of food-restricted rats was 52 μ, compared with 72 μ in controls. After ad libitum feeding was restored, the calorie-restricted rats showed accelerated gain until body weight and adipocyte diameter approximated those of the controls. During this period, overall food intakes and adipocyte diameters were similar for both groups. During the accelerated weight gain, more calories may have been used for growth and less for tissue metabolism.

Neither body weight nor adipocyte size controls voluntary food intake in the rat. If it is found that human appetites are "programmed" in infancy, the results would have important clinical implications for prevention of obesity.

▶ [For a few years, it was held that the overfeeding of infants led to hyperplasia of adipocytes and that the unfortunate child was then forced to eat by his or her collection of hungry adipocytes. Recent investigators have begun to question this concept. The present report on rats notes a discrepancy between adipocyte size and appetite and suggests that the crucial variable is "programming" of appetite in the first 21 days of life. A small litter (or in the human infant, overfrequent breast- or bottle-feeding) gives a lifelong penchant for oral gratification.—R.J.S.] ◄

1–24   **Caloric Restriction and/or Mild Exercise: Effects on Serum Lipids and Body Composition.** Arthur Weltman, Sharleen Matter, and Bryant A. Stamford (Univ. of Louisville) examined the specific effects of caloric restriction (CR), mild exercise (ME), and mild exercise combined with caloric restriction (CR + ME) on alterations in total serum cholesterol concentrations and lipoprotein cholesterol fractions. The alterations in lipoprotein cholesterol were also referenced against weight loss and changes in body composition. Fifty-eight asymptomatic sedentary men, with an average age of 47 years, were studied. The 11 CR subjects were placed on a diet that resulted in 500 kcal per day of caloric restriction. The 11 ME subjects walked briskly (about 3.5 mph) four times per week. The 23 CR + ME subjects combined 500 kcal per day caloric restriction with brisk walking four times per week. Five subjects were controls. Subjects were tested before and after the 10-week program for body weight; body composition; fasting serum cholesterol, fasting high-density lipoprotein (HDL) cholesterol, fasting low-density lipoprotein (LDL) cholesterol, and fasting very-low-density lipoprotein (VLDL) cholesterol concentrations; and caloric intake.

Due to the unequal nature of the four groups, among-group changes

(1–24)   Am. J. Clin. Nutr. 33:1002–1003, May 1980.

were assessed via a 2×4 analysis of covariance and the Scheffe post hoc technique. This procedure was applied to the variables of body weight, percentage body fat, and fat and lean weight. The CR, M, and CR + ME protocols all resulted in significant pre-post changes in body weight, percentage body fat, and fat and lean weight. The CR, ME, and CR + ME protocols all resulted in significant pre-post changes in body weight. Post hoc analysis indicated that the CR + ME treatment resulted in a significantly greater reduction in percentage fat than any other treatment. The CR regimen resulted in significantly greater percentage fat reduction than did the ME treatment. Results were similar for kilograms of fat tissue loss. The CR, ME, and CR + ME regimens all resulted in significant reductions in kilograms of fat after 10 weeks. The CR + ME treatment resulted in 4.27 kg of fat loss, the CR in 2.55 kg of fat loss, and the ME in 0.99 kg of fat loss. The ME treatment resulted in no loss of lean tissue. Both conditions with caloric restriction resulted in significant losses in lean tissue over the 10-week period. Pretreatment serum cholesterol and lipoprotein cholesterol values were not significantly different among the groups. The CR, ME, and CR + ME regimens all resulted in significant reductions of total serum cholesterol concentrations; controls showed no change. The CR regimen resulted in a significant decrease of the HDL cholesterol concentration. The ME and CR + ME regimens did not significantly affect HDL cholesterol values, but only these treatments resulted in significant decreases of LDL cholesterol values. Only the CR + ME treatment resulted in significant decreases of VLDL cholesterol concentrations.

Ten weeks of CR with or without ME lowered total serum cholesterol concentrations. Exercise may be a key factor in lowering LDL cholesterol values. Moderate exercise did not affect HDL cholesterol concentrations over a 10-week period. Ten weeks of CR significantly reduced HDL cholesterol concentrations. A combination of CR and exercise appears to be optimal with respect to body composition alteration.

▶ [There are still dieticians who advocate caloric restrictions rather than exercise to regulate obesity and body composition. The main reason for this erroneous belief is a myopic focus on "weight loss" as the criterion of success. In the present study, a moderate caloric restriction (500 kcal/day) alone or in combination with light exercise produced a substantial weight loss over a 10-week period. However, nearly 2 kg of the 5 kg loss was lean tissue. In contrast, exercise alone gave a smaller fat loss (about 1 kg), but there was no loss of lean tissue. Dieting alone also has no effect on LDL cholesterol, whereas exercise or exercise plus diet reduced LDL and thus improved HDL/LDL ratios. No comment was made on patient attitudes, but a positive form of treatment that is well accepted by the patient is a further argument in favor of exercise rather than dieting.—R.J.S.] ◀

1–25 **Metabolic Response to Moderate Exercise in Obese Man During Prolonged Fasting.** Muscle glycogen is the primary fuel at the onset of exercise. As the course of exercise progresses, increasingly greater amounts of energy are obtained from circulating fuels, including hepatic glucose and fatty acids. Howard I. Minuk, Amir K.

(1–25) Am. J. Physiol. 238:E322–E329, April 1980.

Hanna, Errol B. Marliss, Mladen Vranic, and Bernard Zinman (Toronto, Ont.) investigated the effects of prolonged prior fasting on the metabolic response to exercise in 5 obese, but otherwise healthy, male subjects, aged 19–31 years. They were exercised for 45 minutes on a vertical cycle ergometer at 50%–60% of maximum oxygen uptake after an overnight fast in a postabsorptive state (PAS) and again after 2 weeks of total fasting (TF).

Fasting brought about decreases in glycemia, glucose turnover, pyruvate, alanine, insulin, and respiratory quotient as well as increases in free fatty acids (FFA) and 3-hydroxybutyrate, but lactate or glucagon levels were not altered. Moderate exercise after PAS and TF resulted in the following metabolic changes: Glycemia was constant in both states, but more glucose was available and used in PAS than in TF; respiratory quotients increased in PAS but were unaltered in TF; pyruvate and alanine levels showed less increase in PAS compared with TF; lactate level showed a similar increase in both states; FFA level did not change in PAS but increased in TF; 3-hydroxybutyrate level was unchanged in PAS but decreased in TF; insulin levels were decreased in both states; and glucagon showed only minimal changes.

The results indicate that glucoregulation is preserved in TF during exercise, that less glucose is oxidized during exercise after TF than after PAS, and that metabolic adaptation occurred during TF to use fat-derived substrates preferentially during moderate exercise. It is concluded that exercise as part of a weight-reduction program likely would have specific benefits in terms of fat mobilization.

▶ [The conclusions are well substantiated that (1) glucoregulation is preserved in fasting during exercise in the obese, (2) the glucose utilized during exercise in fasting is oxidized to a lesser extent than in the postabsorptive state, and (3) in this group of subjects, adaptation occurs during fasting that would spare glucose and use fat-derived substrates. This has obvious practical implications in an exercise program for the obese subject.—L.J.K.] ◀

1-26 **Capacity for Moderate Exercise in Obese Subjects After Adaptation to Hypocaloric, Ketogenic Diet.** Optimal function at high submaximal work loads for prolonged periods appears to be promoted by maximizing muscle glycogen content. Eucaloric ketogenic diets have little clinical relevance at present, but supplemented fasting has become common in the treatment of severe obesity. Because physical training has been recommended for weight loss, the effect of ketosis on exercise capacity, if any, must be delineated. Stephen D. Phinney, Edward S. Horton, Ethan A. H. Sims, John S. Hanson, Elliot Danforth, Jr. and Betty M. LaGrange (Univ. of Vermont) examined metabolic changes and work capacity in 6 moderately obese individuals before and during a 6-week course of protein-supplemented fasting (PSF). The test diet provided 1.2 gm of protein per kilogram ideal body weight each day, supplemented by 25 mEq potassium as bicarbonate daily, as well as vitamins and iron. Treadmill endurance

(1–26) J. Clin. Invest. 66:1152–1161, November 1980.

was measured and muscle glycogen concentration determined in vastus lateralis biopsies.

The mean weight loss during the diet period was 10.6 kg. The duration of treadmill exercise to subjective exhaustion was 80% of baseline after 1 week of PSF and 155% after 6 weeks. The final exercise test was performed at a mean of 60% of maximal aerobic capacity, compared to a baseline level of 76%, although weight loss was adjusted for with a backpack. The resting muscle glycogen content fell to 57% of baseline after 1 week of PSF and rose to 69% after 6 weeks, when no decrement occurred after more than 4 hours of uphill walking. The respiratory quotient during steady-state exercise fell from 0.76 to 0.66 after 6 weeks of PSF. The blood glucose level during exercise in ketosis was well maintained. Ketone values on exercise rose from 3.3 to 5.0 mM.

These findings suggest that prolonged ketosis results in an adaptation in which lipid becomes the major metabolic fuel; net carbohydrate utilization is markedly reduced during moderate but ultimately exhausting exercise. Prolonged moderate endurance exercise can be performed by individuals during a protein-supplemented fast if appropriate fluid, mineral, and vitamin supplementation is provided.

▶ [This study provides a solid basis for the view that endurance is not necessarily compromised with protein-supplemented fasting. Alternative substrates other than glycogen become the available and utilized fuel source, presumably due to improved transport of free fatty acids across the mitochondrial membrane or increased capability for fatty acid oxidation within the mitochondria.—L.J.K.] ◀

1–27 **Increased Insulin Receptors After Exercise in Patients With Insulin-Dependent Diabetes Mellitus.** The fall in the blood glucose level that occurs in well-controlled diabetics during exercise has been attributed primarily to an increased uptake of glucose in peripheral tissue; however, the cellular mechanisms involved are not well understood. Oluf Pedersen, Henning Beck-Nielsen, and Lise Heding examined the effects of mild exercise on cellular insulin binding in 9 young men with insulin-dependent diabetes. Changes in insulin receptors on erythrocytes and monocytes were examined in conjunction with bicycle exercise at 33% of maximal aerobic power, in both the fasting and postprandial states. Diabetes was well regulated in these patients, and vascular complications were absent. None was athletically trained.

Insulin binding to red blood cells and monocytes remained constant during postprandial exercise (Fig 1–10). Both postprandial exercise and exercise during fasting significantly increased insulin binding to erythrocytes and monocytes at an insulin concentration of 34 nmol/L compared to control periods. Plasma glucose, free fatty acids, and cortisol levels were reduced with 3 hours of postprandial exercise. Free and total insulin levels, as well as glucagon and lactate levels, were significantly increased. In fasting subjects the plasma glucose and cortisol levels declined significantly, as the free fatty acid and lactate levels increased. A significant overall correlation was found between

(1–27) N. Engl. J. Med. 302:886–892, Apr. 17, 1980.

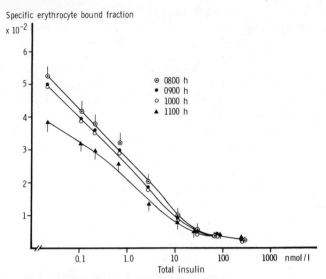

Specific erythrocyte bound fraction

x 10⁻²

⊙ 0800 h
● 0900 h
○ 1000 h
▲ 1100 h

Total insulin

Fig 1–10.—Insulin binding to erythrocytes during postprandial rest. (Courtesy of Pedersen, O., et al.: N. Engl. J Med. 302:886–892, Apr. 17, 1980.)

the specific monocyte- and erythrocyte-bound fractions at the insulin-tracer concentration.

Similar changes probably occur in working muscle cells and contribute to the improvement in glucose tolerance observed with exercise. Accelerated absorption of exogenous insulin from subcutaneous injection sites may contribute. Exercise after eating is a valuable adjunct in the treatment of diabetes.

▶ [Physical exercise is known to improve glucose tolerance and diminish insulin requirements in patients with well-controlled diabetes mellitus. This article nicely demonstrates that these effects of exercise are associated with alterations in insulin binding to erythrocytes and monocytes, and the presumption is made that similar changes occur in working muscle cells, the sum contributing to the improved glucose tolerance induced by exercise. The concept that *postprandial* exercise is a significant adjunct in the treatment of diabetes is not common practice and would appear to have a strong basis of experimental data to recommend it.—L.J.K.] ◀

1–28 **Energy Metabolism in Diabetic Distance Runners.** Diabetics have reported a 30%–40% reduction in their need for insulin during mild exercise training. D. L. Costill, J. M. Miller, and W. J. Fink (Ball State Univ., Muncie, Ind.) studied 10 experienced male juvenile-onset diabetic distance runners and 15 male nondiabetic distance runners to investigate the management of blood glucose levels by using insulin. Blood samples obtained before, during, and after treadmill exercise (70% aerobic capacity) were analyzed for response of blood glucose, ketones, glycerol, free fatty acids, lactic acid, and glucagon. Biopsy specimens from the gastrocnemius muscle were examined for fiber type and glycogen utilization. Perceived exertion was

(1–28) Physician Sportsmed. 8:63–71, October 1980.

AVERAGE BORG SCALE VALUES OF PERCEIVED
EXERTION IN RUNNERS

TIME DURING EXERCISE	WITH INSULIN	NO INSULIN
10 minutes	10.0	8.8
20 minutes	10.4	9.8
30 minutes	10.6	10.2
40 minutes	10.6	10.5
50 minutes	11.0	11.3
60 minutes	11.4	11.8
70 minutes	11.6	12.8
80 minutes	11.6	13.8
90 minutes	11.8	14.2

measured on the Borg scale. The diabetic runners performed 1 run after abstinence from insulin for 24 hours and a second run $2^{1}/_{2}$ to 3 hours after receiving a reduced dose of insulin (6 to 23 units of Lente or neutral protein Hagedorn (NPH) plus 3 to 6 units of regular insulin). All subjects ate a light meal (70% carbohydrate content) 2 hours before the second run.

The diabetics did not become more ketotic during either of the 90-minute runs, despite very high blood glucose levels. At the start of the with-insulin study, blood glucose was approximately three times higher in the diabetic runners than in the nondiabetics. Exercise caused a rapid fall in blood glucose. Blood glucose levels in 1 diabetic remained between 2.2 mM and 2.5 mM during the final hour of the run without a noticeable increase in the level of effort or sensation of fatigue (table). Plasma glucagon levels were similar for each group in the no-insulin run. However, a significant decrease in blood glucagon was observed in diabetics who took insulin ($P<.05$). Diabetic runners without insulin showed considerably higher prerun levels of plasma free fatty acids and glycerol than nondiabetics and diabetics with insulin. Total carbohydrate use was similar for the nondiabetics and diabetics who received insulin.

It is concluded that insulin normalized the uptake and use of glucose during exercise. Without insulin, the muscles appeared to rely more on lipids for energy without a change in the need for glycogen. The differences in free fatty acids may be due to greater hepatic uptake and utilization of glycerol in the diabetics. It is unlikely that glycogen depletion was responsible for the fatigue described by the diabetic runners. Some practical implications of the study for diabetic distance runners are discussed.

▶ [The practical implications of this study for the diabetic distance runner are as follows: To exhibit nearly normal metabolism during running, the diabetic apparently must have some active insulin available to facilitate glucose uptake in muscle. For the diabetic to run in the early morning, at least part of the daily insulin dose should be taken as long-lasting insulin the prior evening. The alternative recommendation is to administer a fraction of the daily dose, between 25% and 50%, some $2^{1}/_{2}$ to 3 hours before the exercise in question. In all cases, a light carbohydrate meal roughly 2 hours before a run is indicated, and little, if any, carbohydrates are taken during the running, with water alone being the oral intake. On such a regimen, the only major risk is hypoglycemia and this appears to be relatively insignificant.—L.J.K.] ◀

1–29 **Muscle Triglycerides in Diabetic Subjects: Effect of Insulin Deficiency and Exercise.** There is indirect evidence that fat stored in muscle may become a major energy source for muscle during exercise in insulin deficiency in diabetics. E. Standl, N. Lotz, Th. Dexel, H.-U. Janka, and H. J. Kolb (Munich) measured muscle triglyceride and glycogen levels in biopsy specimens of the vastus lateralis muscle taken before and after 1 hour of ergometric exercise at 50% to 60% of maximal aerobic power in nonobese men aged 19–35 years. Ten normal persons, 10 insulin-dependent diabetics in good control, and 10 poorly controlled diabetics were studied. Insulin was withdrawn 24 hours before study. Investigations were carried out 1 hour after a morning meal.

The blood glucose level fell with exercise in normal subjects and in well-controlled diabetics, but not in the poorly controlled patients,

Fig 1–11 (above left).—Correlation of resting muscle triglyceride concentration with resting serum triglyceride values in normal persons *(circles)*, in well-controlled, insulin-dependent diabetics *(triangles)*, and in poorly controlled and insulin-deprived insulin-dependent diabetics *(squares)*.

Fig 1–12 (above).—Correlation of decrease of muscle glycogen stores after 1 hour of exercise with resting muscle glycogen value in normal persons *(circles)*, in well-controlled, insulin-dependent diabetics *(triangles)*, and in poorly controlled, insulin-deprived, insulin-dependent diabetics *(squares)*.

Fig 1–13 (left).—Correlation of decrease of muscle triglyceride values after 1 hour of exercise with resting muscle triglyceride values in normal persons *(circles)*, in relatively well-controlled insulin-dependent diabetics *(triangles)*, and in poorly controlled, insulin-deprived, insulin-dependent diabetics *(squares)*.

(Courtesy of Standl, E., et al.: Diabetologia 18:463–469, June 1980: Berlin-Heidelberg-New York: Springer.)

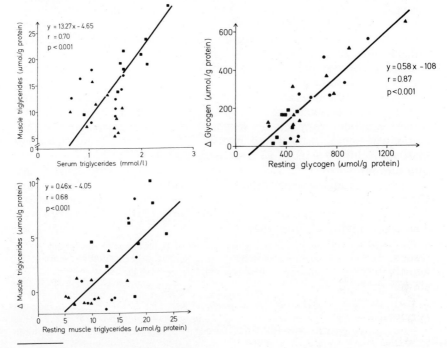

who had very high levels before exercise. Concentrations of serum non-esterified fatty acids initially were elevated twofold in this last group, but mean values after exercise rose only in the normal individuals. Serum glycerol levels rose significantly with exercise in all groups. Ketone body levels did not change significantly in the poorly controlled diabetics. Serum triglyceride concentrations rose with exercise in the normal group and in the well-controlled diabetics and remained at elevated levels in the poorly controlled group. The muscle glycogen concentration was reduced at rest in the latter group; it fell with exercise in all groups but to a significantly smaller degree in the poorly controlled diabetics. Resting muscle and serum triglyceride levels were closely correlated (Fig 1–11). Muscle glycogen or muscle triglyceride levels with exercise were strongly dependent on the resting concentrations (Figs 1–12 and 1–13). The fall in the muscle triglyceride concentration correlated with the increased serum glycerol and nonesterified fatty acid levels during exercise.

The increased muscle triglyceride stores of poorly controlled, insulin-deprived diabetics in this study were mobilized during exercise. These patients appear to rely more on intramuscular triglycerides and less on muscle glycogen during exercise than either relatively well-controlled diabetics or healthy persons.

▶ [This article provides further good data that in poorly controlled and insulin-deprived diabetic patients the increased muscle triglyceride stores are indeed mobilized during exercise and that these patients seem to rely more on intramuscular triglycerides and less on muscle glycogen during exercise than do insulin-treated diabetic patients or healthy persons. This different metabolic behavior occurs at the same absolute work loads and with the same cardiovascular response in all groups.—L.J.K.] ◀

1–30 **Creatine Kinase Elevations in Marathon Runners: Relationship to Training and Competition.** Increased serum creatine kinase (CK) activity may develop in healthy persons after exercise and serves as a marker of injury to skeletal muscle. The risk of rhabdomyolysis is related to adequacy of conditioning and to duration and intensity of exercise. Arthur J. Siegel, Lawrence M. Silverman, and Robert E. Lopez assayed CK activity in 15 male marathon runners before and sequentially after the 1979 Boston Marathon in relation to the finishing times of the participants. Nine men were officially qualified by a time of under 3 hours in those under age 40, or under $3^{1}/_{2}$ hours in older men. Six were registrants in the Doctors' Marathon.

The findings are presented in the table. The overall mean CK level was elevated before the race at 161 units/L, peaked 24 hours after competition at 3,424 units/L, and returned to prerace levels by 4 weeks. Activities observed within 24 hours after the race were significantly higher in the runners who finished under 3:30 than in the slower participants. Mean CK values before and 4 weeks after the marathon were not significantly different in the faster and the slower runners.

Endurance training results in a sequence of biochemical alterations

(1–30) Yale J. Biol. Med. 53:275–279, 1980.

MEAN CREATINE KINASE LEVELS (U/L) FOR ALL RUNNERS AND BY FINISHING TIMES

Elevation of creatine kinase (CK) in serum after exertion is a reliable marker of skeletal muscle injury. Limited data exist on CK levels in conditioned athletes after endurance training and competition. Serum CK was measured by a kinetic UV method (normal $<$ 100 U/L) in 15 long distance runners before (pre-race), 24 hours after (post-race$_1$) and four weeks following (post-race$_2$) the 1979 Boston Marathon. CK levels were elevated throughout the study. Mean values for all runners and for those finishing before and after three hours and 30 minutes are as follows:

	Pre-Race	Post-Race$_1$	Post-Race$_2$
15 Runners	161 (U/L)	3424	157
Under 3:30 (10)	173 (U/L)	4433	166
Over 3:30 (5)	130 (U/L)	1432	135

Post-race$_1$ creatine kinase values were significantly elevated among the 10 faster as compared to the 5 slower runners (P = .025). Elevations of creatine kinase drawn 24 hours after the marathon were inversely related to finishing times among the runners tested.

in skeletal muscle which maximize its capacity for oxidative metabolism and spare muscle glycogen, extending the time during which intense exercise can be sustained. Elite runners may be protected from rhabdomyolysis less by high aerobic endurance than by skeletal muscle specifically endowed for high aerobic performance; this may relate to the proportion of type 2 muscle fibers in these individuals. Runners who can make a sustained intense effort, but in whom skeletal adaptations to training limit efficiency, may be at the greatest risk for the development of rhabdomyolysis. Sustained, intense training may induce some elevation of the CK level as part of a progressive training effect. This may be accompanied by lesser peaks in total CK concentrations after maximal effort, e.g., a marathon race. Additional studies in runners of varying ability are needed to clarify the relation between degree of conditioning and the extent of, or risk for, the development of transient rhabdomyolysis.

▶ [The reader is referred to discussions of enzyme elevation after significant exercise in the 1980 YEAR BOOK OF SPORTS MEDICINE, page 66, and the 1979 YEAR BOOK OF SPORTS MEDICINE, page 161. The present report extends the series and quantitates it more precisely.

Glycogen depletion in marathon runners correlates with the so-called wall. Beyond depletion, oxidative metabolism is very much dependent on ketones and free fatty acids for the regeneration of adenosine triphosphate. Insufficient availability of activated phosphates results in decreased efficiency of muscular work, increasing the likelihood of membrane permeability with the efflux of enzymes into the serum. This is important for two reasons—it may reflect significant muscle inflammation and it may be a forewarning of increased metabolic end-products presenting to the kidney. Further, it may give the false positive elevation of the enzyme that can be mistaken for coronary artery disease. It is very clearly a function of training as well as inherent biologic capacity and perhaps a marker of those who should or should not reasonably engage in vigorous long-distance running.—L.J.K.] ◀

1–31 **Gastric Emptying Characteristics of Glucose and Glucose Polymer Solutions.** Prolonged exercise causes hyperthermia and de-

(1–31) Res. Q. Exerc. Sport 51:299–305, 1980.

pletion of carbohydrate stores. Attempts to attenuate these two effects by ingestion of carbohydrate or fluid, or both, before and during exercise have met with mixed results. The finding of a slightly faster rate of gastric emptying with complex as compared to simple carbohydrate molecules suggests that the optimal carbohydrate molecule for drinks designed for athletes may be more complex than glucose or sucrose.

Carl Foster (Mount Sinai Med. Center, Milwaukee), David L. Costill, and William J. Fink (Ball State Univ.) compared the gastric emptying characteristics of 5%, 10%, 20%, and 40% solutions of glucose and a glucose polymer in 11 healthy male and 4 female subjects (average age, 22½ years) by measuring the volume of gastric residue remaining 30 minutes after ingestion of 400 ml of each of the solutions.

The volume of gastric residue recovered increased progressively with increasing solute concentration. At the lowest carbohydrate concentration the glucose polymer yielded significantly less gastric residue than did glucose. The smaller residue appeared to be due both to a greater rate of exit of the polymer from the stomach and to a lower rate of gastric secretion induced by the polymer. The calculated delivery of carbohydrate to the intestine increased with solute concentration. At the lowest carbohydrate concentration the more rapid gastric emptying of the polymer allowed significantly greater calculated carbohydrate delivery.

At low carbohydrate concentrations (5 gm/100 ml or less), such as used in drinks designed for athletic participants, the glucose polymer might be an advantageous alternative to glucose as a source of carbohydrate.

▶ [Two factors are important in the ingestion of any given solution during competition or vigorous exercise—the need for fluid and the need for carbohydrate calories. In situations where hyperthermia is likely to present the major limitation or hazard, the addition of any carbohydrate to an athletic drink is counterproductive. Where hypoglycemia is likely to be a factor, and especially in events of more than 3 hours' duration, the need for carbohydrate is increased but must be balanced against the need for fluid. For example, in extended cross-country Nordic events, highly concentrated glucose solutions have had an historical and practical basis. There is minimal thermal stress in that situation. In events where both fluid and carbohydrate delivery are of importance, more complex carbohydrate molecules, such as the polymers now available, appear to have merit. At carbohydrate concentrations comparable to those frequently used in athletic drinks, the glucose polymer simultaneously delivers 69% more fluid and 33% more carbohydrate than glucose.—L.J.K.] ◀

1–32 **"Runner's Trots": Gastrointestinal Disturbances in Runners.** "Abnormalities" such as bradyarrhythmia and proteinuria can occur in healthy runners as physiologic adaptations to physical training or as normal responses to extreme exertion. Richard N. Fogoros (Univ. of Pittsburgh) reports that many runners also have gastrointestinal symptoms that are usually mild and consist of abdominal cramping, bloating, and frequent watery bowel movements. These symptoms seem to occur either during a period of rapid increase in daily run-

(1–32) J.A.M.A. 243:1743–1744, May 2, 1980.

ning mileage or during a particularly severe running episode, such as a race. They are occasionally bothersome enough for the runner to consult a physician.

CASE 1.—Man, 31, had suffered for 5 days with cramping periumbilical pain and loose bowel movements that were greatly exacerbated by attempts to run. He had been a runner for 2 years and had been rapidly increasing his mileage in preparation for a marathon. All findings and studies were normal except for bradycardia. The patient tapered his running schedule and symptoms subsided. After a more gradual increase in training, he successfully completed his first marathon without further symptoms.

CASE 2.—Man, 24, complained of 3 weeks of abdominal cramping and watery diarrhea that occurred after hard runs, and for 1 week he had also noted dark red blood mixed with loose stools. He had had occasional episodes of abdominal cramping and watery diarrhea for 1 year, ever since he began running seriously. Six weeks earlier he had markedly increased his training in preparation for his first marathon. Results of physical examination were normal. Proctosigmoidoscopy, barium enema examination, and an upper gastrointestinal roentgenographic series with small bowel follow-through were all normal. He continued his strenuous running schedule and the symptoms gradually disappeared. In the 2 years since then, the patient has maintained a high level of training but has remained asymptomatic except for a few recurrent episodes of diffuse abdominal cramping, watery diarrhea, and, rarely, bloody diarrhea. These episodes have always been associated with particularly strenuous exertion, such as a competitive marathon race.

Gastrointestinal disturbances in runners are most likely due to gut ischemia. During maximal exercise, whether a person is well trained or not, blood flow to the gut is reduced by up to 80%. During prolonged severe exercise, such as a marathon, the runner has the additional stress of hyperthermia, which would predispose to ischemic necrosis. Cardiovascular training results in changes in regional blood flow during submaximal exercise such that, for a given level of submaximal work, blood flow to the gut is much less reduced in the trained than in the relatively untrained person. This training-induced change in regional blood flow can explain why runners have gastrointestinal disturbances when they begin to increase their running and why the symptoms decrease once the training effect has taken hold.

▶ [The various small and large side effects of running have become increasingly known to the medical and lay populace, but gastrointestinal disturbance is one of those not fully appreciated. Further, that this can present as bloody diarrhea has been documented on multiple occasions. It is almost frightening to think that there could be so much relative ischemia as to induce ischemic colitis. Abnormalities of sympathetic and parasympathetic tone are much easier to comprehend as a simple mechanism. Nevertheless, bloody diarrhea must have a more profound basis. It would, in my view, be a relative contraindication to continued running at an intense level. The other possibility not considered is that the extreme exertion might bring about the expression of subclinical inflammatory bowel disease.—L.J.K.] ◀

1–33 **Exercise Effect During Pregnancy on Brain Nucleic Acids of Offspring in Rats.** Reports in the recent literature suggest that more vigorous activities should be added to the treatment of expec-

(1–33)   Arch. Phys. Med. Rehabil. 61:124–127, March 1980.

tant mothers. Robert R. Jenkins and Charles Ciconne (Ithaca College) find this suggestion alarming, since there has been little research into the effect of exercise on the fetus. It has been reported that pregnant women who are exposed to stress (living under an airport landing pattern) give birth to a higher number of offspring with birth defects. Studies in laboratory animals have shown that rough handling results in abnormal adrenocortical activity, that mild foot shock produces increased brain catecholamine turnover, and that minimal electric shock or visual stress results in decreased brain protein and nucleic acid content in offspring.

Recent studies in the pregnant female have shown that this population can tolerate vigorous exercise. Blake and Hazelwood (1971) reported that exercise had no obvious adverse effects on the intrauterine environment in rats. However, others have found that even moderately severe maternal exercise in sheep reduced umbilical circulation, with a resultant decrease in fetal Po_2. Other studies have shown adverse reactions in the neonatal animal as a result of exposure of pregnant dams to stressors specifically related to exercise. The authors, therefore, designed a study to determine the effects of exercise during pregnancy on brain nucleic acids, brain protein, and motor performance of rat offspring.

Eighteen nulliparous female rats were assigned to a sedentary control group, a wheel-running exercise group, or a treadmill-running exercise group. The exercise began at least 1 week before pregnancy and continued to parturition. On the day of birth, the offspring were weighed and all litters were reduced to the 6 largest pups. This standardized the nutrition of those pups that were to perform a motor ability test at weaning (day 21). The other pups were killed. All chemical determinations were performed on brains that had been pooled by litters.

The wheel-running and treadmill-running conditions resulted in significantly lower body weights in the dams. No significant differences were observed between the exercise and control groups in number of pups delivered, brain weight of pups, or pup body weight. No significant group differences were found for DNA, RNA, or protein from the brains of the pups. However, pups of the treadmill-running dams performed significantly poorer on a measure of motor performance on a Rotacone.

This study is in no way definitive for the merits of physical training during pregnancy. It shows that pregnant rats will exercise voluntarily and can be forced to exercise at an intensity sufficient to reduce body weight significantly and with no obvious effect on the brain nucleic acids of their offspring. Ad libitum exercise was as effective as forced exercise, although forced exercise would be expected to exert a more potent emotional stress.

▶ [This article provides a useful review of literature on exercise during pregnancy. Oxygenation of the fetus does become somewhat marginal in the final trimester, and, in consequence, very vigorous exercise could theoretically have some harmful effect on the offspring. Experiments by the authors showed that regular treadmill exercise by pregnant rats had no effect on any measure except the motor performance of the pups. This was assessed by a task where the weanling had to maintain its balance as it walked along a cone rotating at 20 rpm. The offspring of treadmill runners fared only half as well as sedentary controls on this test, but the alarming nature of this result is tempered by the absence of effect in the offspring of rats who exercised in a wheel. Possibly, any bad effects of the treadmill training were related to the more "stressful" nature of this exercise.—R.J.S.] ◄

1–34 **Inhibiting Effect of Atropine on Growth Hormone Release During Exercise.** J. D. Few and C. T. M. Davies (London) found previously that for a given work load the plasma cortisol concentration was higher when atropine had been administered, but paradoxically the growth hormone (GH) concentration was considerably lower. They therefore studied the effect of atropine on the GH response to exercise and simultaneously monitored changes in blood glucose and lactate and plasma cortisol and free fatty acid concentrations. Ten subjects walked on a treadmill at 6.4 km per hour. Two exercise regimens were used. In the progressive exercise, 5 subjects walked as the treadmill gradient that was initially zero was increased (usually in 3% increments) every 10 minutes, until a nearly exhausting load was achieved. In the constant work load exercise, 5 subjects experienced a constant treadmill gradient, but the physiologic work load (oxygen consumption) tended to increase slightly during the experiment. Blood samples were drawn about every 10 minutes throughout the experiment.

At low work loads, atropine had no effect on the changes of cortisol and lactate concentrations, but the normal exercise-induced rise in GH concentration was abolished or markedly reduced. At higher work loads, especially when prolonged, the usual rises in cortisol and lactate concentrations were enhanced by atropine, but the rise in GH values was diminished and delayed. The changes in free fatty acid and glucose concentrations were not significantly affected by atropine. Plasma catecholamine concentrations were measured in six pairs of experiments involving three subjects. In each instance, values were higher in atropine experiments than in control experiments.

Atropine inhibits, partially or completely, the usual GH response to exercise and under appropriate conditions increases circulating cortisol, lactate, and catecholamine concentrations. The effect upon the latter three is consistent with the view that atropine, by diverting a higher proportion of cardiac output to the skin, effectively reduces work capacity in a manner analogous to that of hypoxia. The reduction in GH response, however, is probably a direct result of the cholinergic blocking properties of atropine.

► [The exercise-induced release of growth hormone has interested both exercise biochemists and pediatricians who wish to assess pituitary function in underdeveloped children. α-Adrenergic, serotoninergic, and dopaminergic mechanisms, plus β-adrenergic inhibition, have been suggested during exercise. This article indicated that a cholinergic mechanism may also be involved, particularly at light work loads.—R.J.S.] ◄

1–35 **Anabolic Steroids and Athletes.** Raymond V. Brooks and Robert

(1–34) Eur. J. Appl. Physiol. 43:221–228, April 1980.
(1–35) Physician Sportsmed. 80:161–163, March 1980.

Cottrell discuss the action of anabolic steroids in athletes and methods for their detection. No studies have adequately established that anabolic steroids per se markedly improve athletic performance, perhaps because they are not truly anabolic in healthy adults, but act androgenically. Anabolic steroids, which are synthetic variants of testosterone, supposedly increase the anabolic action of testosterone relative to its androgenic action, promoting muscle growth. However, any improvement in athletic ability should be attributed to the androgenic action, which stimulates the athlete to train harder, instead of to a direct anabolic action on the muscle cell.

Assays for anabolic steroids administered intramuscularly rather than orally were introduced at the 1976 Montreal Olympics. Positive radioimmunoassay results (10% to 20% of samples) were substantiated by identification of the illegal substance with gas chromatography-mass spectrometry. Although there were no positive tests for intramuscular steroid administration at Montreal, there were five positive tests at a major international event 1 year later. One approach to bypassing the tests has been met by the development of an antiserum sensitive to compounds having a 1-methyl group instead of the 17-methyl group usually found in orally active steroids. Further, a test that measures the ratio of testosterone to luteinizing hormone in the blood is being developed for detection of administered natural testosterone.

If athletes risked losing at least one Olympic appearance, they would be discouraged from taking anabolic steroids.

▶ [Antiserums for 1-methyl androgens and testosterone-luteinizing hormone ratios are two new steps in the continuing warfare between the pharmacologic "police" and the unscrupulous advisers of some international athletes. Unfortunately, the enforcers always seem one pace behind, and the excitement of doping control seems merely to encourage new tactics of deceit. Now that competition is between pharmacologists rather than athletes, the time may have arrived for abandoning the concept of national athletic representatives.—R.J.S.] ◀

1–36 **Effect of Testosterone on Compensatory Hypertrophy of Rat Skeletal Muscles.** M. Marchetti, F. Figura, N. Candelor., and S. Favilli (Rome) studied the effect of testosterone, either endogenous or exogenous, on skeletal muscle hypertrophy induced by overload in rats. The tendon of the gastrocnemius on one limb was severed so that its synergists, the soleus and plantaris, were forced to support the full body weight with respect to the corresponding muscles of the contralateral limb, thus avoiding the variability inherent in any interindividual comparison. There were 142 rats (95 males) in the study. At tenotomy the rats were aged 45 days and weighed an average of 100 gm. Sex, natural testicular hormone concentration, testosterone dose, and Δt of hypertrophy (interval between tenotomy and muscle examination) were determined. Two levels of Δt of hypertrophy were established: 87 rats were killed by bleeding 8 days after tenotomy and 55 were killed 15 days after tenotomy. In control rats, sesame oil was injected subcutaneously; experimental rats received a daily injection

(1–36) J. Sports Med. Phys. Fitness 20:13–22, March 1980.

of testosterone phenyl propionate from the day after tenotomy until the day before they were killed. To study the effect of deprivation of natural testicular hormones, 50 male rats were castrated at age 30 days (15 days before tenotomy).

Growth of the rats was not unaffected by castration or testosterone treatment. The lack of testicular hormones in the castrated rats was indicated by a reduction in prostate weight. The effectiveness of the testosterone treatment was indicated by enhancement of prostate weight of treated rats, both castrated and normal, in comparison with placebo-treated rats. No statistically significant difference was found in the water content of the levator ani in the different groups. No statistically significant difference was found among the groups in wet weights of gastrocnemius, plantaris, and soleus muscles of the sham-operated limb, except for a sex difference apparently correlated with the difference in body weight. No statistically significant difference in hypertrophy between male and female rats was observed in the soleus and plantaris muscles, either between castrated and normal rats or between rats observed 7 and 15 days after tenotomy. Testosterone treatment induced a significant increase in hypertrophy of the soleus and plantaris. No difference in muscular hypertrophy related to sex, castration, or time of hypertrophy was observed in testosterone-treated rats. Calculations of hypertrophy from muscle dry weight and wet weight gave the same results, indicating that the observed effect was not due to different hydration of muscles. No significant effect of sex, induction time of atrophy, castration, or testosterone treatment was observed in the gastrocnemius.

When testosterone is administered in high doses, it induces an increase of work-induced muscle hypertrophy. Endogenous testicular hormones have no effect on the work-induced hypertrophy.

▶ [Controversy continues as to whether androgenic hormones are effective in increasing muscle mass. The use of experimental animals allows the examination of the effects of intensive training thrown on the soleus and plantaris by section of the gastrocnemius tendon. Hypertrophy amounted to 22% and 13% without androgen administration and 30% and 17% with large doses of testosterone phenyl proprionate (0.6 mg/day). The effect was seen equally with wet and dry mass; it could not thus be interpreted as a greater hydration of the muscle after testosterone administration. However, daily activity patterns were not controlled. It is thus conceivable that the additional testosterone stimulated movement, increasing the training stimulus to the limb muscles.—R.J.S.] ◀

1–37 **Effects of Androgen Therapy in Physiologic Doses on Physical and Psychic Training Conditions of High-Level Athletes** was investigated by Roger Morvile, Bruno de Lignieres, Jean-Noël Plas, and Fernand Plas (Paris). The prolonged and repeated stress involved in the training program of high-level athletes tends to induce disequilibrium between catabolism and anabolism by progressive development of a testicular endocrine insufficiency. This androgen deficit appears to be a major limiting factor in resistance to stress by its energetic consequences at both the muscular and psychic level.

In the present double-blind study, 10 athletes submitted voluntar-

(1–37) Med. Sport 54:303–308, September 1980. (Fre.)

ily to 2 months of androgen therapy, with regular clinical and hormonal surveillance. All subjects (aged 25 to 30 years) were experienced athletes of national or international reputation, aware of their capacities and thus particularly apt to note any improvement in their performance.

The study suggested that there is indeed a causal relationship between the decrease of plasma androgens and the sensation of fatigue, the lessening of muscular energy and lengthening of the recuperation phase. During androgen therapy (dihydrotestosterone, 12.5 mg a day administered percutaneously, and hydroalcoholic gel of DHT, 5 gm spread daily on the skin) most subjects were able to increase the intensity and duration of training with a shorter recuperation period, the phase of equilibrium between anabolism and catabolism having been prolonged. This beneficial effect was obtained with relatively low doses of the hormone, without development of plasma hyperandrogenism, and afforded better final results after an equal number of training days.

▶ [This is a somewhat disturbing report from Paris, because it seems to imply that some French clinicians regard the "stress" of competition as clinical grounds for supplementing natural androgens. The postulated hypothesis is that with an overvigorous training program, the catabolic action of cortisol outweighs the anabolic action of testosterone.—R.J.S.] ◀

1–38 **Investigation of Secretion and Metabolism of Cortisol During a 100-Km Race Using 4-^{14}C- and 11α-^{3}H-Cortisol.** J. D. Few and M. W. Thompson (London) used a long-distance race as an experimental situation to study the effects of exercise on cortisol metabolism. A mixture of 4-^{14}C-cortisol to study cortisol metabolism in the conventional manner and 11α-^{3}H-cortisol to study interconversion of cortisol and cortisone was used. When 4-^{14}C,11α-^{3}H-cortisol is metabolized to cortisone, the 11α-tritium atom is lost, so that when the resulting ^{14}C-cortisone is reduced back to cortisol the ^{3}H-^{14}C ratio is lowered. The decline of this ratio becomes an index of the degree of cortisone-cortisol interconversion. Eight participants in the race drank 1 ml of an ethanolic solution containing 5 μCi of 11α-^{3}H-cortisol and 1 μCi of 4-^{14}C-cortisol. Four subjects who were not running received an identical dose of ^{3}H,^{14}C-cortisol, and urine was collected for 24 hours (basal controls). Three subjects followed the same protocol as the resting controls but also received 20 mg of cortisol orally at the same time as the labeled cortisol and subsequently at 90-minute intervals until a total of 100 mg was ingested (high-cortisol controls). Six racers provided useful collections of urine. Three subjects (group A) could not supply samples after leaving the race, but follow-up samples were obtained from the other 3 (group B). All runners except 1 produced some urine during the race. All samples produced by each of the group A subjects were pooled. From the group B runners and the control subjects two pools were obtained, one corresponding to about 8 hours, for comparison with the group A runners, and one of 24 hours or as near as could be obtained.

(1–38) Acta Endocrinol. (Copenh.) 94:204–212, June 1980.

Neither the runners nor the controls showed significant differences in the specific activities or radionuclide ratios of 5α-tetrahydrocortisol (5α-THF) or tetrahydrocortisol (THF). The radionuclide ratio of tetrahydrocortisone (THE) was extremely low and the specific activity of THE was higher than that of the two 11β-hydroxy metabolites. The relative distributions of ^{14}C among the three major tetrahydro metabolites of cortisol indicated that, relative to the resting controls, there was a shift from THE to the 11-hydroxy metabolites, THF and 5α-THF.

After exploring the use of 11α-^{3}H,4-^{14}C-cortisol to calculate the total quantity of cortisol oxidized to cortisone in a given time, the authors conclude that they have not developed a model satisfactory for this purpose. A less sophisticated analysis of the data reveals that a major determinant of the ^{3}H-^{14}C ratio is the magnitude of the cortisol pool. Exercise has little if any effect. As the quantity of cortisol secreted or administered increases, the fractional conversion to cortisone decreases.

▶ [Whereas it is well recognized that sustained and strenuous exercise can increase blood cortisol concentrations, the balance among secretion, metabolism, and excretion of cortisol is less clearly established. The authors attempted to answer this question by administering two radioactive forms of cortisol orally. This is a possible weakness in the experiment, since the long-distance running may have modified absorption of cortisol by the oral route. One important observation is that the twofold to fourfold increase of cortisol secretion was reflected in the urinary excretion of cortisol, but not in the urinary 17-hydroxyketosteroids, which are often interpreted in this sense.— R.J.S.] ◀

1–39 **Influence of Exercise and Diet on Myoglobin and Metmyoglobin Reductase in the Rat.** Louis Hagler, Robert I. Coppes, Jr., E. Wayne Askew, Arthur L. Hecker, and Robert H. Herman (Letterman Army Inst. of Res.) evaluated the influence of exercise and diet on selected aspects of heme protein metabolism in the rat, including myoglobin (MB) and metmyoglobin (MetMB) reductase of rat muscle.

Male rats, aged 6½ weeks and weighing about 130 gm, were divided into six treatment groups with 11 to 17 rats per group. Groups 1 and 2 were trained by treadmill running and group 3 served as a sedentary pair-fed control. Groups 4 through 6 remained sedentary in cages and received different quantities of diet. Rats were trained at high (group 1) and moderate (group 2) exercise levels. Group 1 rats consumed food ad libitum, and groups 2 and 3 were each pair-fed at the intake level of group 1. Group 4 was allowed to consume food ad libitum. Group 5 received a diet restricted to 75% of that consumed by group 4, and group 6 received a diet restricted to 65% of that consumed by group 4. At the end of the 12-week period of training and diet, the rats were decapitated. Before being killed, trained rats were rested for 24 hours and all rats were fasted for 12 hours. At death, blood was collected for the MetMB reductase assay.

Neither training nor diet had any effect on erythrocyte reduced nicotinamide adenine dinucleotide (NADH)-methemoglobin reductase.

(1–39) J. Lab. Clin. Med. 95:222–230, February 1980.

The group undergoing the higher level of treadmill exercise had a significantly lower hemoglobin (HB) concentration. The activity of NADH-MetMB reductase was increased in the group undergoing the highest level of training and decreased in the groups whose diets were restricted by 25% and 35%. These changes were seen only in the soleus muscle. Other muscles, including the heart, psoas, and quadriceps, were unaffected by either exercise or diet. Both levels of exercise were effective in increasing muscle MB concentration, but only in the quadriceps and soleus.

The data illustrate the adaptive nature of muscle MB and NADH-MetMB reductase. Exercise apparently signals the increase in MB concentration only in those muscles that are being stressed by the training regimen. The increase in MB concentration is not a nonspecific or generalized response to exercise, because it is not seen in all muscles.

▶ [It has been fairly widely accepted that vigorous training enhances muscle myoglobin concentrations. The experiments discussed in this article show that the change is restricted to the active muscles (quadriceps and soleus only). In contrast to some earlier reports, intracardiac myoglobin concentration is unchanged. A new feature of the present research is the study of NADH-metmyoglobin reductase, the enzyme that prevents the gradual conversion of myoglobin into the physiologically inactive "met" form. This enzyme is also increased in the trained muscles.—R.J.S.] ◀

1–40 **Adenylate Deaminase Deficiency in a Hypotonic Infant** is reported by Jack B. Shumate, Kenneth K. Kaiser, James E. Carroll, and Michael H. Brooke (Washington Univ.).

Girl, aged 18 months, was referred because of delayed motor and speech development. She was born to a gravida 2, para 1, aged 24, after a pregnancy complicated by repeated urinary tract infections, which were treated with nitrofurantoin and ampicillin. Fetal movements were said to have been reduced. Birth weight was 3.54 kg and delivery was uneventful. Although the infant fed well, the mother noticed she was "like a rag doll." She rolled over at 6 months, sat unassisted at 10 months, and was unable to pull to stand at 18 months. Speech was poorly developed. The infant was hospitalized for pneumonia at age 6 months. A sibling, aged 6 months, was normal, but a maternal uncle was severely retarded and a female maternal cousin had spina bifida.

The child was hypotonic, tended to slip through the hands when held, and could not stand unsupported. Height, weight, and head circumference were at the tenth percentile. Cranial nerves and funduscopic examination were normal. There was no muscle wasting. Tendon reflexes were brisk bilaterally, and plantar reflexes were flexor. Sensation was normal. Laboratory test results were normal. Muscle biopsy with histochemistry showed only an increased proportion of the number of type I fibers seen on adenosine triphosphatase staining. Special studies showed that muscle adenylate deaminase (AMPDA) activity in the patient was about 40 times less than normal.

Although the finding of muscle AMPDA deficiency in a hypotonic infant would, in light of the proposed adenosine triphosphate-adenosine diphosphate regulatory function of the enzymes suggest a causal relation, the authors have reservations that it is causal. Long-term

(1–40)   J. Pediatr. 96:885–887, May 1980.

follow-up of muscle function in this child, search for AMPDA deficiency in children undergoing muscle biopsy for reasons other than hypotonia, and better definition of the physiologic function of AMPDA are needed before AMPDA deficiency can be labeled a disease.

▶ [The enzyme adenylate deaminase (AMPDA) is thought to play a role in the generation of the immediate energy stores of muscle (adenosine triphosphate and adenosine diphosphate). Deficiency of AMPDA could thus be one cause of congenital hypotonia. However, the authors are commendably cautious in reaching such a conclusion from a single report, pointing the need for further cases and for longitudinal study of the infant described.—R.J.S.] ◀

1–41 **Marathon Run III: Effects on Coagulation, Fibrinolysis, Platelet Aggregation, and Serum Cortisol Levels; Three-Year Study** was conducted by T. Mandalaki, A. Dessypris, C. Louizou, C. Panayotopoulou, and C. Dimitriadou. Thirty-five Finnish amateur runners, aged 27 to 56 years, and 3 men, aged 65, 67, and 82 years, respectively, who had run a noncompetitive marathon in 1975, 1976, and 1977 were studied. Blood samples were taken within 20 minutes of completion of the marathon.

In each of the 3 years, kaolin-activated partial thromboplastin time (APTT) was significantly shortened, whereas prothrombin time and plasma fibrinogen concentration were not markedly changed. Euglobulin lysis time was also significantly shortened and fibrin degradation products were increased. Each subject had a positive protamine sulfate precipitation test, but the ethanol gelation test was negative. Platelet count and aggregation were significantly increased after the 1975 marathon when the environmental temperature was 25 C; this was not the case in 1976 and 1977 when the temperatures were 15 to 18 C. Serum cortisol concentrations were significantly increased after each of the runs, especially after the 1975 race. The responses were the same for both sexes.

A noncompetitive marathon could be of value in the prevention of thromboembolic disease by increasing plasma fibrinolytic activity. However, this beneficial effect would have to be watched because of the activation of platelet aggregation when high temperatures prevail.

▶ [The acute effect of sustained exercise on the blood is that complex fibrinolysis is accelerated, but the tendency to coagulation of blood specimens is increased. The present report suggests that the net effect is normally favorable to the individual with vascular disease, but that if the day is warm (>25 C), the potential benefit may be more than offset by an increase of platelet count and aggregation.—R.J.S.] ◀

1–42 **Plasma AVP, Neurophysin, Renin Activity, and Aldosterone During Submaximal Exercise Performed Until Exhaustion in Trained and Untrained Men.** B. Melin, J. P. Eclache, G. Geelen, G. Annat, A. M. Allevard, E. Jarsaillon, A. Zebidi, J. J. Legros, and Cl. Gharib (Lyons, France) note that during severe and prolonged exercise, the different hormonal systems involved in sodium- and water-saving mechanisms are strongly stimulated, as judged by the increase

(1–41) Thromb. Haemost. 43:49–52, Feb. 29, 1980.
(1–42) Eur. J. Appl. Physiol. 44:141–151, August 1980.

in plasma hormonal levels. Therefore, they investigated the mechanism of appearance of such changes in hormonal concentration and the differences between trained and untrained subjects.

TECHNIQUE.—Fourteen male subjects, aged 19–27, all undergoing regular physical activity, were studied during intense muscular work (80% of maximal oxygen uptake) performed on a cycle ergometer until exhaustion. Experiments were carried out in an environmental chamber where temperature, relative humidity, and wind speed were constant at 25 C, 30%, and 1.2 m·second^{-1}, respectively. Pulmonary gas exchange, heart rate, rectal and skin temperature, and weight loss were measured. Brachiovenous catheters were inserted, and blood was taken before and in the first minute after the end of the exercise. Urine samples were collected during the 1-hour period just before and 10 minutes after the end of the exercise. The subjects were divided into three groups: well-trained (group I), trained (group II) and untrained (group III).

In each group, there was a significant increase in plasma protein concentration as a result of exercise. Osmolality rose significantly in group I only. Osmolality did increase in all three groups, but in groups II and III individual values were scattered. Trained subjects, at rest, had the highest hematocrit reading (group I) and showed no significant variation at the end of the exercise, whereas the hematocrit reading increased significantly in the other two groups (Fig 1–14). The comparison between the importance of weight loss and hematocrit variation indicates that in the group where the variation of hematocrit was smallest the weight loss was greatest; weight loss was significantly different between group I (trained) and group III (untrained). Plasma renin activity (PRA) and aldosteronemia displayed highly significant increases after exercise: a 4.5-fold increase for PRA (Fig 1–15) and a 13-fold increase for plasma aldosterone (Fig 1–16). Nevertheless, there was no correlation between the changes in PRA

Fig 1–14.—Changes in hematocrit and body weight: *clear columns,* before exercise; *shaded columns,* after exercise. Asterisk denotes significance (*P*<.05). It is noteworthy that subjects in group I (endurance-trained subjects) have the slightest change in hematocrit reading and the most important weight loss. (Courtesy of Melin, B., et al.: Eur. J Appl. Physiol. 44:141–151 August 1980; Berlin-Heidelberg-New York: Springer.)

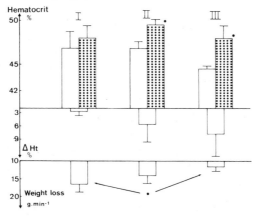

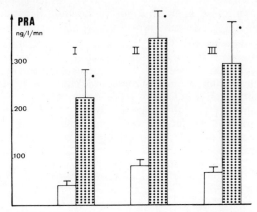

Fig 1–15.—Mean PRA before and after exercise: *clear columns,* before exercise; *shaded columns,* after exercise. (Courtesy of Melin, B., et al.: Eur. J. Appl. Physiol. 44:141–151, August 1980; Berlin-Heidelberg-New York: Springer.)

and those in plasma aldosterone level, nor between aldosterone level and plasma sodium or potassium level. For antidiuretic hormone (AVP or vasopressin) and neurophysin, the pattern was similar, with a significant increment increase after exercise when compared with levels at rest (between-group comparison).

In conclusion, these data demonstrate a different hormonal behavior between trained and untrained subjects as a result of strenuous prolonged exercise. Plasma concentrations of AVP, neurophysin, renin, and aldosterone increase markedly in both, but such changes are of lesser magnitude in the well-trained subjects. This could be related to the observed changes in hematocrit reading and body weight. The authors propose that water is shifted from previously ac-

Fig 1–16.—Mean plasma aldosterone concentrations before and after exercise: *clear columns,* before exercise; *shaded columns,* after exercise. (Courtesy of Melin, B., et al.: Eur. J. Appl. Physiol. 44:141–151, August 1980; Berlin-Heidelberg-New York: Springer.)

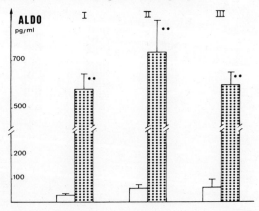

tive muscular tissues to plasma during exercise, this being more marked in trained than in untrained subjects.

▶ [At one time, industrial physiologists maintained that well-trained workers sweated less than sedentary employees; however, this view was based on a fixed work rate. If all subjects exercise at a comparable fraction of their Vo_2 (max), the trained subjects produce more sweat than the untrained. The fluid losses involved, up to 2 L per hour, pose a substantial threat to the plasma volume, and it is hardly surprising that a vigorous response is evoked from the hormonal mechanisms concerned in the regulation of plasma fluid volumes. This article is interesting in showing that despite greater sweat production, trained subjects are better able to preserve plasma volume during exercise. The explanation suggested is a greater availability of fluid (due to larger intramuscular stores of glycogen and associated water molecules). The consequence is a lesser activation of the renin-aldosterone axis in well-trained subjects.—R.J.S.] ◀

1–43 **Effect of Dichloroacetate on Plasma Lactic Acid in Exercising Dogs.** Strenuous physical exercise is associated with an increase in plasma lactic acid (LA) concentration. Dichloroacetate sodium (DCA) has recently been reported to reduce the lactacidemia associated with some disorders. Gary F. Merrill, Edward J. Zambraski, and Steven M. Grassl (Rutgers Univ.) undertook to determine what effect DCA has on plasma LA accumulation during treadmill exercise in a conscious model. Eight adult female dogs were trained to run on a motor-driven treadmill. A jugular catheter was inserted for injection of saline or DCA while each dog was tested. Group 1 dogs were tested with light, moderate, and heavy exercise and group 2 with prolonged, moderate exercise.

In group I, DCA treatment at rest had no effect on heart rate. During light and moderate exercise, the increase in heart rate was attenuated by DCA, compared with saline. Heart rates were 10% and 18%

Fig 1–17.—Changes in plasma LA concentration in group II controls *(solid circles)* and dogs given 100 mg of DCA per kg intravenously *(open circles),* when DCA was administered after first 10 minutes of 50-minute run; N = 6. (Courtesy of Merrill, G. F., et al.: J. Appl. Physiol. 48:427–431, March 1980.)

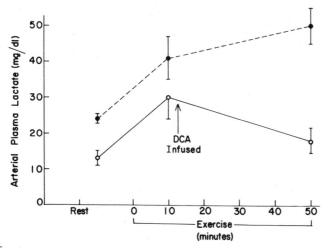

(1–43) J. Appl. Physiol. 48:427–431, March 1980.

lower during light and moderate exercise, respectively. There was no difference between control and DCA-treated dogs for the heavy exercise heart rate. Plasma LA concentrations increased during the three work loads. In the same dogs, when identical treadmill tests were conducted after DCA injection, the rise in LA concentrations was significantly attenuated. In group 2, dogs receiving saline showed increased LA concentrations. However, during repeat tests with DCA, the mean LA concentration was 60% lower 50 minutes after DCA administration than the concentration during the control run (Fig 1–17).

Because DCA markedly reduced plasma LA concentrations, it would be tempting to consider the use of DCA as an ergogenic aid. Although DCA has been used clinically for treatment of lactic acidosis, recent reports have showed that long-term administration can cause temporary hindlimb paralysis and permanent degenerative histologic changes in the central nervous system. However, DCA is a potentially valuable tool for study of LA metabolism during exercise.

▶ [Physicians involved in "doping" controls have been concerned for many years that attempts might be made to extend human performance through the administration of buffering agents. At one time, there was a flurry of experimentation on bicarbonate, but it was concluded that other effects generally outweighed any gains from the countering of lactacidosis.

A new agent on the clinical lactacidemia scene has been the weak carboxylic acid dichloroacetate sodium (DCA). This apparently acts by inhibiting the pyruvate dehydrogenase kinase that converts pyruvate dehydrogenase to the inactive, phosphorylated form. Whereas the acute use of DCA may be justified in clinical treatment of severe lactacidemia, the risk of chronic toxicity is sufficient that athletes should be warned strongly against any experimentation with this compound.—R.J.S.] ◀

1–44 **Use of Phenylbutazone in Sports Medicine: Understanding the Risks.** Although phenylbutazone is widely used, its safety is controversial. Phenylbutazone is now the most common cause of fatal, drug-related aplastic anemia and agranulocytosis. Since the drug is frequently used in sports medicine, Howard M. Black, Jay S. Cox, and William Rex Straughn (US Naval Academy Hosp., Annapolis, Md.) reviewed the medical records of about 3,000 midshipmen who had received a total of about 3,300 courses of phenylbutazone to evaluate its toxicity.

The review failed to reveal any adverse reactions. Reexamination of 446 midshipmen after 1 week of treatment with phenylbutazone showed several side effects: 19 patients (4%) had mild gastrointestinal disturbances but continued treatment; 3 patients had severe nausea or epigastric pain that necessitated discontinuance of medication; and 1 patient discontinued medication because of blisters that developed in the mouth. The gastrointestinal symptoms and oral lesions resolved promptly after phenylbutazone was withdrawn. No significant hematologic abnormalities were observed.

It is estimated that the risk of a severe reaction to phenylbutazone is less than 1/100,000 among young, healthy persons who take the drug for 1 week or less. Longer treatment and advanced age signifi-

(1–44) Am. J. Sports Med. 8:270–273, July–Aug. 1980.

cantly increase the risk. A history of an allergic reaction to phenyl-butazone is an absolute contraindication to treatment. Little is known about the effects of phenylbutazone on athletic performance. However, its capacity to cause significant fluid retention, with an increase of as much as 50% in plasma volume and a corresponding dilutional anemia, could impair overall performance if the drug were continued after the athlete returned to competition.

▶ [This paper is somewhat reassuring for the sports physician. Although phenylbutazone is now the most common cause of aplastic anemia and agranulocytosis, such conditions seem to arise when it is given to the elderly for long periods to treat chronic conditions such as osteoarthritis. In sports medicine, the administration is more short-lived, to help in resolving inflammatory conditions such as tendinitis and bursitis, and the risk of a serious reaction in a young person is then only about 1/100,000. Nevertheless, the authors did not reply to a question posed by a commentator in the original publication, "Have they compared it to aspirin for similar conditions?" It is easy to use wonder drugs with serious complications without checking the value of simpler remedies.—R.J.S.] ◀

1–45 **Reflections on a 100-Mile Run: Effects of Aspirin Therapy.** Herbert L. Fred (St. Joseph Hosp., Houston) reports the effects that aspirin had on him while running a 100-mile ultramarathon race. Because of knee pain, he took 10 grains of a buffered aspirin preparation (Ascriptin) every 4 hours for 7 days before and throughout the run. On the basis of his own observations, he concluded that the aspirin increased his sweat rate, body temperature, and urinary output; inhibited his desire for liquids; abolished the knee pain; and dulled his sense of fatigue. As a result, he had heat illness in the 92nd mile of the race. It is concluded that the therapeutic use of aspirin may be dangerous when combined with physical exertion in the heat, and that it may reduce the extreme thirst associated with hyperreninemia.

▶ [A single case report is presented here, and, obviously, it is conjectural in part. Nevertheless, aspirin is such an ubiquitous drug that we should appreciate that it can cause increased sweating, that it does not block the rise of body temperature from physical activity, and that it can induce diuresis by inhibiting renal tubular reabsorption of bicarbonate, promoting the excretion of sodium, potassium, and water. This will be extremely variable in different people, but the potential for significant diuresis is present.—L.J.K.] ◀

1–46 **Influence of Therapeutic Doses of Amoxicillin on Aerobic Work Capacity and Some Strength Characteristics.** Athletes are often reluctant to take antibiotics, because they are believed to impair athletic performance. Harm Kuipers, Frans T. J. Verstappen, and Robert S. Reneman (Univ. of Limburg) investigated the effects of therapeutic doses of amoxicillin on maximal aerobic work capacity and some strength characteristics in 15 male volunteers, aged 21 to 38 years.

The subjects were tested once a week for 4 consecutive weeks. The results of the first two tests were used to establish baseline values. After the second test, the subjects randomly received placebo capsules or capsules containing 375 mg of amoxicillin to be taken three times

(1–45) Med. Sci. Sports Exerc. 12:212–215, 1980.
(1–46) Am. J. Sports Med. 8:274–279, July–Aug. 1980.

a day for 5 days. After the third test, the medications were crossed over. The subjects were tested on each occasion for maximum work load attained on the cycle ergometer, maximum heart rate, maximum serum lactate concentration, heart rate and serum lactate concentration after 10 minutes of workout at 80% of the maximum work load attained, maximum isometric extension force of the legs, vertical jump height, and body weight.

Two-way analysis of variance revealed no significant difference between any of the variables and measurements during tests two, three, and four. More frequent and less firm stools was the most common side effect. However, this did not last for more than 2 days; diarrhea was never a problem.

Therapeutic doses of amoxicillin have no demonstrable effect on maximum aerobic work capacity and on the measured strength characteristics of physically active men.

▶ [It is hard to know why athletes developed the idea that antibiotics impair performance. Possibly, the disease for which the antibiotic was administered led to depression and/or impaired performance. Toxic doses of penicillin can influence synaptic transmission in the central nervous system, but this is hardly relevant to normal pharmacology, where no effect is observed. If bacterial flora were upset to the point of severe diarrhea, this could conceivably reduce blood volume and thus physical performance.—R.J.S.] ◀

PHYSIOLOGY OF SPECIFIC SPORTS

1-47 **Exercise Heart Rate as a Predictor of Running Performance.** Peter A. Farrell, Jack H. Wilmore, and Edward F. Coyle studied the predictive power of exercise heart rates for performance in road racing, because a reduced heart rate at a standard exercise intensity is a well-established result of endurance training.

TECHNIQUE.—Eighteen experienced male distance runners volunteered for the study. Body density, residual lung volume, and relative body fat were determined. An average of 8 treadmill runs at various speeds were performed by each subject. Heart rate was determined during the last 15 seconds of each minute. After the subjects had completed 3 or 4 steady-state runs, $\dot{V}O_2$ max was determined on two separate occasions. Performance data consisted of road races from 3.2 to 42.2 km (table). Whenever a subject ran a competitive race during the time span of steady-state treadmill tests, his time was recorded and the distance verified using a calibrated measuring wheel. In addition, each subject ran 2 races at each of the following distances: 3.2, 9.7, and 19.3 km. These races were over a flat course specifically designed for this study.

Subjects showed the characteristically high $\dot{V}O_2$ max and low relative body fat of distance runners. The heart rates required to run at a treadmill velocity of 268 m/minute ranged from 151 to 218 beats/minute, which corresponds to 77% and 111% of the individual's maximal heart rate, respectively. It should be noted that some heart rates calculated by using regression equations for heart rate vs. treadmill velocity were in excess of the subject's maximal heart rate. The relationship between heart rate and treadmill velocity was linear.

(1–47) Res. Q. Exerc. Sport 51:417–421, May 1980.

ZERO ORDER CORRELATIONS FOR HEART RATE, PERCENT MAXIMAL HEART RATE AT 268 M/MINUTE, AND RACE PACE FOR DISTANCE ROAD RACES

	Distance				
	42.2 km	19.3 km	15 km	9.7 km	3.2 km
Heart Rate	$-.87^*$	$-.86^*$	$-.87^*$	$-.86^*$	$-.81^*$
	$y = -2.037(x)$	$y = -1.652(x)$	$y = -1.581(x)$	$y = -1.566(x)$	$y = -1.543(x)$
	$+ 597$	$+ 545$	$+ 540$	$+ 546$	$+ 566$
	$Sx \cdot y = 18$ m/min	$Sx \cdot y = 19$ m/min	$Sx \cdot y = 17$ m/min	$Sx \cdot y = 19$ m/min	$Sx \cdot y = 22$ m/min
Percent Maximal	$-.89^*$	$-.89^*$	$-.91^*$	$-.89^*$	$-.86^*$
Heart Rate	$y = -2.038(x)$	$y = -3.165(x)$	$y = -3.022(x)$	$y = -3.003(x)$	$y = -3.047(x)$
	$+ 598$	$+ 546$	$+ 541$	$+ 547$	$+ 575$
	$Sx \cdot y = 17$ m/min	$Sx \cdot y = 17$ m/min	$Sx \cdot y = 15$ m/min	$Sx \cdot y = 16$ m/min	$Sx \cdot y = 19$ m/min

*Significant at $P<.05$.

The correlations between performance and most of these variables are not in excess of the correlations found in this study. Thus, as a predictive tool, heart rates at a standardized treadmill velocity may be preferable because of the ease of data collection.

▶ [Many sports scientists propose very sophisticated tests for the ranking of athletes. Runners, for example, are evaluated in terms of glycogen stores, mechanical efficiency, muscle fiber composition, temperature regulation, and lactate buildup. The present authors make the useful point that the simple procedure of measuring pulse rate at a fixed speed of treadmill running provides just as effective a method of classification. Nevertheless, none of the available procedures is really satisfactory; for example, in a 15-km event, the error in prediction of speed is ±35 m/minute, about 15% of the typical speed of 265 m/minute.—R.J.S.] ◀

1–48 **Effects of Wind Assistance and Resistance on the Forward Motion of a Runner.** The aerobic energy cost of level and gradient exercise has been studied often, but the effects of wind assistance and resistance on oxygen consumption ($\dot{V}O_2$) have received little attention. To learn more about the effects of a head and following wind on the forward motion of a runner, C. T. M. Davies (London School of Hygiene and Tropical Medicine) investigated the aerobic energy cost ($\Delta \dot{V}O_2$) of running at different speeds with and against various wind velocities (W_v) in 3 healthy male subjects. The wind experiments were conducted in a wind tunnel, and the results were compared with those for uphill and downhill gradient running on a motor-driven treadmill.

Comparison of the treadmill and wind tunnel results showed that in terms of equivalent vertical and horizontal forces, the two modes of exercise were physiologically identical for exercise gradients and W_v ranging from -10% to $+5\%$ and 1.5 to 15 m · second^{-1}, respectively. The apparent efficiency of work with and against the wind was approximately $+0.35$ and -1.2. When the W_v was greater than 15 m · second^{-1}, running against the wind and at the corresponding gradient on the treadmill was more efficient. A possible explanation for this greater efficiency could be that at high W_v, the subjects adjusted their posture to lean into the wind, thus possibly converting potential

(1–48) J. Appl. Physiol. 48:702–709, April 1980.

drag into body lift. The $\Delta\dot{V}O_2$ of overcoming wind resistance outdoors on a calm day was calculated to be 7.8% for sprinting (10 · second^{-1}), 4% for middle distance running (6 m · second^{-1}), and 2% for marathon running (5 m · second^{-1}). The experimental results and the implications for athletic performance are discussed.

▶ [Sports scientists often make the unwarranted assumption that laboratory treadmill experiments can be translated directly into track performance. These data look at the added mechanical variable introduced by a head or following wind in a wind tunnel. On the track, air resistance is encountered even on a still day, and the magnitude of this depends on the forward profile of the runner; the head may be held lower against wind and/or rain. Other differences on the track are: (1) the coefficient of ground friction, (2) more ready evaporation of sweat due to air currents created by forward movement, and (3), on a clear day, solar radiation.—R.J.S.] ◀

1–49 **Body Temperature, Respiration, and Acid-Base Equilibrium During Prolonged Running.** Previous studies suggest that respiratory responses related to acid-base equilibrium during prolonged, high-intensity exercise may be influenced by body temperature. Michael N. Sawka, Ronald G. Knowlton, and Roger M. Glaser studied respiratory responses related to acid-base equilibrium at different body temperatures during two bouts of high-intensity, prolonged running. Seven males who ran at least 50 miles a week and had completed marathon races in less than 3 hours in the past year were studied. Mean age was 28 years, and mean maximal aerobic power was 66 ml/kg per minute. Two bouts of treadmill running lasting 80 minutes were performed, with water intake limited to 100 ml during each run. A 280-ml drink was allowed during the 90-minute interval between the exercise bouts.

The subjects exercised at mean relative intensities of 70% and 71% of maximal aerobic power during the two runs, corresponding to mean oxygen uptakes of 3.12 and 3.16 L per minute. Mean plasma volume was reduced by 8% at 30 minutes into the first run. Rectal temperature increased significantly during each run and was higher during the second run at all respective time periods. Plasma volume, arterial lactate and hydrogen ion concentrations, $PaCO_2$, and bicarbonate concentration were constant throughout each run, as were pulmonary ventilation and ventilatory equivalent of carbon dioxide. The $PaCO_2$ was lower and the ventilatory equivalent of carbon dioxide was higher during respective periods of the second run.

After initial adjustments, most of the variables studied were fairly constant despite increasing rectal temperature during prolonged running by highly trained subjects. Greater pulmonary ventilation responses in untrained subjects have been attributed to higher body temperature during exercise. If increased temperature provides a stimulus for the hyperpnea of muscular exercise, it is apparently attenuated in trained subjects during prolonged running.

▶ [Rectal temperature is elevated during prolonged running and appears to act as a stimulus for the hyperpnea of muscular exercise. This study documents that in the trained person this is an insignificant change and that respiration and acid-base equi-

(1–49) Med. Sci. Sports Exerc. 12:370–374, 1980.

librium remain fairly constant, presumably as a function of training and irrespective of the elevation of rectal temperature.—L.J.K.] ◄

1–50 **Anatomical and Physiologic Characteristics to Predict Football Ability: Report of Study Methods and Correlations, University of Arkansas, 1976.**Little has been done to develop tests predictive of football ability. James A. Arnold, Barry Brown, Ralph Peter Micheli, and Tom P. Coker (Univ. of Arkansas) conducted a prospective study of 56 scholarship football players during the 1975 season. Fourteen anatomical and physiologic measurements were made to assess the correlation of strength, power, and balance factors with the coaches' subjective ratings of football playing ability.

A correlation matrix for the criterion measure and 14 predictor variables was devised. Genu varum and tibial torsion had the highest correlations with the criterion variables. The average tibial torsion was 42.6 degrees, compared with 27.4 degrees reported for a nonscholarship group. Of the strength measures, hip abduction had the highest correlation with the criterion variables, but the relation was not significant. Horsepower in the Margaria-Kalamen power test showed a correlation of 0.255. Horsepower and time were related significantly to the 40-yd dash, and the 40-yd dash was highly correlated with hip abduction, knee extension, plantar flexion, height, and weight. The Margaria-Kalamen power test was highly correlated with hip abduction, knee extension, knee flexion, the 40-yd dash, height, and weight.

Tibial torsion, genu varum, height, body weight, the Margaria-Kalamen anaerobic power test, and knee flexion are the best predictors of football playing ability. Strength tests that use a cable tensiometer and Fleishmann's static balance test are not good predictors of football ability.

► [There have been several previous physiologic descriptions of football players (see: Shephard, R. J.: *Human Physiological Work Capacity*, Cambridge University Press, 1978), but this is probably the first attempt to develop an equation for the prediction of playing ability. As might be predicted in an orthopedic journal(!) the two most useful measures found were genu varum and tibial torsion. Both had relatively low correlation coefficients (0.45 and 0.34, respectively), and although they were statistically significant they would not be of great help in identifying successful players. Surprisingly, body mass and body build did not emerge as predictors, although the average mass (216 pounds) was quite high (professional football players are, of course, even heavier).—R.J.S.] ◄

1–51 **Cardiovascular Stress Associated With Recreational Tennis Play of Middle-Aged Males.** Many physical activities that require a high energy cost and cause appreciable discomfort are commonly prescribed to improve cardiovascular-respiratory fitness, whereas more popular lifetime sports such as tennis are viewed with skepticism by some, because they are thought to provide relatively mild physiologic stress. Tennis is an increasingly popular lifetime sport that has a reputation for being too intermittent for the recreational player to receive adequate cardiorespiratory stimulation. J. E. Mis-

---

(1–50) Am. J. Sports Med. 8:119–122, Mar.–Apr., 1980.
(1–51) Am. Correct. Ther. J. 34:4–8, Jan.–Feb., 1980.

ner, R. A. Boileau, D. Courvoisier, M. H. Slaughter, and D. K. Bloomfield (Univ. of Illinois, Urbana-Champaign) assessed the intensity of tennis-playing in 28 men aged 23 to 52 years who were "club" players, primarily at intermediate or advanced ability levels. Heart rate and the ECG were monitored before, during, and after a tennis match played at the customary pace.

Mean heart rates during match play averaged 63% of estimated age-adjusted maximum exercise heart rate reserve, compared with 46% during warm-up. The estimated intensity of the match was 6.1 on a scale of 0 to 10. Individual heart rates were relatively stable during both warm-up and game play. Factors that appeared to be important in heart rate included ambient temperature, estimated exercise intensity, exercise time, and percentage of time the ball was in play. One subject had isolated premature ventricular contractions during recovery. Three subjects had slight S-T flattening and depression during peak exercise, but they were asymptomatic and had normal ECGs at rest and during recovery. Twelve subjects showed J-point depressions during peak exercise.

Young adult and middle-aged recreational tennis players of intermediate to advanced ability can engage in singles tennis match play at an intensity that generally provides adequate stimulation for maintenance and improvement of cardiorespiratory function. Tennis warm-up and noncompetitive rallying usually are not equivalent conditioning activities. Prudence on hot days appears to be advisable for competing tennis players.

▶ [The data reviewed make the solid case that tennis, at least singles, and as practiced by the middle-aged club athlete, is a reasonable and reasonably vigorous exercise. It seems to be academic to argue whether it serves as cardiovascular conditioning because, as a potential overuse sport, a strong case can be made for the need to condition prior to the tennis play for the sake of joints and muscles as well as for the intrinsic cardiovascular conditioning itself. This is another way of saying that those of us who enjoy racket sports would be wise to warm up extensively, to carry out alternative strength building and cardiac conditioning, and to implement the activity of the tennis match by a significant additional exercise commitment.—L.J.K.] ◀

1–52 **Maximal Oxygen Uptake During Free, Tethered, and Flume Swimming.** Maximal oxygen consumption ($\dot{V}O_{2\,max}$) appears to be highly specific to the musculature used during maximal exercise and specific to the mode of training. A. Bonen, B. A. Wilson, M. Yarkony, and A. N. Belcastro compared the $\dot{V}O_{2\,max}$ in 21 swimmers during free, tethered, and flume swimming and evaluated the efficacy of a laboratory arm ergometer test in assessing the aerobic capacity of swimmers.

Extremely high correlations between $\dot{V}O_{2\,max}$ during tethered and flume swimming and tethered and free swimming were observed. The differences between these tests were negligible and were well within the range of variations expected for repeated measurements of $\dot{V}O_{2\,max}$ with the same ergometer. The respiratory rate for tethered swimming was greater than the rates for flume and free swimming, but the differences were not significant because of large differences in several

(1–52) J. Appl. Physiol. 48:232–235, February 1980.

subjects. The $\dot{V}O_{2\ max}$ during arm ergometry was significantly lower than during the swimming tests, despite a high correlation between the measurements; this was attributable in part to the range of the data. Predictions of tethered and flume swimming $\dot{V}O_{2\ max}$ based on the results of arm ergometry were in considerable error, $\pm 7.4\%$ and $\pm 7.1\%$, respectively.

Measurements of $\dot{V}O_{2\ max}$ that use free, tethered, and flume swimming are virtually identical. Estimates of $\dot{V}O_{2\ max}$ in swimmers based on arm ergometry, bicycle ergometry, or treadmill running should not be made because $\dot{V}O_{2\ max}$ is specific to the exercise protocol involved.

▶ [After the popularization of the swimming flume by Holmér, there was a tendency to assume that this expensive piece of equipment was essential to assessment of the swimmer. The present results show that, at least in moderate swimmers, closely similar results can be obtained by tethered or by free swimming. As might be expected, the usual arm ergometer gives lower results. Although the authors criticize use of the treadmill for swimmers, their own results given no specific information on the relationship between treadmill and in-water results.—R.J.S.] ◀

1–53 **Respiratory and Heart Rate Responses to Tethered Controlled-Frequency Breathing Swimming.** Swimming coaches have recently emphasized the controlled-frequency breathing (CFB) training method, in which swimmers are required to reduce the total number of inspirations for a given distance swum in the hope of enhancing exercise performance through cellular adaptations to reduced oxygen delivery to the tissues. Scott G. Dicker, Geraldine K. Lofthus, Norton W. Thornton, and George A. Brooks (Univ. of California, Berkeley) obtained data on the effects of CFB during tethered swimming from 9 members of a college varsity swim team. All but 1 were Olympic competitors or had competed at a national or international level. Stroke frequency was regulated by an electronic pacing device as the subjects swam against various resistances for 4-minute periods using the freestyle stroke.

Oxygen consumption did not change significantly as subjects breathed at every five rather than every two arm strokes. Minute ventilation fell significantly during CFB, but oxygen extraction rose sufficiently to compensate for this. The PaO_2 decreased and the $PaCO_2$ increased significantly with CFB. The respiratory exchange ratio, carbon dioxide production, and heart rate did not change significantly. Both oxygen consumption and carbon dioxide production increased linearly with resistance to swimming. The heart rate increased as a direct function of the weight pulled. No significant changes in PaO_2 or $PaCO_2$ were observed from increments in weight pulled during CFB.

These observations indicate the occurrence of hypercapnia rather than hypoxia during CFB in swimming. If specific physiologic adaptations occur in response to CFB training, they may more likely be associated with improved tolerance of high alveolar carbon dioxide cencentrations than of systemic hypoxia.

▶ [During the 1978 World Swimming Championships, 14 world records were broken.

(1–53) Med. Sci. Sports Exerc. 12:20, Spring 1980.

Since this article came to press, 25 world marks in swimming have been established. As the authors suggest, these improvements in performance are undoubtedly attributable in part to training methods. If the training model was the East African who achieved outstanding performance in distance running because of high-altitude environment, then this is the correlative training method that would require athletes to decrease the total number of inspirations for a given distance swim. Thus, instead of breathing with every arm cycle, swimmers would breathe at every third, fourth, or fifth arm stroke. This has been called "hypoxic training" or "controlled-frequency breathing" (CFB). The claim has been that cellular adaptations then ensue that enhance exercise performance and that this is a consequence of CFB. It has also been used as an alternative to the hard sprint training that might induce more muscle soreness. The words have been used loosely to say that CFB swimming permits both "aerobic" and "anaerobic" conditioning from exercise of submaximal intensity.

It may well be that this technique enhances performance. The physiologic argument is whether this is due to true tissue hypoxia or whether there are compensatory changes that permit the maintenance of Vo_2 by increasing oxygen extraction and tidal volume. This article would support the latter. Carbon dioxide retention during CFB may constitute the main stress during CFB swim training.—L.J.K.] ◀

1–54 **Ventilatory Response to Hypercapnia in Sprint and Long-Distance Swimmers** was compared with that in untrained subjects by Tetsuo Ohkuwa, Noriaki Fujitsuka, Toshikazu Utsuno, and Miharu Miyamura (Nagoya, Japan). Ten untrained students, 17 sprint swimmers, and 11 long-distance swimmers were studied. To estimate aerobic work capacity, maximum oxygen uptake ($Vo_{2\,max}$) was determined by an incremental loading technique. Maximal exercise was performed on the cycle ergometer with a constant pedaling rate of 60 rpm. The ventilatory response line to carbon dioxide was obtained by the rebreathing method of Read.

The table summarizes the average values and standard deviations for $Vo_{2\,max}$, maximum oxygen uptake per kilogram body weight ($Vo_{2\,max}/W$), and ventilatory response to hypercapnia in the untrained and swimmer groups. The mean slope of the ventilatory response line of the swimmers was lower than that of the untrained group, and the

DATA* ON MAXIMUM OXYGEN UPTAKE AND VENTILATORY RESPONSE TO CARBON DIOXIDE IN UNTRAINED AND SWIMMER GROUPS

	$Vo_{2\,max}$ (l/min)	$Vo_{2\,max}/W$ (ml/kg · min^{-1})	S (l/min/mm Hg)	S/BSA (l/min/mm Hg/m^2)	B (mm Hg)
Untrained (n = 10)	2.87 ± 0.16 †	0.1 ± 4.1†	2.03 ± 1.40	1.19 ± 0.81	38.3 ± 8.7
Sprint swimmer (n = 17)	3.08 ± 0.33‡	48.4 ± 3.2‡	1.72 ± 0.75	0.96 ± 0.42	40.3 ± 11.6
Long-distance swimmer (n = 11)	3.36 ± 0.54	54.0 ± 6.2	1.43 ± 0.63	0.83 ± 0.33	43.0 ± 5.7

*Values are mean ± SD. S, slope of ventilatory response line expressed as change in ventilation per unit change in alveolar P_{CO_2}; S/BSA, slope divided by body surface area; B, extrapolated intercept on alveolar P_{CO_2} axis.
†N = 3.
‡N = 13.

(1–54) Eur. J. Appl. Physiol. 43:235–241, April 1980.

mean slope of the long-distance swimmers was lower than that of the sprint swimmers, though these differences were not statistically significant.

Whether the ventilatory responsiveness to inhaled carbon dioxide changes with physical training is uncertain, because decreased ventilatory responses in athletes have never been shown to be the consequence of conditioning. However, hypercapnic ventilatory drive may be decreased by severe physical training prolonged until the maximum possible oxygen uptake is reached, but this possibility requires further study.

▶ [Although not statistically significant, the present findings support the generally held view that carbon dioxide responsiveness is moderately reduced in athletes relative to sedentary persons. The phenomenon has been described both in distance runners and in swimmers. A longitudinal (training) study is still necessary to show that the difference is not due to athletic selection rather than conditioning.—R.J.S.] ◀

1–55 **Metabolic Changes in Man During Long-Distance Swimming.** G. Haralambie and L. Senser observed 16 young men before, immediately after, and 24 hours after exercise. All subjects were asked to swim at a speed that they considered would allow them to perform 5,000 m in 90 minutes. Central and skin temperatures, blood chemistry, neuromuscular excitability of the vastus medialis and deltoid muscles, pulse rate, and weight were determined at rest. A blood sample was drawn from the hyperemic ear lobe for lactate and glucose determination. Measurements were repeated after the swimming exercise.

Mean weight loss after swimming was 0.7 kg. Mean pulse rate at the end of the exercise was 151 beats per minute. Skin and rectal temperatures were slightly increased. Except for marked leukocytosis, no changes were observed in hematologic values. Serum enzyme activities, except for triose phosphate dehydrogenase, showed marked increases; creatine kinase and malate dehydrogenase activities did not return to preexercise values on the next day. No hypoglycemia occurred. Blood lactate values increased markedly. Free fatty acid, free glycerol, 3-hydroxybutyrate and serum urea and uric acid values rose markedly after swimming, whereas α-amino nitrogen, triglyceride, and serum magnesium values significantly decreased. The electric excitability of the vastus medialis and deltoid showed opposite changes: the deltoid showed significantly higher threshold values after swimming, and the vastus medialis showed an increase in excitability. These differences are ascribed to the muscles' different involvement during swimming.

Changes in blood substrates observed in this study suggest that after a short phase, during which anaerobic glycolysis plays a role in energy delivery, the oxidative breakdown of lipid substrates covers the main part of the energy demands. The better-performing (and therefore probably better-trained) subjects were able to adapt more rapidly to oxidative metabolism and thus showed markedly lower lactate concentrations at the 15th minute of exercise. This and other

(1–55) Eur. J. Appl. Physiol. 43:115–125, March 1980.

experiments suggest lipid mobilization and partial breakdown at a high rate. Endurance swimmers are able to use fat and probably can spare glycogen, provided that the work intensity is not exaggeratedly high. The changes in enzyme activities are the same as those seen in long-distance ski races of similar duration, but they are markedly lower than the modifications observed in impact-type sports such as running.

► [There have been many metabolic studies of long-distance runners and of cross-country skiers, and it is interesting to see comparable analyses for 90 minutes of swimming. The water temperature selected was fairly warm, and because the weight loss (0.71 kg) was larger than predicted from metabolism, some sweating presumably occurred. Serum enzymes were generally increased, although less than in runners; the authors attribute this to the absence of impact, although better perfusion of the active muscles might also be a contributing factor. Blood glucose level is well maintained, and much of the energy needs are met from fat; again, there is ease of tissue perfusion when the task is widely distributed over the body muscles, and body mass is supported.—R.J.S.] ◄

1–56 **Physiologic Profiles and Selected Psychologic Characteristics of National Class American Cyclists** are presented by J. M. Hagberg, J. P. Mullin, M. Bahrke, and J. Limburg (Univ. of Wisconsin). The data were compared with those on European cyclists. Whether endurance cyclists are introverted and whether they possess a Profile of Mood States (POMS) similar to that of other high-level athletes were also investigated. After psychologic inventories were administered, 9 national class American cyclists completed a questionnaire to determine training methods and gear preferences. Maximal oxygen consumption was determined with a cycle ergometer. Maximal power determinations were made on a modified cycle ergometer. Blood samples were obtained from a prewarmed fingertip before the test and 3 minutes after exercise to determine the lactic acid concentration.

The mean maximal oxygen consumption for the group was 70 ml/ kg. The eventual World Team members and nonmembers could not be differentiated on the basis of maximal oxygen consumptions. No other statistically significant differences were found in any of the psychologic, physiologic, or training variables between these two groups. The 9 cyclists were within the normal range on the neuroticism-stability dimension of the Eysenck Personality Inventory. However, on the extraversion-introversion dimension, they were significantly more introverted than normal adults. The cyclists also scored significantly lower than college norms on the tension, depression, anger, and confusion scales of the POMS inventory. They scored significantly higher than normal adults on the vigor scale but no differently on the fatigue scale.

American cyclists have essentially the same maximal oxygen consumption values as top Europeans. Therefore, it appears that other factors must contribute to producing high-level cycling performances. Though they have well-developed aerobic systems, road cyclists also have the capacity for high power outputs over short periods as evi-

(1–56) J. Sports Med. Phys. Fitness 19:341–346, December 1979.

denced by their output of 0.84 horsepower for slightly less than 1 minute. Their psychologic profile reveals that they are introverted; they also possess a POMS profile similar to those of elite marathon runners, oarsmen, and wrestlers.

▶ [Cycling might seem one of the more mechanical sports, with little scope for techniques. However, this report suggests that the relatively unsuccessful United States team has a physiologic profile similar to their European counterparts. (Caution must be shown in accepting this conclusion, because the tests were conducted in different laboratories, and this factor can in itself have a substantial influence on the results reported.) One interesting feature of the report is the stated preference of pedal speed for hills (80 rpm) and level ground (101 rpm). The figures are somewhat puzzling. In an average person, efficiency is maximal at 50–60 rpm. A higher speed might be needed to facilitate muscle perfusion at high power outputs, but why is a lower speed chosen for hills than for level riding? This is the reverse of the gearing used on a recreational cycle! Possibly, the riders stand on the pedals when climbing hills, and this modifies the optimum frequency of pedaling.—R.J.S.] ◀

1–57 **Relationship Between Anaerobic Power and Olympic Weight Lifting Performance.** Michael H. Stone, Ronald Byrd, John Tew, and Michael Wood (Louisiana State Univ.) studied the effects of training for Olympic weight lifting competition on power as measured from the vertical jump and from stair climbing among novice trainees. The two methods of estimating power were also compared as to their ability to predict Olympic weight lifting success. Thirteen healthy male subjects enrolled in an advanced weight training course. Training consisted of exercises with free weights 3 days per week. Variables were measured at the beginning of training, at the end of the seventh week, and at the end of the fourteenth week.

The training program produced significant increases in the subjects' ability to perform the snatch and clean. Significant increases across time were also found in vertical jump power and in stair-climbing power. No differences were found in stair-climbing time or body weight. Increase in the subjects' ability to produce power appeared to be a major factor for the improvements in the snatch and clean. Correlations between the snatch and clean and the vertical jump power increased across the trials.

Vertical jump power is apparently a better predictor of Olympic weight lifting success than stair-climbing power. Within a body weight class, the vertical jump alone may be a good predictor of Olympic weight lifting success, at least among more-experienced lifters.

▶ [The authors suggest that vertical jump distance and vertical jump power provide useful indications of ability to perform the snatch and clean manuevers. They fail to stress sufficiently that the magnitude of the correlations observed (0.7 to 0.8) has statistical rather than practical significance—the tests are describing not much more than one half of the variation in weight lifting performance.—R.J.S.] ◀

1–58 **Heart Rates in Boat Racers.** Clifford Johnson (Edmonds, Wash.) measured the heart rates of 6 powerboat racers before and during competition. The subjects were aged 28 to 48 years (mean age, 35), were normotensive and had resting heart rates of 75 beats per minute

(1–57) J. Sports Med. Phys. Fitness 20:99–102, March 1980.
(1–58) Physician Sportsmed. 8:86–93, June 1980.

or less. The air temperature was 60 to 65 F at the time of the races.

Because powerboat racing requires little physical strength, the heart rates were affected only by psychologic stress. Heart rates ranged from 112 to 180 beats per minute (mean, 149) while racers waited in the boat. One minute before the start of the race, heart rates had increased to 160 to 195 beats per minute (mean, 178) and went as high as 210 in 1 subject during the race. Experience was not a factor in these elevated heart rates.

The findings support other studies on the impact of psychologic stress on heart rate. Blood pressures as high as 220/120 mm Hg have been reported up to 3 hours before a race in otherwise normotensive subjects. The high heart rates are due to excessive catecholamine release. The medical significance of this tachycardia is not known. However, the brief time span of powerboat races and the small work load imposed may lessen the likelihood of ventricular fibrillation.

▶ ["Sedentary" sports are no guarantee against cardiac stress. Similarly, high heart rates and blood pressures have been observed in car-racing drivers prior to a start and in referees. Because high standards of physical fitness are not needed for such pursuits, the persons concerned may sustain a "heart attack" (ventricular fibrillation) while awaiting the starter's signal or officiating. Surprisingly, this does not seem to cause accidents—usually, the car or boat is brought to rest, and Johnson notes that there were no cardiac incidents in 600 boat-racing accidents.—R.J.S.] ◄

1–59 **Body Composition, Endurance Capacity, and Strength of College Lacrosse Players.** Larry G. Shaver (Vanderbilt Univ.) studied physical and physiologic characteristics of 30 male intercollegiate lacrosse players, aged 18 to 20 years. Each position (midfielder, attacker, defense, and goalie) was represented in the sample. Body composition was determined by the hydrostatic weighing technique of Wilmore and Behnke. Maximal pulmonary ventilation, maximum oxygen uptake, and maximal heart rate during treadmill running were used as measures of cardiorespiratory endurance capacity. Three strength trials with each hand were given with the grip dynamometer. The leg and back strength tests were given with leg and back dynamometers. The players were divided into three groups: midfielders, attackers, and defensive players (including goalies).

The results showed that although lacrosse athletes as a whole are generally taller and heavier than other persons of similar age, they are also leaner. Body fat ranged between 5% and 17% of composition, weight between 58.6 and 82.7 kg, lean body weight between 55 and 78 kg, and height between 168.5 and 190.2 cm. Vital capacity ranged between 2.98 and 6.50 L and total lung capacity between 3.93 and 8.76 L. Residual volume varied between 0.95 and 2.26 L. Maximal pulmonary ventilation ranged from 137.3 to 199.5 L per minute (BTPS) and maximum oxygen uptake from 32.5 to 72.4 ml/kg per minute. Grip strength varied between 20 and 68 kg and back and leg strength between 122.7 and 209 and between 336.3 and 645.4, respectively.

Intercollegiate male lacrosse players are generally taller, heavier,

(1–59) J. Sports Med. Phys. Fitness 20:213–220, June 1980.

stronger, and leaner than male nonathletes of similar age. They also have slightly greater lung and cardiorespiratory endurance capacity. Attackers and defensive players (including the goalie) have similar body builds and are stronger, whereas midfielders are taller and lighter, have less fat, and have greater cardiorespiratory endurance capacity.

▶ [Lacrosse is one of the few indigenous North American sports, vividly described by Father Breboeuf and other early missionaries to the "New France." This article is useful, because there has been almost no previous information on the characteristics of lacrosse players. One would anticipate a physique similar to that of the soccer player, but with a greater height and a greater upper body strength, and the present data, in general, support this view. The authors show commendable honesty by including one $Vo_{2\,max}$ value of only 32.5 ml/kg/minute. In view of the associated respiratory minute volume (137.3 1/minute), one is inclined to expect an error in this oxygen consumption determination; it is a pity the subject concerned was not retested. The mean $Vo_{2\,max}$ of 59.5 ml/kg/minute nevertheless looks quite feasible.—R.J.S.] ◀

2. Biomechanics

2–1 **Body Segment Contributions to Sport Skill Performance: Two Contrasting Approaches** are described by Doris I. Miller (Univ. of Washington). Although phrases such as "transfer of momentum" and "sequential buildup of limb velocities" commonly are used, implying that segmental contributions to sports skills are obvious, biomechanics researchers have just begun to explore this important area. One approach, joint immobilization or restraint, relies on an external measure of performance. Another, resultant muscle torque patterns, involves detailed computations of the internal (muscular) forces responsible for performance. There appears to be renewed interest in the joint immobilization or restraint paradigm. This approach has been used to analyze such activities as throwing, jumping, and springboard diving. Some general insights into segmental contributions to performance may result, but this approach probably will never prove particularly fruitful since it is assumed that the restriction of one or more joints will not alter the coordinated action of the unaffected body segments, an assumption that is tenuous at best.

Analysis of muscular torque patterns is a more promising approach, since the initiation, execution, and control of motor skills lie at the level of the neuromuscular system. The free body diagram, a simplified representation of the "system" isolated from its surroundings and showing all external forces acting on it, is the key to this type of analysis. Adequate linear and angular acceleration values are needed as input to the equations of motion. Segmental moments of inertia must be estimated, and the time histories of contact forces must be determined. The muscle torque pattern approach has been used to analyze the kicking limb, and running. More information on muscle torque patterns may be expected within the next few years. It is unlikely that a single approach will provide enough information to answer all questions relating to the role of body segments in motor performance, but an understanding of muscular torque patterns is central to the issue. Segmental inertial forces, angular momenta, kinetic energy, and linear and angular velocity patterns can be by-products of the determination of muscle torque histories.

▶ [For those not familiar with the biomechanical methods for analysis of sports skills performance, this may be a bit too complicated. Just accept that what Miller is talking about is basic to the biomechanical approach that is being used in helping us to better understand the mechanical movement of the human body. It is obvious that the study of the laws of physics is central to understanding these techniques.—J.L.A.] ◀

(2–1) Res. Q. Exerc. Sport 51:219–233, March 1980.

2–2 **Surface EMG and Muscle Force at Low Force Levels: A Model-Based Theoretic Study** is reported by V. Pollak (Univ. of Saskatchewan). It has been found empirically that, under a fairly wide range of conditions, the absolute integral of the surface electromyogram (EMG) of a muscle can be used as a measure of its mechanical tension. A similar relationship exists for the root mean square value of the EMG and even for the simple spike frequency of the EMG. However, the nature of the relationship between muscle tension and the EMG is not clear. A close correlation between the EMG and force is theoretically far from obvious. The biophysical foundations of the observed relationships have now been examined and a model developed, the response characteristic of which would mirror the experimental observations.

The simplest model for simulation of the extracellular action potential of an excitable fiber is an axial dipole located in the fiber axis at the transition between the two states of the membrane. The dipole model assumes an abrupt transition between the polarized and depolarized sections of the fiber membrane, which is not the case in reality. Because the wave shape of the action potential expands with increasing distance, the spectrum of the action potential is compressed toward the low-frequency end of the spectrum. The model predicts that motor units with differing strengths are approximately uniformly distributed across the muscle. The mean cross-sectional area of the active motor units is a constant regardless of the recruitment threshold reached. At low firing frequencies the effect of fusion between successive twitches of the same unit is small, and the overall relationship between the EMG and muscle tension is determined largely by the proportion in which units with different speeds are represented in the recruited ensemble. A linear relationship is noted when this proportion is approximately constant. The scale factors involved may vary from one case to another, necessitating individual calibration when absolute force values are required.

▶ [This study is recommended for those who are serious students or practitioners of electromyographic techniques.—J.L.A.] ◀

2–3 **Synergy of Elbow Extensor Muscles During Static Work in Man.** Synergy in elbow flexion has been analyzed quantitatively, but only some qualitative data are available on elbow extension. S. Le Bozec, B. Maton, and J. C. Cnockaert (France) undertook a quantitative electromyographic (EMG) comparison of activity in the three heads of the triceps brachii and the anconeus muscle during static work in 13 healthy subjects aged 18–30 years, who maintained different extension torques with the arm and forearm in a horizontal plane. Subjects exerted a constant extension torque of 0.6 kg/m at elbow angles of 40–120 degrees. The triceps exerted a constant muscular force of 420 N at the above-elbow angles, with the external torque varying from one angle to another.

The integrated EMGs of the three heads of the triceps increased

(2–2) Am. J. Phys. Med. 59:126–141, June 1980.
(2–3) Eur. J. Appl. Physiol. 43:57–68, February 1980.

quadratically with torque. The integrated EMG of the anconeus muscle increased more rapidly than those of the triceps for low values of torque; for higher values, it increased in the same way as for the triceps muscle. With a constant external torque at any elbow angle, the EMG of the heads of the triceps remained about constant. With the force of the triceps constant with any elbow angle, a significant decrease in the integrated EMG was noted, of the same amount for the three heads of the muscle. Similar results were obtained whatever the position of the arm.

It appears that, in static contractions, the "equivalent muscle" concept can be applied to the extensor muscles of the elbow for a large range of external extension torques. There is a common motor control for the three heads of the triceps muscle, and the shape of the force-length relationship is about the same for the three heads. Variations in the lever arm of the muscle with the elbow angle appear to compensate for force variations due to variations in muscle lengths.

▶ [This is an excellent example of the importance and the complications involved in using biomechanical techniques to study the functions of various body parts—in this case, the elbow extensors. Electromyography (EMG) is very convenient and sensitive, but it indicates muscle tension indirectly by measuring when the muscles are electrically active. Because biomechanics is largely concerned with mechanical actions, it is important to determine the relationships between mechanical and electric activity. Elbow extension is primarily the action of the anconeus muscle and the triceps brachii which arises from the medial head, lateral head, and long head. This investigation of the functional roles and coordination is the same type of study that should be done by competent researchers for all of the interacting muscle groups of the body if we are to gain a detailed understanding of how the body moves.—J.L.A.] ◀

2–4 **Angle-Angle Diagrams in the Assessment of Locomotion** are discussed by Cecil Hershler and Morris Milner (McMaster Univ., Hamilton, Ont.). A number of workers have used the angle-angle diagram representation of data in which two selected leg joint angle variations are plotted against one another for corresponding points in time. Subjects are fitted with electrogoniometers to measure hip angle and knee angle histories in the sagittal plane during locomotion. Foot-switches are fitted to measure heel and toe contact times. Single loops reflect kinematic data for a single footstep. Multiple loops provide a visual impression of the repeatability of gait, but other information confuses the issues, and ranges of variability must be estimated to quantify the repeatability of gait. Typical diagrams are shown in Figures 2–1 and 2–2.

Hip and knee angle histories were collected from 5 normal subjects, from electrogoniometer systems at the hip and knee joints, usually on both sides. The hip was seen to flex continuously but relatively slowly during the change from knee flexion to extension in the swing phase. The abrupt change in shape of the loop after the onset of stance demonstrated the nature of the control mechanism that allows the subject's musculature rapidly to absorb the impulsive shock at the knee and hip joints. Conjoint angular motion was seen to be shared in a ratio of 1:2 between the stance and swing phases of a footstep. A

(2–4) Am. J. Phys. Med. 59:109–125, June 1980.

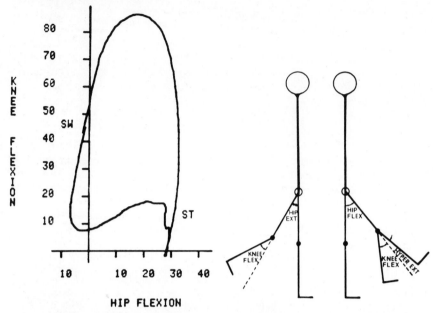

HIP FLEXION

Fig 2–1 (left).—A typical normal knee-angle/hip-angle diagram. Angles are in degrees. ST indicates onset of stance; then, "reading" the loop in a clockwise direction; SW indicates onset of swing.

Fig 2–2. (right).—Direction of flexion and extension.

(Courtesy of Hershler, C., and Milner, M.: Am. J. Phys. Med. 59:109–125, June 1980.)

substantially greater amount of perimeter appeared to be associated with the stance segmental area than with the swing area. Apparently, more control and coordination are called for during stance than during swing.

This type of analysis provides a more complete assessment of locomotor function. Quantitative analyses could be done on a number of distinct gait pathologies in both the sagittal and frontal planes to determine whether characteristic patterns can be identified. Pattern recognition techniques may prove useful in clinical assessments of locomotor function.

▶ [This is an excellent method to measure the change in gait that is caused by fatigue. Maybe we can determine whether overuse injuries such as those suffered by marathon runners may really be the result of poor mechanics brought on by fatigue. In this study, the authors used five subjects. It is hoped that this work will be continued with more subjects to identify and analyze distinctive gait patterns for skilled as well as unskilled subjects.—J.L.A.] ◀

2–5 **The Development of Mature Gait.** Both learning and maturation of the central nervous system contribute to evolution of the mature gait. David H. Sutherland, Richard Olshen, Les Cooper, and Savio L.-Y. Woo (San Diego) performed gait studies on 186 normal children aged 1–7 years to determine the normal gait patterns in childhood.

(2–5) J. Bone Joint Surg. [Am.] 62-A:336–353, April 1980.

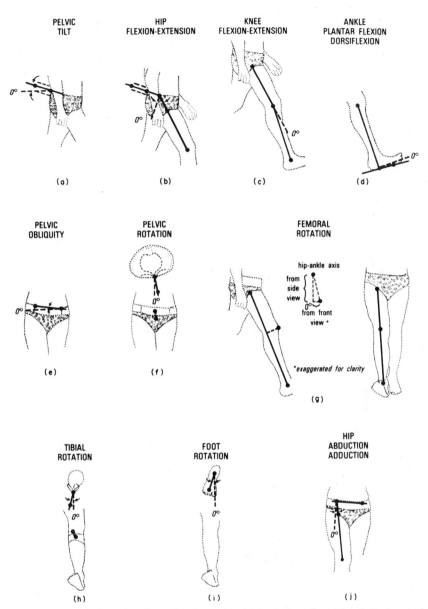

PELVIC TILT

(a)

HIP FLEXION-EXTENSION

(b)

KNEE FLEXION-EXTENSION

(c)

ANKLE PLANTAR FLEXION DORSIFLEXION

(d)

PELVIC OBLIQUITY

(e)

PELVIC ROTATION

(f)

FEMORAL ROTATION

hip-ankle axis

from side view

from front view *

*exaggerated for clarity

(g)

TIBIAL ROTATION

(h)

FOOT ROTATION

(i)

HIP ABDUCTION ADDUCTION

(j)

Fig 2–3.—Methods used to determine the various joint rotations. Large dots indicate actual measurement points, and broken lines show the 0-degree reference for each angle. The drawings for femoral rotation show neutral rotation. Hence, the center of the front of the patella falls on the hip-ankle axis, and no perpendicular line segment is visible in the front view. (Courtesy of Sutherland, D. H., et al.: J. Bone Joint Surg. [Am.] 62-A:336–353, April 1980.)

High-speed movies, a Graf-Pen sonic digitizer, a computer, a plotter, and electromyograms were used to analyze rotations of the leg joints in the sagittal, frontal, and transverse planes, step length, cadence, walking velocity, and the duration of single-limb stance as a percentage of the gait cycle (Fig 2–3).

Sagittal plane angular rotations in children aged 2 years and older were very similar to those of normal adults. Younger subjects had greater knee flexion and more ankle dorsiflexion in the stance phase, and their knee flexion wave, or stance-phase knee flexion after foot-strike and subsequent knee extension before toe-off, was diminished. External rotation of the hip was pronounced in the younger subjects. Most children exhibited reciprocal arm-swing and heel-strike by age 18 months. The chief determinants of a mature gait were found to be duration of the single-limb stance, walking velocity, cadence, step length, and the ratio of pelvic span to ankle spread. Cadence decreases as maturity advances, while walking velocity and step length increase. Increasing limb length and limb stability contribute to a mature pattern and are manifested by an increasing duration of single-limb stance. A mature gait pattern is well established at age 3 years.

These normative data can be used to compare the gait patterns of abnormal children with those of normal children of the same age, in order to elucidate the pathomechanics of gait disorders in childhood. The present observations confirm the relatively short time needed for gait maturation to take place. A longer step length, not a greater step frequency, is responsible for the increase in walking velocity with growth and maturation. The greatest change in the step factor occurs before age 3 years. Elaborate laboratory methods are not necessary to establish the presence of a mature gait pattern in a normal child. The presence of heel-strike and reciprocal movements of the arms and legs are quite easily observed, and the narrow base of support of the mature walker is readily distinguished visually from the wide base of the toddler.

▶ [The understanding of the mature gait and its development is important in evaluating gait disorders in children. However, it is also important that we continue to follow and study the gait in greater detail than what the authors show as the chief determinants: duration of single-limb stance, walking velocity, cadence, step length, and the ratio of pelvic span to ankle spread. Foot placement and changes in the gait variables as velocity increases from slow walk to fast walk to running are important, as are the changes in the variables with the onset of fatigue. It may be that increased speed and the onset of fatigue change the gait pattern to the extent that overuse injuries are the result. It is my observation that a large number of novice runners or joggers have poor running mechanics even though they had developed a mature gate before their third birthday. These are also the people who complain the most about leg injuries.— J.L.A.] ◀

2–6 **Force-, Power-, and Elasticity-Velocity Relationships in Walking, Running, and Jumping.** Pekka Luhtanen and Paavo V. Komi (Univ. of Jyväskylä) examined force- and power-velocity relationships in 6 ordinary-level track and field athletes as they walked

(2–6) Eur. J. Appl. Physiol. 44:279–289, September 1980.

at maximal velocity with a normal or racing gait, ran at varying proportions of maximum velocity, and made a maximal running long jump. Six national-level triple jumpers and 4 long jumpers also were investigated. Ground reaction forces and mechanical power were assessed, and the apparent spring constants of the support leg in the eccentric and concentric phases were estimated during the running long jump takeoff and in the triple jump. A cinematographic technique and a mathematical model of hopping were used.

As the angular velocity of the knee changed with faster running, most mechanical power was used to change the linear velocity of the body. Relationships between resultant force and horizontal velocity and between mechanical power and horizontal velocity for different activities are shown in Figure 2–4. Force and power values declined from the long jump takeoff through maximal running speed and submaximal running, to racing gait and normal gait. The parameters were greatest in the long jump takeoff by the long jump athletes. The increase in force and mechanical power output was generally related to the value of the apparent spring constant of the support leg in the eccentric phase. The spring constant in the eccentric phase increased with the velocity of motion in running, the long jump takeoff, and the triple jump.

It may be possible to use the spring constant in the eccentric phase as a measure of mechanical performance, because it may reflect the combined elasticity of the muscles, tendons, and bones of the human

Fig 2–4.—**A,** resultant force (mean ± SE) and **B,** mechanical power (mean ± SE) in walking, running, and long jump at different horizontal velocities. (Courtesy of Luhtanen, P., and Komi, P. V.: Eur. J. Appl. Physiol. 44:279–289, September 1980; Berlin-Heidelberg-New York: Springer.)

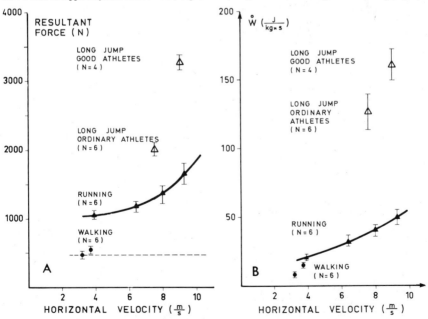

mechanical system. In general, this constant is large when the resultant force at center gravity is high, the peak-to-peak oscillation and horizontal displacement of the center of gravity are small, and the contact time is short. Its relationship with mechanical power in the eccentric phase is significant. However, the basic assumption of harmonic oscillation of the path of the center of gravity may not hold in all conditions. In addition, it is expected that the point value of the spring constant changes continuously during contact, because the length of the muscles and tendons of the support leg change in a complex manner.

▶ [It seems intuitively obvious that the spring constant in the eccentric phase may be the single most effective measure of mechanical performance short of measuring the performance itself, which is cheaper in terms of time and resources. Therefore, the importance of the knowledge of the correlation between spring constant and mechanical performance is so that trainers can better analyze how to increase the magnitude of the spring constant and thus attain better performance. From what is known at this time, or at least what coaches use, as horizontal velocity increases, the spring constant increases and mechanical performance increases. The best example of this is the performance of Carl Lewis of the University of Houston, who won both the 100-m dash and the long jump at the 1981 National Collegiate Athletic Association Track and Field Championships.—J.L.A.] ◀

2–7 **Biomechanics of Walking, Running, and Sprinting.** Roger A. Mann and John Hagy report a biomechanical study of 2 male sprinters, 5 experienced joggers, and 6 elite long-distance runners. Six of the runners and joggers were female. The elite runners were college athletes who routinely ran races longer than 1,500 m. Sagittal plane motion in the lower extremity was analyzed by a photometric technique based on biplane high-speed photography. Electromyography also was carried out.

The length of the stance phase decreased progressively as the speed of gait increased, from 62% for walking to 31% for running and 22% for sprinting. Sagittal plane motion increased with speed of gait. The body generally lowered its center of gravity with increasing speed by increased flexion of the hips and knees and magnified dorsiflexion at the ankles. Electromyographic studies about the knee showed increased quadriceps and hamstring activities with increased speed. Recordings about the ankle showed that the posterior calf muscles, which normally function in the midstance phase of walking, became late swing-phase muscles and were active through the first 80% of stance phase, compared with 15% in walking. The anterior compartment muscles of the calf underwent a concentric contracture at initial floor contact during running and sprinting but an eccentric contraction during walking.

The body tends to lower its center of gravity as the speed of gait increases. The calf muscles exhibit a longer period of electric activity as the speed of gait increases. Knee function reflects impact absorption of ground contact by increased flexion, followed by a second period of extension, in walking and jogging. In sprinting the second period of extension is not observed. Hip flexion appears to be an

(2–7) Am. J. Sports Med. 8:345–350, Sept.–Oct., 1980.

important part of running, but one about which little is known. The speed of hip flexion increases with the speed of gait. Further research is needed to determine what actually propels the body through space during running and sprinting.

▶ [We could have more confidence in the data from this study if the sample size were larger. That would help us in deciding on the ideal amount of flexion or extension of the knee or hip. It would also be helpful if studies such as this would pay attention to foot placement from the standpoint of toeing-in or toeing-out. Professor Karl Klein of the University of Texas has reported that the efficiency of the propulsion is significantly affected, especially if the foot placement is excessively toed-out. I have noticed that toeing-out is a common foot placement of many large athletes such as football linemen.—J.L.A.] ◀

2–8 **Some Fundamental Aspects of the Biomechanics of Over-ground Versus Treadmill Locomotion** are discussed by G. J. Van Ingen Schenau (Free Univ., Amsterdam). The motor-driven treadmill frequently is used in biomechanical and exercise physiology studies of locomotion and for training and rehabilitation purposes. It often may be used to simulate overground walking or running, but there are widely differing views of the validity of extrapolating treadmill data to the overground environment, or vice versa. Many workers have found differences in the kinematics or energy consumption, or both.

When a subject walks on a treadmill with a slope, the swinging foot is placed higher than the supporting foot, as in walking up a hill, but in treadmill walking the power from knee extension is not used in the same way because the supporting leg is going down with the belt. It might be concluded that a mechanical difference in terms of power output exists because potential energy is gained in walking uphill, but kinetic and potential energy calculations indicate that this conclusion is incorrect. Descriptions of treadmill locomotion with respect

Fig 2–5 (left).—External forces in walking uphill.
Fig 2–6 (right).—External forces in treadmill walking.
(Courtesy of Van Ingen Schenau, G. J.: Med. Sci. Sports 12:257–261, 1980; copyright 1980, the American College of Sports Medicine. Reprinted by permission.)

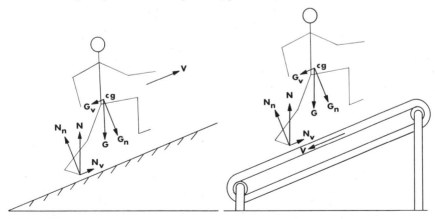

to a fixed coordinate system can lead to faulty conclusions. As long as the belt speed is constant, a coordinate system that moves with the belt should be used. In such a system, no mechanical difference exists in comparison with overground locomotion with respect to a fixed coordinate system (Figs 2–5 and 2–6). Therefore, all differences in locomotion patterns must arise from other than mechanical causes.

The mechanical equality of overground and treadmill locomotion follows from the Galilean principle of invariance, which states that the laws of motion are identical in all reference frames that move with uniform speed with respect to one another. Visual information is a possible source of differences in treadmill and overground locomotion. Many children exhibit fear of walking on a treadmill and show much longer double support phases than when walking overground. This effect might be less with a treadmill built so that the belt seems to be an integral part of the floor.

▶ [It is good that the authors have demonstrated that besides testing and validating our conclusions, we should also test and validate our methods, even those long in use.—J.L.A.] ◀

2–9 **Joint Looseness: Function of the Person and the Joint.** John L. Marshall, Norman Johanson, Thomas L. Wickiewicz, Henry M. Tischler, Bertram L. Koslin, Susan Zeno, and Al Meyers (Hosp. for Special Surgery, New York) sought to determine whether joint looseness is a characteristic of the person or whether the concept is applicable only to particular joints. If it is a trait, looseness should be identifiable in several joints, and a total measure of looseness should be related to some predicted consequences or known effects. Study was made of 124 boys and girls, aged 6 to 18 years, at a tennis camp. A set of anatomical states such as varus and valgus was scored, and a set of reliable judgmental measures was shaped to assess joint looseness. Agility and strength also were assessed, and anthropometric measurements were recorded.

The tests for joint looseness were correlated with one another and with total scores. Wherever test results were significantly related to one another, they were positively correlated. Moderately strong correlations were generally absent. The correlation of each joint looseness test with total score was significantly different from zero. Where there was significant correlation between joint looseness and performance, poorer performance was associated with greater looseness. The pattern of correlations suggested that joint looseness as a trait, as well as looseness in a particular joint, could explain poor performance. Sex was correlated with some joint looseness tests, but not with total score. Wherever joint looseness tests correlated with age or weight and height, or both, the relation was always negative.

The observations indicate that joint looseness is a trait. It remains to be determined whether joint looseness plays a differential role in predicting performance when a task does or does not require changing direction and acceleration under conditions of load.

(2–9) Med. Sci. Sports 12:189–194, 1980.

▶ [In reading this study, one has to wonder if history of physical activity or lack of physical activity would have had an impact on these findings. For example, is joint looseness associated with lack of physical activity? It seems intuitively obvious that lack of activity would be positively correlated with poor performance. That also may explain why it appeared in this study that joint looseness is a trait. This is fascinating information and must be followed up!—J.L.A.] ◀

2–10 **Electromyographic Investigation of Muscle Stretching Techniques.** Many stretching techniques have been developed by athletes, dancers, and physical therapists, including ballistic or "bouncing" methods, slow movements such as those used in dance, static stretches, and proprioceptive neuromuscular facilitation (PNF) procedures. Classic Sherringtonian views regarding the stretch reflex and reciprocal inhibition underlie assumptions that the static and PNF methods are advantageous. However, contrary to traditional views, a muscle is initially more resistant to change in length after a static contraction. Marjorie A. Moore and Robert S. Hutton determined the level of muscle relaxation achieved during static and modified PNF stretch procedures electromyographically (EMG) in 21 women aged 17–23 years, actively involved in gymnastics for an average of 6 years. The experimental setup is shown in Figure 2–7. Subjects produced hamstring stretch by static, contract-relax (CR), and contract-relax with agonist contraction (CRAC) methods.

In 12 subjects, the CRAC method elicited significantly greater hamstring EMG activity than the other methods. The static method produced a higher level of muscle activation in only 1 subject. No significant differences were found in EMG activity across stretch conditions in 8 subjects. Involuntary paroxysmal tremor activity occasionally was observed in most subjects at low levels of muscle activation. The CRAC technique, while apparently contributing to increased muscle stiffness, produced the largest gains in hip flexion.

A modified PNF-CRAC technique resulted in higher hamstring EMG activity in most subjects than the CR and static stretch methods

Fig 2–7.—Experimental conditions. (Courtesy of Moore, M. A., and Hutton, R. S.: Med. Sci. Sports 12:322–329, 1980; copyright 1980, the American College of Sports Medicine. Reprinted by permission.)

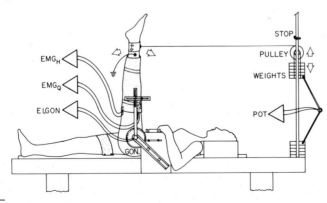

and produced the greatest increase in range of motion. Full muscle relaxation was not necessary for effective muscle stretching. The subjects tended to rate as most effective the stretch that elicited the least EMG activity and pain; they did not use the extent of hip flexion achieved as the chief criterion. The CRAC technique appears to be best for achieving maximum flexibility in experienced, well-motivated subjects when enough time is available to practice the procedure. If comfort and limited training time are major considerations, the static method appears to be more desirable.

▶ [I am convinced that there is much that we do not understand about muscle stretching and increasing joint flexibility. How effective can we expect to be with the various methods that are being espoused? What part do genetics play? How much time is necessary to show a significant increase in flexibility? How important is muscle stretching in preventing injuries? . . . in improving performance? This study is an assist in helping us to understand.—J.L.A.] ◀

2–11 **Comparative Study of Reaction Time in Indian Sportsmen Specializing in Hockey, Volleyball, Weight Lifting and Gymnastics.** Individual differences in speed of reaction and speed of movement depend to a considerable degree on neuromuscular coordination abilities. Athletes have better reaction times than nonathletes, and reaction times improve with an increasing level of skill in some activities. J. L. Bhanot and L. S. Sidhu (Punjabi Univ., Patiala, India) compared hand and foot reaction times in Indian sportsmen participating in hockey, volleyball, weight lifting, and gymnastics. A total of 59 subjects were studied. All had competed at the national

Fig 2–8.—Histogram showing mean values in milliseconds of hand visual and auditory reaction times of players of hockey, volleyball, weight lifting, and gymnastics. (Courtesy of Bhanot, J. L., and Sidhu, L. S.: J. Sports Med. 20:113–118, March 1980.)

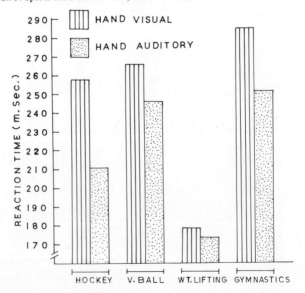

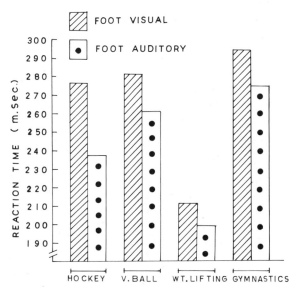

Fig 2–9.—Histogram showing mean values in milliseconds of foot visual and auditory reaction times of players of hockey, volleyball, weight lifting, and gymnastics. (Courtesy of Bhanot, J. L., and Sidhu, L. S.: J. Sports Med. 20:113–118, March, 1980.)

level. Visual and auditory reaction times of the hand and foot were recorded on a kymograph.

The findings are shown in Figures 2–8 and 2–9. Both visual and auditory reaction times of the hand and foot were shortest in the weight lifters. Hockey players were faster than the volleyball players and gymnasts for both visual and auditory reactions of the hand and foot, but the differences were significant only for auditory reaction times. Volleyball players had shorter visual and auditory reaction times of the hand and foot than did gymnasts, but the differences were not significant.

In this study, weight lifters were found to have shorter reaction times than hockey players and volleyball players, whereas gymnasts were the slowest group. Weight lifters require good neuromuscular coordination to lift capacity weights successfully. Hockey players compete for possession of the puck, while this situation does not arise in volleyball or gymnastics. In volleyball, a player must coordinate his body with the falling ball.

▶ [This study is placed here to help dispel the myth that weight lifters become "muscle bound" and clumsy. It should be noted that this study does not show that the four sports—weight lifting, hockey, volleyball and gymnastics—are the causal factors in developing the reaction times. Rather, it simply shows that of the athletes tested the weight lifters had the fastest reaction times, followed by the hockey players, the volleyball players, and the gymnasts, respectively.—J.L.A.] ◀

2–12 **Mechanics of Translation in the Fosbury Flop.** Dick Fosbury won the high jump event at the 1968 Olympic Games using a new

(2–12) Med. Sci. Sports 12:37–44, Spring 1980.

technique termed the "Fosbury flop," which involves a curved approach run that proved difficult to analyze by the usual two-dimensional cinematographic methods. Ecker theorized that the curved approach offsets the natural tendency to lean toward the bar at takeoff, insuring a more vertical takeoff and increasing the force exerted against the ground. Jesús Dapena (Univ. of Iowa) examined the mechanics of the translations involved in the Fosbury flop technique of high jumping in 6 subjects, all experienced jumpers, using a three-dimensional cinematographic method. The subjects were filmed both during an official track meet and during a training session.

The curved run-up was found to cause the athletes to lean toward the center of the curve at the start of the takeoff phase. The center of gravity of all subjects had a negative vertical velocity at this point (Fig 2–10). The lateral deviation of the path of the center of gravity during takeoff was small. The initial trajectory of the parabolic path of the center of gravity after takeoff made an angle of 40–48 degrees with the horizontal plane. The takeoff leg flexed at least as much as previously reported for jumpers using the straddle style. One subject was able to clear the bar, although the peak height of the parabolic path followed by his center of gravity was at the same level as the bar.

Centripetal forces involved in the Fosbury flop technique of high jumping are small. At least part of the purpose of the curved run-up might be to cause a lean toward the center of the curve. The advantages of a jump involving a fast run-up and a large residual horizontal velocity over one involving a slower run-up and a smaller residual horizontal velocity remain unclear. The maximum flexion of the takeoff leg is similar for athletes using the Fosbury flop and the straddle techniques. With the Fosbury flop technique, the bar can be cleared

Fig 2–10.—Forces applied on an athlete while running on a curve: **A,** athlete is leaning toward the center of the curve; **B,** athlete is not leaning. (Courtesy of Dapena, J.: Med. Sci. Sports 12:37–44, Spring 1980; copyright 1980, the American College of Sports Medicine. Reprinted by permission.)

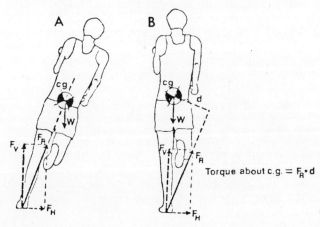

while the subject's center of gravity rises no higher than the level of the bar.

▶ [This is a typical example of the use of cinematographic techniques to analyze athletic performances. Ultimately, the analysis should lead to a better understanding of the mechanics of the particular activity and thus help to develop better teaching techniques.—J.L.A.] ◀

2–13 **Mechanics of Rotation in the Fosbury Flop.** The use of the curved run-up used by most athletes who practice the Fosbury flop technique of high jumping is not understood. It has been suggested that it facilitates production of centrifugal force during takeoff, offsets the natural tendency to lean toward the bar, or produces "rotation" or kinetic energy of rotation before the start of the takeoff phase. Jesús Dapena (Univ. of Iowa) compared components of the angular momentum vector before and after takeoff by three-dimensional cinematography in six subjects who used the Fosbury flop technique. Two different orthogonal coordinate systems fixed to the ground were used.

At the start of takeoff the subjects had little angular momentum. Most of the angular momentum needed to clear the bar properly was produced during the takeoff phase. A curved approach run appeared to favor production of "somersaulting" angular momentum, the component that mainly serves to lower the shoulders and lift the knees during the flight phase, and of a greater vertical range of motion of the center of gravity during the takeoff phase.

The findings do not support the view that the purpose of the curved run-up is to produce angular momentum. They favor the hypothesis that its main purpose is to make the jumper lean away from the bar. One subject with particularly small somersaulting angular momentum made effective use of a hitch-kick motion to achieve efficient bar clearance. This approach has considerable potential for detecting problems related to the airborne motion of individual athletes.

▶ [Although the sample size of six is not large enough to be statistically inferential, this is the kind of information that coaches need to help them to understand the mechanics of complicated skills such as the Fosbury flop. With a sample size of six, each jumper demonstrated slightly different techniques. It is then difficult to decide which technique or combination of actions will provide the correct technique. However, until more data are available, this study is an example of useful, albeit incomplete, data.—J.L.A.] ◀

2–14 **Kinetic and Kinematic Factors Involved in Execution of Front Aerial Somersaults.** The front aerial somersault is a basic gymnastics movement for any gymnast of reasonable ability. The ground reaction forces (GRF) developed during takeoff are important in performance, determining the projection velocity and increase in total body angular momentum necessary for a successful somersault. Zinovy Kinolik, John Garhammer, and Robert J. Gregor (Univ. of California, Los Angeles) examined variations in GRF during takeoff for the front aerial somersault in 9 highly skilled female gymnasts aged 13 to 19 years. Six somersaults were performed from a hurdle

(2–13)   Med. Sci. Sports 12:45–53, Spring 1980.
(2–14)   Med. Sci. Sports 12:352–356, 1980.

step with the rear or the front foot touching a force platform, and the movements were photographed. The total body center of mass position was used to calculate angular impulse during rear, double, and front leg support.

Similar angular impulse patterns were observed in these subjects, but various kinetic and kinematic variables were introduced. Rear foot horizontal components were always positive, whereas the pattern for the front foot revealed two peaks of opposite sign. A negative or braking force was observed on initial front foot support, followed by a propulsive force. Peak GRF during front foot support were about 1.5 times larger than those during rear foot support. With respect to center of mass, the mean angular impulse for all subjects was 61.7 Nms in the forward somersaulting direction. The rear leg contributed about 70% of this impulse. The velocity of the swinging limb during front foot support contributed to the velocity of the center of mass as well as to the angular velocity of the body about its center of mass. At maximum force production, the hip angle averaged 33 degrees and the knee angle 139 degrees.

A combination of kinetic variables suited to the given performer's strength and body size must come into play in the proper sequence for superior performance to be realized. Further study is needed of this combination.

▶ [One of the problems of biomechanical analyses of physical performance variables is knowing how to interpret what it is that we have found. Theoretically, if we collect enough data from enough superior performers, we can then develop a pattern for the "normal" performer, but as these authors have found, the combination of kinetic variables must be suited to each performer's strength and body size. In addition, this combination of variables must come into play in the proper sequence to give the most efficient summation of forces that will lead to superior performance. Excellent, knowledgeable coaches will always be needed to help the athlete to accomplish this.— J.L.A.] ◀

2–15 **Biomechanical Analysis of Olympic-Style Flat Water Kayak Stroke.** Ralph V. Mann and Jay T. Kearney (Univ. of Kentucky) studied the biomechanics of flat water kayaking by analyzing the techniques of 9 Olympic-caliber K-1 paddlers by cinematographic and computer procedures. The subjects were aged 17 to 31 years. They were filmed at least twice while they paddled through the test area attempting to maintain maximum velocity. Displacements, velocities, and accelerations of the wrists, elbows, shoulders, and body center of gravity were evaluated, as were relations between body segment movements and pattern of kayak movement, and the time and phase characteristics of the stroke.

During paddle-water contact the horizontal arm action was one of push-then-pull, with the push coming from the arm further from the water, followed by pull by the arm closer to the water. The center of paddle rotation shifted up the paddle shaft as the stroke progressed, increasing the time the paddle was in the power phase of the stroke. The push was accompanied by an integrated movement of the thrust wrist and elbow, with minimal shoulder participation. The pull was achieved by an integrated movement of the draw wrist, elbow, and shoulder and the thrust shoulder. The paddle was rapidly withdrawn from the water to avoid dragging. Subject stability in the frontal plane was maintained by shifting the body mass toward the water contact side at paddle entry and away from it at exit. This action opposed the vertical forces produced as a byproduct of the stroke. The result was maintenance of the body center of gravity velocity while the boat oscillated beneath the paddler. Both "fluid" and "explosive" styles of paddling were observed. Many subjects exhibited considerable bilateral asymmetry.

Olympic-style flat water kayak paddling is a complex skill involving repetitive application of horizontal force to produce or maintain boat velocity. The balance of the craft is maintained by shifting the mass of the paddler to oppose unwanted forces that could upset the delicate lateral stability maintained during paddling. The asymmetry observed might be due to the blade on the control side naturally being in a proper orientation for immersion, whereas on the noncontrol side it must be rotated before entry.

▶ [This is an excellent example of the use of biomechanical analysis of a physical performance skill in order to understand better the most important facets of an efficient stroke. Whereas it is important to be able to collect and report these data, it is equally important to be able to use the findings in order to improve the performance of future paddlers.—J.L.A.] ◀

2–16 **Knee Anatomy: Brief Review** is presented by Turner A. Blackburn and Emily Craig. An understanding of the anatomy of the knee is necessary for proper management of knee problems. The knee usually is viewed as consisting of the tibiofemoral and patellofemoral joints, the former divided into medial and lateral compartments. The extensor mechanism, or quadriceps femoris, consists of six muscles, the quadriceps femoris tendon, and the patellar ligament or tendon. The patella itself is a critical component of the extensor mechanism; its location allows greater mechanical advantage for extension of the knee. The patella is stabilized by the patellofemoral and patellotibial ligaments, thickenings of the extensor retinaculum that covers the anterior part of the knee. The prepatellar and infrapatellar bursae are subject to inflammation from trauma or overuse.

The medial compartment of the knee is supported by part of the extensor retinaculum. The pes anserinus group of muscles crosses the posterior medial area of the joint and attaches to the anterior medial part of the tibia. The medial meniscus is intimately attached to the capsular ligaments at its periphery. The posterior cruciate ligament is often referred to as the main stabilizer of the knee.

In the lateral compartment, muscular support is provided by the iliotibial band and tract, which attach anterolaterally into Gerdy's tubercle. The insertion of the popliteal muscle reinforces the posterior third of the lateral capsular ligaments. The lateral capsular ligaments attach to the lateral meniscus. The anterior cruciate ligament is included in the lateral compartment; its function is unclear, but it

(2–16) Phys. Ther. 60:1556–1560, December 1980.

is an important stabilizer of the knee. The structure of this ligament allows for several different areas of stability, and whether it should be repaired after injury is controversial.

▶ [To the knowledgeable reader, this review is extremely basic—too basic. However, for those who have been away from the anatomy book for a while, this is a nice review of the anatomy of the knee. Hopefully, the controversy over the repair of the anterior cruciate ligament will be settled, because more and more restorations are being done. It is not satisfactory to simply tell the weekend athlete that he or she will have to live with the unstable knee and not participate in that favorite sport.—J.L.A.] ◀

2–17   **Biomechanical Analysis of the Knee: Primary Functions as Elucidated by Anatomy** are discussed by William D. McLeod and Stewart Hunter. The knee can be viewed as consisting of the patellofemoral and femorotibial joints. Under weight-bearing conditions the tibial spine inserts into the femoral intercondylar notch, creating an effective bony stabilizer and providing self-centering during the transition to full weight-bearing. The patella serves as a bearing surface to keep the femur from sliding forward off the tibia. The tendinous connection of the patella and tibia, with the active quadriceps femoris mechanism, serves as a shock absorber in buffering the patellofemoral joint from high deceleration forces. The knee ligaments also keep the relative positions of the femur and tibia within bounds. The thigh muscles control rotation and deceleration and function as primary movers.

The patellofemoral joint absorbs compressive forces from the femur, transforming them into tension forces in the quadriceps femoris and patellar tendon. This permits the powerful quadriceps femoris to act as a retainer for the femur. The knee is basically unstable in the anteroposterior direction between a position of maximum hyperextension and that in which a load is applied to the tibial surface at an angle of at least 9 degrees anteriorly. The anterior cruciate ligament helps keep the femur from sliding back off the tibia, aided by the menisci and the meniscotibial ligaments. The posterior cruciate ligament helps keep the femur from sliding too far anteriorly on the tibia, although the primary force for this function is the patella and the quadriceps femoris mechanism.

Ligament strength appears to increase with exercise. Properly adjusted bicycle exercise permits progressive strengthening of the anterior cruciate ligament and the meniscotibial ligaments for rehabilitation. Any rehabilitation of the lower limb that requires minimal patellofemoral force should be done with the leg as close to full extension as possible, since patellofemoral irritation can result from flexion-to-extension exercises.

▶ [Blackburn and Craig presented the basic anatomy of the knee in the preceding article, whereas McLeod and Hunter add to the basic anatomy the primary mechanical functions as derived through a biomechanical analysis. This was done with the clinician in mind; thus, we have the clinical approach to biomechanical analysis that can be used to select positions of exercise that can increase or minimize stress to the various components within the knee.—J.L.A.] ◀

(2–17)   Phys. Ther. 12:1561–1564, December 1980.

2–18 **Thickness of Articular Cartilage in the Normal Knee.** Ferris M. Hall and Grace Wyshak (Boston) carried out a prospective arthrographic study of the thickness of the articular cartilage of the medial and lateral femoral condyles in 370 patients undergoing standard double-contrast arthrography of the knee. The cartilage of the medial condyle was found to be thicker than that of the lateral condyle. Minimum negative correlations were found between cartilage thickness and age. Cartilage thickness correlated best with patient weight, which as an independent variable accounted for 24% of the variation in thickness. Correlation of cartilage thickness with weight was much greater for women than for men. Weight was comparable with that of American adults between 1971 and 1974, but patients in the third decade of life were overrepresented, and those over age 60 were underrepresented, compared with the general adult population.

The relationship observed between articular cartilage thickness and patient weight is consistent with the hypothesis that cartilage thickness varies with the load applied across the joint. Although it usually is assumed that thicker articular cartilage affords greater protection to a joint, an increase in cartilage thickness may contribute to the development of degenerative arthritis. Both increased cartilage thickness and degenerative joint disease are seen in acromegaly. Suboptimal diffusion of nutrients from the joint to chondrocytes in the deeper layers of thickened cartilage might lead to sublethal cell injury and impaired ability to repair cartilage damage. The higher correlation of cartilage thickness with weight in women than in men is not understood, but it may be related at least in part to the presumed greater level of general physical activity in men. A marked decrease in activity could theoretically increase the importance of weight in providing the compressive forces needed for cartilage nutrition.

▶ [These data are interesting and might be useful as baseline data to study the effects of age, height, weight, and activity on cartilage thickness. A longitudinal study would be valuable in measuring changes in the thickness as a result of the above variables. Although the authors gave up on their attempt to collect data on individual levels of physical activity, that information would have added significantly to this study if it could have been collected accurately.—J.L.A.] ◀

2–19 **Strength of Isometric and Isokinetic Contractions: Knee Muscles of Men Aged 20 to 86.** Measures of isometric strength provide only partial information on muscle function. The strength generated during isotonic contraction is also an important measure of muscle performance. M. Patricia Murray, Gena M. Gardner, Louise A. Mollinger, and Susan B. Sepic (VA Med. Center, Wood, Wisc.) used the Cybex II isokinetic dynamometer to obtain normal standards of knee flexor and extensor muscle performance in groups of 24 normal men aged 20–35, 50–65, and 70–86 years. Torque generated by isometric and isokinetic contractions was measured on a dynamometer as knee position was monitored with an electrogoniometer. Each subject per-

(2–18) J. Bone Joint Surg. [Am.] 62-A:408–413, April 1980.
(2–19) Phys. Ther. 60:412–419, April 1980.

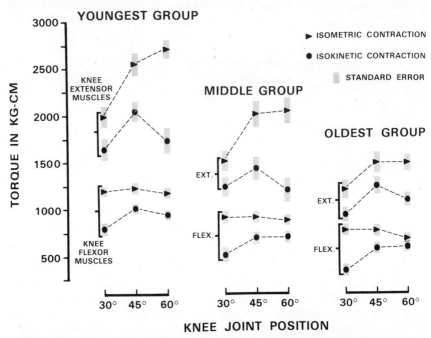

Fig 2–11.—Torque vs. knee joint position for isometric and isokinetic contractions of the knee flexor and extensor muscles in 3 groups of healthy men. For each type of contraction and joint position, the mean maximum torque values shown represent the strongest of 2 successive trials during the first test week. The shaded areas represent 1 SE above and below the mean values. Isokinetic contractions were performed at a speed of 36 degrees/second (6 rpm). Full knee extension was considered 0 degrees. (Courtesy of Murray, M. P., et al.: Phys. Ther. 60:412–419, April 1980.)

formed two consecutive cycles of maximum isokinetic contractions consisting of knee extension followed by knee flexion. The isokinetic contractions were done at 36 degrees/second, and the isometric contractions were sustained for 5 seconds.

Strength of the older men was significantly less than that of the youngest subjects. The strength of isokinetic contractions was significantly less than that of isometric contractions for all joint positions (Fig 2–11). The oldest men generally took longer than the younger subjects to reach peak torque during isometric contractions. For all joint positions combined, mean flexor muscle torque was about half that of the extensor muscles for all age groups and for both types of contractions. For isokinetic contractions, average torque was generally significantly higher on the second of two consecutive trials.

Decreasing muscle strength with advancing age is a common clinical observation and was documented in the present study. Factors that must be considered in measuring knee muscle strength include sex; knee joint position; the type, rate, and duration of muscle contraction; and the response to repeated efforts at generating maximal torque. Expectations of strength levels to be achieved in rehabilitative efforts must be modified by the age of the male subject.

▶ [The findings of this study agree in a relative degree with the work that we have done in the rehabilitation of athletes. The authors used "normal" healthy men who were not participating in a regular exercise program. Naturally, better conditioned, active athletes can be expected to have relatively higher torque values. We agree with the 2:1 ratio in favor of the extensor muscles over the flexor muscles. However, assuming that only one knee is being rehabilitated, there is no need to modify the expectation of the strength levels to be achieved if you follow a protocol that requires the subject to work at strengthening both the affected and the unaffected knees. The expected strength level of the affected knee should be within 10% of that of the unaffected knee. With this protocol, in our program it is not unusual for the affected knee as well as the unaffected knee to be stronger at the end of rehabilitation than the unaffected knee was before rehabilitation began.—J.L.A.] ◀

2–20 **Muscle Fiber Type Composition and Knee Extension Isometric Strength Fatigue Patterns in Power- and Endurance-Trained Males.** Walter Kroll, Priscilla M. Clarkson, Gary Kamen, and Jean Lambert (Univ. of Massachusetts, Amherst) investigated muscle fiber type composition in the vastus lateralis muscle and patterns of knee extension isometric strength fatigue in 8 endurance-trained and 8 power-trained men. The former were active in long-distance racing, while the latter were long-time weight lifters. Twenty-five repeated maximal isometric contractions, each lasting 10 seconds, were performed, with intertrial rest periods of 5 or 20 seconds.

Fatigue patterns for the power- and endurance-trained groups under the 10-second contraction, 5-second intertrial rest period regimen are shown in Figure 2–12. The power group fatigued nearly 4 times faster than the endurance group in this condition. In the 10:20 exercise condition, the endurance group showed no fatigue pattern, whereas the power group showed a significant strength decrement of 32%. In both exercise conditions, the power-trained group showed more complex fatigue patterns in terms of significant trend components. Maximal isometric strength correlated positively with percent-

Fig 2–12.—Isometric knee extension strength fatigue patterns for the power and endurance groups under the two exercise regimens. (Courtesy of Kroll, W., et al.: Res. Q. Exerc. Sport 51:323, May 1980.)

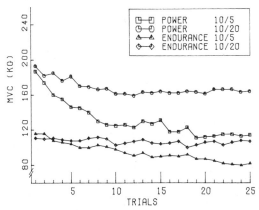

age of slow twitch fibers in both groups, but negatively with linear trend coefficients in both groups. Maximum isometric strength correlated more closely with fatigue-curve trend coefficients than did muscle fiber type composition. Strength correlated with body weight for the two groups combined.

These findings support the view that there is a degree of uniqueness in fatigue patterns, particularly between differing levels of absolute maximum strength. The mechanism responsible for isometric strength fatigue patterns appears not to be determined solely by muscle fiber type characteristics. Although these do play an important role in controlling isometric strength fatigue patterns, maximum isometric strength and muscle mass may be even more important factors.

▶ [This excellent study confirms some of the generally held ideas concerning endurance and power training and slow-twitch and fast-twitch muscle fibers. Continued studies of this type with standard protocols are needed to help us to understand better the meaning of the data that are gathered.—J.L.A.] ◀

2–21 **Breaststroke Swimmer's Knee: A Biomechanical and Arthroscopic Study.** Knee complaints are fairly common in breaststroke swimmers, but the cause of breaststroke swimmer's knee with medial pain in the joint has not been established. Kari Keskinen, Ejnar Eriksson, and Paavo Komi (Stockholm) performed arthroscopy in 9 breaststroke swimmers with knee pain and carried out biomechanical analyses by cinematographic techniques on 6 patients swimming in a special flume at 90% of their best competitive speed (Fig 2–13). Three swimmers without knee symptoms were also filmed.

The subjects with knee pain had pain bilaterally along the medial side of the knee. All had clinically stable knees, and arthroscopy of

Fig 2–13.—Schematic diagram of the swimming flume used in the biomechanical part of the study. Reproduced with permission of the *Journal of Applied Physiology*. (Courtesy of Keskinen, K., et al.: Am. J. Sports Med. 8:228, July–Aug. 1980.)

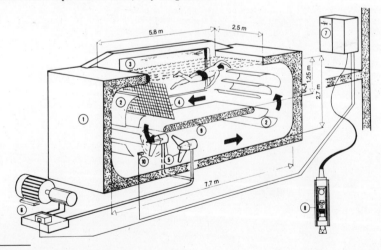

the most painful knee showed only relatively marked medial synovitis in 7 subjects. None had meniscal, cruciate ligament, or other injuries. No pathologic features were found in the popliteal fossa or in the suprapatellar pouch. Biomechanical analysis of the whip-kick movement showed slightly higher peak velocities of knee extension and flexion. The range of velocities was rather high. No clear differences were seen in velocity curves for hip abduction and adduction. However, in the patient with the most severe symptoms, the hip-knee angle-angle diagram differed clearly from the average, particularly from that of the best control swimmer. This subject began and finished the kick action with a very high degree of hip abduction, between 42 and 54 degrees.

A combination of high angular velocities at the hip and knee and external rotation of the tibia relative to the femur, repeated to excessive degrees, may be the chief cause of medial synovitis in breaststroke swimmers. Breaststroke swimmer's knee appears to be an overuse syndrome. Weekly training in breaststroke swimming may involve 20,000 or more whip-kick repetitions.

▶ [A survey of 2,496 Canadian swimmers by J. C. Kennedy and R. J. Hawkins showed that approximately 3% suffered from "breaststroke swimmer's knee." If we accept the findings of this study—as small as the sample of subjects was—that "breaststroke swimmer's knee" appears to be an overuse syndrome, then about 97% of the swimmers do not experience the pain. Maybe we should attempt to identify what training methods are used by the 97% of breaststroke swimmers who do not suffer pain. Will strengthening of the hip and leg muscles help prevent the overuse syndrome?— J.L.A.] ◀

2–22 **Knee Ligament Tests: What Do They Really Mean?** Frank R. Noyes, Edward S. Grood, David L. Butler, and Linda Raterman outline biomechanical concepts that govern the successful interpretation of clinical ligament laxity tests. Ligaments can be divided by their function into primary and secondary stabilizers, which must be recognized for every plane of knee stability or motion. The amount of laxity in the knee depends on the force applied, and only small forces are applied during clinical laxity evaluation compared with what the knee is subjected to with activity.

Laxity tests are highly subject to the amounts of joint opening and the types of motion produced, and by themselves do not provide a reliable prediction of functional stability. Many workers still disagree on which ligaments are being tested with standard laxity tests. For each plane of knee motion, only one or two ligaments act as the primary passive restraints. The others provide only a secondary restraint, although they do aid in providing stability. Both the primary and secondary restraints work together to provide stability. In 12 young cadaver knees, the anterior cruciate accounted for 85% of the restraining force at 30 degrees of knee flexion, and all other ligaments combined provided a secondary restraint of 15% of the total restraining force. Only a small force, often in the range of 20 lb, is applied in clinical drawer tests. The secondary structures may later

(2–22) Phys. Ther. 60:1578–1581, December 1980.

stretch when a primary restraint is lost, but the degree of laxity seen may initially be limited by the weak secondary restraints once the primary restraint has ruptured. Isolated ligament ruptures seldom, if ever, occur. Joint surfaces also may be affected in cases of ligament injury.

A "little" laxity is significant in an acute knee injury. Examination under anesthesia and arthroscopy may be necessary to determine the extent of ligament damage. Functional stability of the knee may not be long-lasting if it depends on muscle control alone, without the fine tuning action of the ligamentous system. Abnormal laxity on clinical examination is predictive of increased risks for joint wear, cartilage deterioration, and arthritis. Any serious ligament injury requires close follow-up, adequate rehabilitation, and correct advice on permissible activities.

2-23 **Ligamentous Restraints to Anterior-Posterior Drawer in the Human Knee: A Biomechanical Study.** One problem in previous ligament-cutting studies is that the increased laxity depends on the order in which the ligaments are cut. David L. Butler, Frank R. Noyes, and Edward S. Grood (Univ. of Cincinnati Med. Center) have overcome this difficulty with a new test method that allows the restraining force of each ligament to be determined. A precise displacement is applied while measuring the restraining force, and the reduc-

Fig 2–14.—Changes in anterior and posterior laxity in 1 knee preparation before and after loss of the cruciate ligaments. Laxities are shown for increasing activity force. Note the small increase in anterior laxity for a clinical anterior drawer test performed with a forward pull. A large increase in laxity occurs for posterior drawer when the posterior cruciate ligament is cut. (Courtesy of Butler, D. L., et al.: J. Bone Joint Surg. [Am.] 62-A: 259–270, March 1980.)

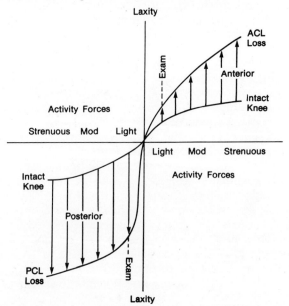

tion in force that follows severance of a ligament defines its contribution. Fourteen cadaveric knee preparations from subjects aged 18–65 years were tested with the knee at 90 and 30 degrees of flexion up to 5 mm of anterior and posterior drawer in the intact knee, and tests were repeated at larger drawer displacements to estimate backup restraints with the cruciate ligaments cut.

In anterior drawer, the anterior cruciate ligament is the primary restraint, providing an average of 86% of the total resisting force. Other structures each provided typically less than 3%. For straight posterior drawer, the posterior cruciate ligament provided a mean of 95% of the total restraining force. Secondary restraints were the posterior lateral capsule and popliteus complex combined (58%), the medial collateral ligament (16%), and many other structures to a lesser extent. The anterior cruciate ligament did not resist posterior drawer, not was the reverse true. Changes in one knee preparation before and after loss of the cruciate ligaments are shown in Figure 2–14.

Numerous passive secondary restraints operate when the cruciate ligaments of the knee are torn or ruptured and may block a positive drawer test. Effusion and muscle spasm also may act as restraints in acute injuries. The anterior drawer test, done under small clinical loads at 90 degrees of flexion, may not always be a sensitive indicator of insufficiency of the anterior cruciate ligament, especially in acute injuries. Other tests such as the flexion-rotation drawer and Slocum tests and arthroscopy with the use of anesthesia may be necessary to detect loss of this structure.

▶ [This article and the preceding one, by the same authors, are valuable to all athletic team doctors and athletic trainers to help them understand the benefits and limitations when they apply drawer tests to determine knee stability.—J.L.A.] ◀

2–24 **Biomechanics of Knee Rehabilitation With Cycling.** The bicycle has proved to be a simple and effective tool in rehabilitating the injured knee or the knee operated on. William D. McLeod and T. A. Blackburn (Columbus, Ga.) hypothesized that, by riding a bicycle, one eliminates the normal body weight and the high deceleration forces needed to modify body motion from the knee, making the loads transmitted through the knee controllable. When the load imposed on the knee is relatively low, the femur can be allowed to slide to the posterior side of the joint (Fig 2–15), gently stressing the anterior cruciate ligament and the meniscotibial ligaments.

Cinematographic studies were made of 6 persons aged 21–30 years riding a cycle ergometer at different seat-height settings. Two subjects underwent electromyography. The quadriceps became active at about 300–320 degrees of crank angle and dropped out at about 120–140 degrees. In general, the gastrocnemius was more active during pedaling with the ball of the foot and when the leg was extended by a higher bicycle seat. The hamstring was relatively inactive under normal conditions. With the seat low and the rider using the ball of the foot, the patellofemoral force is relied on to stabilize the femoral

(2–24) Am. J. Sports Med. 8:175–180, May–June 1980.

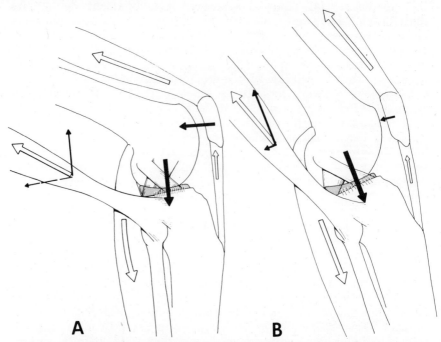

Fig 2–15.—**A** and **B,** lines of action of forces in and around the knee. Hamstring force resolved to show force parallel to tibial plateau. (Courtesy of McLeod, W. D., and Blackburn, T. A.: Am. J. Sports Med. 8:175–180, May–June 1980.)

tibial position. The more posterior the angle of the tibia, the greater is the tendency for the femur to slide off the posterior side, and the greater is the load applied to the ligaments. Hamstring activity was enhanced when the subject pedaled by pulling the pedal through at the bottom of the stroke.

Patients being rehabilitated can be instructed in how to pedal an exercycle to achieve the results desired and protect ligaments from stress. As ligament healing proceeds, use of the gastrocnemius can be enhanced while that of the hamstrings is reduced. This approach to rehabilitation eliminates the large inertial forces required in running or jogging and permits the force input to the joint to be easily controlled. The well-conditioned athlete can be placed on a 10-speed bicycle and ride about 20 miles a day in about 1 hour within 4–6 weeks. The level of activity for the nonathlete will be much less.

► [I agree with the authors concerning the value of cycling in rehabilitating the injured knee. We certainly use the bicycle as a part of our rehabilitation program. However, we find that we get faster results by also using isokinetic lifting to exercise both the hamstrings and quadriceps before cycling on a stationary bicycle. We have not used the 10-speed bicycle in our rehabilitation program but do recommend it as an excellent method to develop a long-term maintenance program. It should not be overlooked that the bicycle, whether free cycling or stationary, also helps the patient to build and maintain aerobic conditioning while the knee is healing.—J.L.A.] ◄

2–25 **A New Method of Quantitative Measurements of Abdominal and Back Muscle Strength.** The abdominal and back muscles have an important role in the supporting function of the spine. Mitsuo Hasue, Masatoshi Fujiwara, and Shinichi Kikuchi (Fukushima Med. College) used the Cybex machine for quantitative measurements of abdominal and back muscle strength in 50 normal subjects of each sex who had no complaints referable to the spine and in 12 men and 14 women with chronic low back pain. A muscle fatigue curve was made from data for 50 normal subjects. After trunk flexion isometrically and isokinetically, the subject was turned prone and trunk extension was carried out in the same way (Fig 2–16), as curves of muscle torque were recorded continuously.

Normal subjects of both sexes had the same maximal muscle torque values in isometric and isokinetic contractions. The ratio of abdominal to back muscles was less than unity in most subjects, especially women. Subjects with strong abdominal muscles also were apt to have strong back muscles. Both abdominal and back muscles tended to become weaker with increasing age, especially after age 40. In

Fig 2–16.—Examination of torque curve of trunk muscles. **Top,** examination of abdominal muscles. **Bottom,** examination of back muscles. (Courtesy of Hasue, M., et al.: Spine 5:143–148, Mar.–Apr. 1980.)

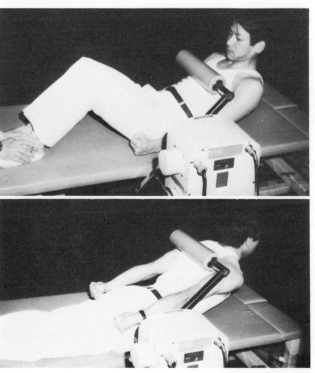

women, the abdominal muscles may weaken more than the back muscles with advancing age. Most values for subjects with low back pain were below the normal range, but wide individual differences were apparent. Muscle fatigue curves generally showed larger values in isometric than in isokinetic contraction in both the abdominal and back muscles and in both sexes, indicating readier fatigue of the trunk muscles by a sustained contraction. In addition, the abdominal muscles were more easily fatigued than the back muscles. No significant age relationship was observed.

These studies indicate that the abdominal muscles are ordinarily weaker than the back muscles and that the trunk muscles more easily are fatigued by a sustained contraction than by repeated contractions. The role of the trunk muscles in pain production and prevention remains to be clarified.

▶ [This excellent study provides much-needed information about one of our most significant medical problems. Although the authors concluded that we still do not fully understand the role of the trunk muscles in pain production and prevention, they have given us other information of significant value. Intuitively, we would expect that the antigravity back muscles would be stronger than the abdominal muscles, and these authors have confirmed this. They showed that subjects with strong abdominal muscles also have strong backs and that both muscle groups weaken with age. Again, intuitively, one would think that physical activity is the key to developing strong abdominal muscles and strong backs and, therefore, physical activity can be used to slow down the aging process. That women's abdominal muscles weaken faster than their backs should lead us to the conclusion that women must spend more time strengthening the abdominal muscles, especially after childbirth. We need more longitudinal research using subjects who have had low back pain and been placed on an exercise program, to see if a measurable gain of strength in the trunk muscles will relieve the pain.—J.L.A.] ◀

2–26 **Biomechanics of Hyperextension Injuries to the Cervical Spine in Football.** The practice of using the helmet as the primary impact area in blocking and tackling in football has been extensively criticized. Schneider suggested that impingement of the posterior rim of the helmet on the posterior cervical spine, through an initial impact on the face mask, may cause hyperextension injuries of the cervical spine. Dennis R. Carter and Victor H. Frankel (Univ. of Washington, Seattle) examined the guillotine mechanism of injury proposed by Schneider. Static-free body analyses were carried out to assess forces on the cervical spine when the face guard is struck so as to create hyperextension of the cervical spine. Three loading conditions created by different helmet designs (Fig 2–17) were evaluated. Either the helmet rim was cut high enough posteriorly so as not to impinge on the posterior cervical spine, or the helmet rim impacted at the level of C4 or on the shoulder pads.

The most dangerous hyperextension situation was observed with the helmet rim cut high enough posteriorly so as not to impinge on the posterior cervical spine. This leads to high forces and possibly serious upper spine injury. Impact of the posterior helmet rim at C4 reduced the forces significantly.

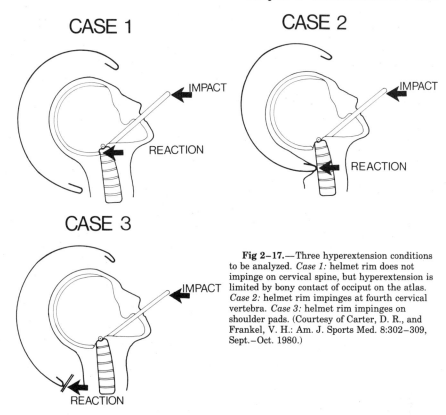

CASE 1

IMPACT

REACTION

CASE 2

IMPACT

REACTION

CASE 3

IMPACT

REACTION

Fig 2–17.—Three hyperextension conditions to be analyzed. *Case 1:* helmet rim does not impinge on cervical spine, but hyperextension is limited by bony contact of occiput on the atlas. *Case 2:* helmet rim impinges at fourth cervical vertebra. *Case 3:* helmet rim impinges on shoulder pads. (Courtesy of Carter, D. R., and Frankel, V. H.: Am. J. Sports Med. 8:302–309, Sept.–Oct. 1980.)

These findings directly contradict the so-called guillotine hypothesis of hyperextension injury of the cervical spine. Impact of the posterior rim of the football helmet on the shoulder pads was found to create the least hazardous loading conditions. Injury may result from hyperextension bending moments when these exceed local bending strength, but the exact site of such injury is difficult to predict. Hyperextension and other cervical spine injuries can be minimized by neck conditioning, the use of properly fitted helmets and shoulder pads, neck rolls, and good coaching.

▶ [This is an example of the need for sound research to test intuitive deductions or prior research. The results of this study directly contradict Schneider's findings. However, we must understand that this study is limited because the action of the muscles were not considered in this analysis. The authors have shown how biomechanical research techniques can be used to analyze causes of injuries. Our concern should be to understand the causes of injuries and take steps through rule changes, better equipment, and proper conditioning in order to prevent them. It is not satisfactory to say, "Stop the game. There are too many injuries."—J.L.A.] ◀

2–27 **Radiographic Measurements of the Normal Adult Foot.** Unusual bony relationships in foot x-ray films can be quite striking despite an asymptomatic foot. Maxwell W. Steel III, Kenneth A. John-

(2–27) Foot Ankle 1:151–158, November 1980.

son, Myrna A. DeWitz, and Duane M. Ilstrup (Mayo Clinic) studied the range of the normal foot in standard x-ray films providing data applicable to the clinical setting. Study was made of 41 pairs of feet of women aged 40–60 years. Standard anteroposterior (AP) and lateral x-ray films were obtained, both being weight-bearing views. A total of 28 measurements were taken from the AP view (Fig 2–18) and 31 from the lateral view (Fig 2–19).

Significant variations in bony relationships were documented in the normal painless adult foot. When recognized criteria of radiographic measurements were evaluated, some were found to be too narrow or inaccurate. Some of the present x-ray films would be considered to have an abnormal Bohler angle of the os calcis from conventional figures. The findings for the first ray, or "bunion," area of the foot were similar to Barnett's wider limits. The position of the tibialward sesamoid was quite variable. Wide variation also was found in the angle between the first metatarsal axis and its proximal phalanx. The first metatarsophalangeal angle varied along with other forefoot measurements, but was independent of the midfoot and hindfoot bony configurations. There generally was little difference between measurements in the two feet.

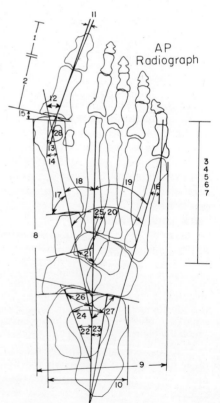

Fig 2–18.—Location of measurements on anteroposterior x-ray film of weight-bearing normal foot. (Courtesy of Steel, M. W., III, et al.: Foot Ankle 1:151–158, November 1980.)

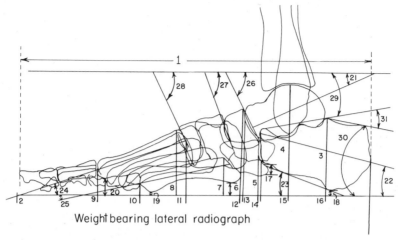

Weight bearing lateral radiograph

Fig 2–19.—Location of measurements on lateral x-ray film of weight-bearing normal foot. (Courtesy of Steel, M. W., III, et al.: Foot Ankle 1:151–158, November 1980.)

The normal adult foot exhibits significant variations in bony relationships. The present observations confirm the validity of using contralateral foot x-ray films for comparison. Surgical procedures are not indicated to produce radiographic homogeneity in the foot, because the foot is a heterogeneous structure. Treatment should be directed specifically toward areas of pain, not radiographic appearances.

▶ [With the increase in athletic activity, the feet are getting more and more attention—and they should, when we consider the number of complaints there are from all of our weekend athletes. These data, although not complete by themselves, provide some guidance concerning the wide range of normality in radiographic measurements of the human foot.—J.L.A.] ◀

2–28 **Vibration-Induced Decrease in the Muscle Force in Lumberjacks.** The vibration syndrome is an entity of symptoms arising from vessels, peripheral nerves, bones, and muscles of the arms. M. Färkkilä, I. Pyykkö, O. Korhonen, and J. Starck (Univ. of Helsinki) examined muscle fatigue produced during a maximal handgrip force-relaxation task for 2 minutes, with and without vibration exposure. Isometric maximal handgrip force was measured with a strain gauge dynamometer in 91 lumberjacks and 31 control subjects, with respective mean ages of 35.8 and 37.4 years. The lumberjacks had used a chain saw for a mean of 9,760 hours. A dynamic shaker was used to produce vibration at 80 Hz.

The muscle forces of older subjects were smaller than those of younger men, apart from vibration exposure. The fatigue curves of lumberjacks and control subjects had the same shape. During vibration exposure, forces decreased significantly in the left hand in the lumberjacks but not in control subjects. The force level of fatigue curves was lower in the lumberjacks with a history of decreased grip force

(2–28) Eur. J. Appl. Physiol. 43:1–9, February 1980.

and was reduced more during vibration exposure than in those with a history of normal grip force. Handgrip force was reduced in 18 of the lumberjacks. This was not related to Raynaud's phenomenon, but numbness and pain in the hands were associated with a history of reduced grip force. The decrease was associated with occupational vibration exposure, being absent in those who had sawn for less than 5,000 hours, and increasing in prevalence and severity with exposure time.

Prolonged exposure to vibration from operating a chain saw in some lumberjacks can reduce handgrip force. This appears to be related to lesions of peripheral nerves, and possibly to activation of the so-called tonic vibration reflex. A relation of muscle force reduction with circulatory changes appears unlikely, although hand numbness is associated with reduced grip force.

▶ [This study is interesting and may have some implications for athletes, especially in baseball, tennis, race car driving, speedboat racing, and perhaps handball.—J.L.A.] ◀

2–29 **Skeletal Muscle Strength During Exposure to Hypobaric Hypoxia.** Human beings exposed acutely to high altitude have decreased aerobic work capacity because of inadequate compensation for the reduction in ambient oxygen tension, but little is known of the effects of hypoxia on muscle strength capacity. A. Young, J. Wright, J. Knapik, and A. Cymerman (US Army Res. Inst. of Environmental Medicine, Natick, Mass.) examined the effects of a 48-hour stay at a simulated altitude of 15,000 ft on the static and dynamic strength of several functional skeletal muscle groups. Studies were done in 10 men aged 19 to 23 years. All were physically active but not involved in a strength training program. The isokinetic strength of the knee extensors, the isometric strength of the upper part of the torso, knee, and trunk extensors, and the strength endurance of the knee extensors and elbow flexors were assessed before, during, and after exposure to simulated altitude.

The 8 evaluable subjects showed no significant differences in strength at sea level and after 2 and 24 hours of hypoxic exposure. Mean strength measurements after 48 hours of exposure were increased over sea level values, but the difference was significant only for isometric strength of the upper part of the torso. Strength endurance was unchanged throughout exposure to simulated altitude. Symptoms of acute mountain sickness were most marked after 24 hours of exposure and remained significant, although somewhat reduced, after 48 hours of hypoxia. Many subjects reported "weakness" after 24 and 48 hours of exposure.

Skeletal muscle strength was not impaired during acute exposure to hypobaric hypoxia in these young men, even when symptoms of acute mountain sickness were most pronounced and despite the subjects' perception of muscle weakness. Several tests showed increased strength, compared with sea level values, although the differences were generally not significant. That a significant training effect occurred during the study is unlikely. Other possible explanations of increased muscle strength are motivation, alkalosis, and increased sympathetic activity. Further studies are warranted to determine whether muscle strength increases with more prolonged hypoxic exposures.

▶ [The findings of this study appear to agree with various experiences of athletes when they compete at altitudes somewhat higher than they are trained for. There is no valid experience of loss of strength, although aerobic work capacity is affected adversely. Of course, this study was done at an altitude where only the mountain climbers perform.—J.L.A.] ◀

2–30 **Neurophysiologic Inhibition of Strength Following Tactile Stimulation of the Skin.** Afferent cutaneous stimulation has been used in physical medicine and rehabilitation regimens for developmental disabilities and neuromuscular disorders. It is used as a component of proprioceptive neuromuscular facilitation techniques to restore flexibility and strength and improve sensorimotor integration. Such techniques recapitulate neurologic development, cephalocaudal and proximal to distal, by strengthening the entire linkage between the proximal and distal segments of a limb. James A. Nicholas, Meredith Melvin, and Anthony J. Saraniti (Lenox Hill Hosp., New York) used a shoulder abduction manual muscle test to demonstrate strength changes after tactile stimulation of the skin. Resistance was applied to the distal radioulnar joint as a scratch stimulus was applied inferior to the clavicle on the clavicular head of the pectoralis major after maximum contraction, and isotonic measurements were quantified electromechanically. Isometric strength was measured with a standard dynamometer system.

Studies were done in 23 normal subjects and 17 strong, athletic subjects. The normal group showed a 19% decrease in strength after tactile stimulation, whereas the athletic subjects showed a 17% reduction in strength as measured by the manual muscle-testing unit. With isometric measurements, the normal group had an 8% decrease in mean strength after stimulation, whereas the athletic subjects showed no significant decrease in strength.

This study demonstrated neurophysiologic inhibition of strength in the shoulder abductors after tactile stimulation of the overlying skin dermatome. Isometric tests were less sensitive than a manual muscle test. This phenomenon is not observed if there is a history of pathologic change in the limb being tested. Facilitation and inhibition of strength can be viewed as both protective and detrimental. The possibility that such neurophysiologic mechanisms contribute to the cause of injuries by affecting recruitment remains open. Quantitative manual muscle tests may clarify the processes of radiation and recruitment that transmit strength from proximal to distal segments.

(2–30) Am. J. Sports Med. 8:181–186, May–June, 1980.

3. General Medicine

GENERAL

3–1 **Migraine Precipitated by Head Trauma in Athletes.** Donald R. Bennett, Samuel I. Fuenning, George Sullivan, and Jerry Weber (Univ. of Nebraska) examined 3 members of a university football team for transient neurologic symptoms after minor head trauma and analyzed the clinical data from 8 previously reported cases of migraine associated with head trauma.

It was found that the head trauma was usually minor and not associated with amnesia. After a symptom-free period, usually of several minutes, visual, motor, sensory, or brain stem signs and symptoms began and usually lasted for about 15–30 minutes. These symptoms were followed by headache, often accompanied by nausea and vomiting. In 9 of the cases, subsequent head trauma resulted in migraine attacks. Four of the athletes indicated that they had spontaneous migraine episodes. However, the incidence of spontaneous episodes may be higher because of the relatively short follow-up period. The use of prophylactic, antimigrainous drugs does not seem to be warranted. The possible long-term complications of minor head trauma followed by migraine attacks are not known because this entity has only recently been recognized.

Even though migraine occurs frequently in the general population, the possibility that it exists as a significant sports medicine problem has not been established.

▶ [Migraine, as neurologically defined, has an appreciable prevalence rate of 15%–20% in the male general population and 23%–29% in the female general population. Further, roughly three fourths of persons with migraine will have the onset of their episodes between 11 and 30 years of age. That some of these attacks will follow trauma in the age group participating in athletics is not too surprising. Perhaps the greatest concern is that migraine occurring during a contact sport could readily simulate a major neurologic crisis such as intracranial bleed and represents a significant differential.—L.J.K.] ◀

3–2 **Neuralgiform Facial Pain in Motorcyclists.** L. Pöllmann reports the occurrence of bilateral neuralgiform facial pain in motorcyclists. The patients had ridden motorcycles for extended periods in cold weather (down to less than 10 C). While warming up after the ride, they experienced severe facial pain, primarily in areas innervated by the second and third branches of the trigeminal nerve. The pain was first felt about 2–4 hours after the ride and in no case was it intermittent. Several patients reported that the pain extended to the

(3–1) Am. J. Sports Med. 8:202–205, May–June 1980.
(3–2) Quintessence Int. 11:99, May 1980.

teeth. Acute symptoms subsided after 2–4 days. Conduction anesthesia without vasoconstrictor gave immediate relief. It is concluded that motorcyclists should be made aware of this potential problem so that appropriate preventive measures can be taken.

▶ [The uniqueness of the motorcycle syndrome is that it is bilateral, as opposed to unilateral trigeminal neuralgia. It is apparently quite disabling, a cold stress injury, and dependent on moderately extended exposure. Prevention should not be too difficult. However, in a population group that eschews helmets for the prevention of far more serious injury, one should not be too optimistic.—L.J.K.] ◀

3–3 **Retinal Detachment and Jogging.** It is estimated that about 22,000 retinal detachments occur in the United States annually, and middle-aged men are most commonly affected. Because of the increased interest in jogging and the possibility of an associated increase in the incidence of retinal detachment, David M. Worthen (VA Med. Center, San Diego) surveyed the membership of the United States Retina Society regarding their experience and opinions about the likelihood of this association.

Of the 112 members sent questionnaires, 92 (82%) responded. Seventy-three percent of the respondents were in retina practice exclusively and reported seeing an average of 180 retinal detachments a year. The total number of retinal detachments seen by all the respondents was 13,500. Symptoms of retinal detachment developed during jogging or running in 11 of these patients. A worsening of symptoms during jogging or running was noted in 7. None of the respondents believed that the number of retinal detachments associated with jogging or running had increased. Sixty-four percent thought there was no relationship whatsoever between jogging and retinal detachment, and 36% were unsure. However, 82% of the physicians surveyed recommended avoiding running or jogging after treatment of retinal detachment, the most common time period being 1–3 months.

It is concluded that there is no greater incidence of retinal detachment attributable to jogging or running and that jogging may be one of the safer activities for physical fitness.

▶ [Although apparently 10% of respondent ophthalmologists state that they had seen patients developing symptoms of retinal detachment while jogging or running, there appear to be only 11 such cases among 13,500 detachments. It would appear that running and jogging are not associated with a very high order of risk to the retina and that the only correlation of consequence is that if there is retinal detachment for other reasons, jogging or running generally would be contraindicated for 1 to 3 months thereafter.—L.J.K.] ◀

3–4 **The Runner's High** is discussed by Herbert Wagemaker, Jr., and Leonide Goldstein (Univ. of Louisville). Some runners experience a feeling of euphoria after running for 25–30 minutes. This could be related to the antidepressant effect of running and may be attributable to increases in norepinephrine levels. Changes in EEGs have indicated that right-left confusion, or the inability to change from right-sided image thinking to left-sided verbal thinking, is resolved by running. Subjects report that they can think more clearly, the

(3–3) Ophthalmic Surg. 11:253–255, April 1980.
(3–4) J. Sports Med. Phys. Fitness 20:227–229, June 1980.

ability to concentrate is improved, and they can verbalize better after running. It may be that the subjective changes experienced by some runners are reflected in these EEG changes.

▶ [Most articles addressing this psychologic phenomenon tend to be subjective odes to the glories of running. This article is little different, other than the author's mentioning without data and without controls the fact that right- and left-sided EEG confusion may clear in these same people. The normal spectrum of EEG changes still must be defined. Of some interest, perhaps, would be an additional study that evaluated patients with anxiety, before and after running and that discussed those same patients in terms of the use of β-blockade drugs to alleviate anxiety.—L.J.K.] ◀

3–5 **Strategies for Modifying Type A Behavior** are outlined by Margaret A. Chesney and Ray H. Rosenman (Stanford Res. Inst., Menlo Park, Calif.). The marked rise in coronary heart disease in most industrialized societies amounts to an epidemic that can no longer be attributed simply to a greater population of older persons, improved diagnostic methods, or wholly to the classic risk factors. Persons with the type A behavior pattern that has been reported to be causally associated with coronary heart disease strive to achieve in a constant struggle against others. They are work oriented and chronically hurried and exhibit enhanced aggressiveness, competitiveness, and adrenergic arousal. Early studies, though incomplete, indicate possible benefits from modifying type A behavior in preventing primary coronary heart disease and recurring morbidity. It is more often possible to modify a person's perception of environmental stressors than the environment itself. Subjects must be assured that type A behavior is not responsible for their major achievements and that alternate behaviors will not threaten their socioeconomic well-being or control of their environment.

Self-observation is a critical first step in modifying type A behavior. Patients should keep a log of incidents that arouse anger, anxiety, frustration, and time-urgency. Self-contracting is an effective means of bringing about change. Patients may, for instance, contract in writing to avoid rushing in various ways, practice deep relaxation, or exercise. Only a few changes should be proposed in each contract. The most effective way of learning a new set of behaviors is to watch a successful "model" carry out the desired behavior. Other successful persons whom the patient knows can serve as models. Relaxation methods can help reduce excessive adrenergic arousal. No means of altering hostility has been devised, but a structured group therapy format may be useful. Groups provide an opportunity for subjects to role-play and practice new behaviors, and they provide models. No negative effects of modification of type A behavior have appeared to date. Attempts to modify type A behavior may enhance understanding of the psychologic factors related to coronary heart disease risk.

▶ [After more than two decades of research, the type A behavior pattern (TABP) was granted recognition as a new coronary heart disease risk factor by a panel of experts convened by the National Heart, Lung and Blood Institute, which panel concluded: "This increased risk is over and above that imposed by age, systolic blood pressure, serum cholesterol, and smoking and appears to be of the same order of magnitude as

(3–5) Consultant, pp. 216–222, June 1980.

the relative risk associated with any of these factors." The Western Collaborative Group Study of 3,524 men concluded that the type A male has twice the rate of primary coronary heart disease and a higher rate still of recurring coronary artery disease compared with his type B cohort after adjustment for all other risk factors. The question is then, "Can we really change the leopard's spots?"

Certainly, the goal is worthy. But if we exclude the minor aspects of the diffuse energy activities of the type A person and concentrate on the basic aggression and hostility that is the makeup of the core of this personality, there is not much room and reason for optimism at this time. Damping the adrenergic arousal has great appeal, and here there is the great likelihood that exercise is effective in those who will accept this on a regular basis. If we are honest, we are going to have to grant that this may very well have a significant pharmacologic future via adrenergic blockade.—L.J.K.] ◄

3-6 **Sudden Cardiac Death.** Peter L. Frommer (Natl. Inst. of Health) states that sudden cardiac death (SCD) kills about 350,000 Americans each year. An estimated half of ischemic cardiac disease deaths occur within 1 or 2 hours of the onset of acute symptoms, including the one-third that occur essentially instantaneously or unwitnessed. Ischemic heart disease is the overwhelming cause of SCD. In 10% to 20% of persons who develop ischemic heart disease, SCD is the first manifestation. The cardiac risk factors are essentially the same as in patients with other initial manifestations, and few or no risk factors may be present. In patients with established ischemic heart disease, the severity of underlying coronary artery disease and heart disease is the chief factor in any subsequent cardiac event, including SCD. Ventricular fibrillation is the pathophysiologic mechanism most commonly associated with SCD. Persistence or appearance of ventricular ectopy late in the course of infarction is a risk factor, especially when coupled with poor ventricular performance.

For the vast majority of patients with detectable heart disease who have asymptomatic or only mildly symptomatic arrhythmias, there is no clear answer to the question of whether antiarrhythmia prophylaxis improves longevity. The few clinical trials of long-term antiarrhythmia drug administration after myocardial infarction have given negative results, and side effects are not infrequent with these agents. Some studies of β-blocking drugs have yielded completely negative results and some, equivocally positive results. Many large-scale clinical trials are in progress. Sulfinpyrazone is also being considered for use after myocardial infarction. It is important to identify trigger factors and to gain understanding of the pathophysiologic mechanisms that lead to SCD.

▶ [This summary on sudden cardiac death is timely in putting the problem in fair perspective and pointing out that much of the early enthusiasm for β-blockade, antiarrhythmic agents, and sulfinpyrazone has not reached the point where statistical validity can be granted to any concrete pragmatic regimen. It is recognized that ventricular ectopic activity is a very significant factor, provided there is coexisting cardiac disease. It is stressed that this ectopic activity, hardly uncommon in younger people, does not have the implications of sudden cardiac death if there is no underlying cardiac disease, which should be defined by extremely thorough medical testing and evaluation. This review would certainly support the position that no regimen can be recommended now as prophylaxis for sudden cardiac death syndrome other than those that relate to the general wisdom of diet, leanness, and reasonable activity.—L.J.K.] ◄

(3–6) J. Cardiovasc. Med. 5:788–790, Sept. 15, 1980.

3-7 **The Acute Cardiac Risk of Strenuous Exercise.** There is some evidence, though not conclusive, that regular vigorous exercise helps to protect against coronary heart disease. Larry W. Gibbons, Kenneth H. Cooper, Betty M. Meyer, and Curtis Ellison (Inst. for Aerobic Res., Dallas) reviewed the computer logs of amount and intensity of exercise performed by 2,935 adults (mean age, 37 years) during a 65-month period to estimate acute cardiac risk of strenuous exercise. The computer logs represented 374,798 person-hours of exercise, which included 2,726,272 km of running and walking.

During the study period, there were 2 cardiovascular complications; both subjects survived and resumed regular exercise. Based on age-specific categories, the maximum risk estimates (MRE) consistent with the upper 95% confidence limits for the data range from 0.3 to 2.7 cardiac events per 10,000 person-hours of exercise for men and 0.6 to 6.0 events per 10,000 person-hours for women. The higher MRE for women is attributable to the relatively low number of women in the study. It is calculated that if exercise were performed 3 times a week for 30 minutes per session for 52 weeks, the MRE would be .002 to .027 events per person-year for men and .005 to .05 events for women. However, actual risks are likely to be lower.

The combination of exercise and preexistent coronary disease, rather than exercise alone, appears to pose the major risk factor. Factors that may increase the risk of cardiac episodes occurring as a result of exercise are smoking, the element of competition, and lack of regularity of exercise.

▶ [This report confirms earlier evidence that the risk of a cardiac attack *during* exercise is greater than that of sitting in a chair reading a book. However, this is not an argument against exercising, because risks for the active person seem lower between exercise bouts.—R.J.S.] ◀

3-8 **Mural Left Anterior Descending Coronary Artery, Strenuous Exercise, and Sudden Death.** Azorides R. Morales, Renzo Romanelli, and Robert J. Boucek (Univ. of Miami) present the case reports of 2 ostensibly healthy men, aged 54 and 34, respectively, and one girl, aged 17, who died suddenly during or after jogging (2 cases) or swimming (1 case). Postmortem studies showed an unobstructed but mural left anterior descending artery, diminished vascularity to the posterior left ventricle and ventricular septum, and morphological evidence of patchy, ischemic necrosis of the ventricular septum in different stages of healing.

These morphological findings, coupled with reports that cyclic compression of a mural left anterior descending artery produces ischemia, strongly suggest that in selected subjects a mural left anterior descending coronary artery may be critically constricted during systole and produce myocardial ischemia and fibrosis. This intramyocardial location of the left anterior descending artery may represent a potentially lethal anatomical variant.

The incidence of mural left anterior descending artery is 27% in

(3–7)   J.A.M.A. 244:1799–1801, Oct. 17, 1980.
(3–8)   Circulation 62:230–237, August 1980.

autopsy series and 0.51%–1.6% in arteriographic series. Perhaps a mural left anterior descending artery might be suspected in young patients with angina-like pain, the ECG syndrome of septal fibrosis, and a positive exercise stress ECG response. These patients may warrant coronary arteriography and myocardial scintigraphy to document systolic compression of the left anterior descending artery and reduced perfusion of the posterior septum and left ventricle. The study should include atrial pacing and coronary sinus lactate measurements. Recognition of a mural left anterior descending artery with associated myocardial ischemia and fibrosis as a potentially lethal variant should direct attention to possible left ventricular myotomies.

▶ [There is no question that some patients die of myocardial ischemia and/or ventricular fibrillation during exercise. However, it will take a much larger series of observations than this to distinguish particular features predisposing persons to exercise-induced deaths.—R.J.S.] ◀

3–9   **Regional Distribution of Cardiac Output in Conscious Rats at Rest and During Exercise: Effects of Diltiazem.** Diltiazem hydrochloride and several other calcium-blocking agents constitute a new class of drugs that are rapidly gaining prominence as a new tool to relieve symptoms of coronary artery spasm. However, few in vivo studies of diltiazem have been conducted. Stephen F. Flaim and Robert F. Zelis (Pennsylvania State Univ.) tested the effects of intravenously administered diltiazem on cardiovascular hemodynamics in conscious rats at rest and during submaximal treadmill exercise. The effects of diltiazem on total distribution of cardiac output and regional systemic vascular resistance at rest and during exercise were also studied.

Normal, conscious male rats were studied a minimum of 3 hours after instrumentation for measurement of left ventricular and mean arterial pressures. Radioactive microspheres were used to measure regional blood flow. Control data were obtained in resting rats before intervention. Saline solution or diltiazem was infused intravenously, the latter at 6 mg/kg per hour, then 30 mg/kg per hour, and then 50 mg/kg per hour. In another study, diltiazem (30 mg/kg per hour) or saline solution was administered at identical intravenous infusion rates for 15 minutes while the rats were at rest. Data were collected during the last minute of infusion and the rats were subsequently subjected to submaximal treadmill exercise for 5 minutes.

Cardiac output generally increased during diltiazem infusion. This increase was most prominent at the highest dosage. Heart rate and stroke volume did not change significantly during drug administration, but mean arterial pressure was consistently increased by the highest dosage of diltiazem. Diltiazem reduced systemic vascular resistance; the effect was greatest with the highest dosage. Average coronary blood flow was consistently increased and average coronary vascular resistance reduced by infusion of diltiazem in a dose-respon-

(3–9) Chest 78 (Suppl.):187–192, July 1980.

sive fashion. Similar responses to diltiazem were observed in the cerebral and renal circulations. Infusion of diltiazem did not result in consistent changes in arterial pH or PCO_2, but arterial PO_2 was increased by infusion of diltiazem at the highest dosage. During exercise, infusion of both saline solution and diltiazem increased cardiac output, heart rate (slightly), and stroke volume. Infusion of saline or diltiazem had no effect on mean arterial pressure, but it did reduce systemic vascular resistance. During infusion of saline solution or diltiazem, exercise increased blood flow to the skeletal muscle, cerebral, and coronary beds, but it had little or no effect on hepatic artery or renal blood flow. There was no consistent difference in blood gas values during infusion of saline or diltiazem at rest or exercise, except that the PO_2 was consistently higher during diltiazem infusion.

Diltiazem does not produce uniform reduction in vascular resistance throughout the peripheral circulation. The effects of this agent on the peripheral circulation at rest are different from its effects during exercise. However, infusion of diltiazem results in a net reduction in systemic vascular resistance both at rest and during exercise. The redistribution of peripheral blood flow away from the cutaneous and gastrointestinal regions, which normally occurs in rats during exercise, is magnified by treatment with diltiazem.

▶ [Over the past six years, calcium antagonists have gained increasing popularity in the treatment of patients with angina. The success or otherwise of such therapy has generally been thought to depend on the relative effects in reducing coronary spasm and in reducing myocardial muscle tone; in patients with a tendency to myocardial failure, the calcium blockers may be a disaster. This article is interesting in suggesting a differential effect on the peripheral vasculature, so that during exercise there is a greater than normal redistribution of blood flow from the liver and kidneys to the muscles. Again, this is a mixed blessing. In a cool environment it will likely be an advantage, but under warm conditions it could conceivably provoke renal failure.—R.J.S.] ◀

3-10 **Molsidomine in Ergometric Tests** was studied by D. Röhl and K. H. Lehmann. The aim of this study was to prove the effect of molsidomine in coronary insufficiency and the correlation of the effect with the simultaneously measured blood plasma levels.

Nine patients (5 women and 4 men, median age 59.4 years) with stable angina pectoris were examined. In 6 patients the ECG at rest was normal. Three patients had signs of a healed myocardial infarct. All patients had lowering of the S-T segment equal to or greater than 1 mm in the exercise ECG. The cardiothoracic index was under 50% in all patients.

In a double-blind crossover study, patients received 2 mg sublingual molsidomine or placebo and, with use of the cycle ergometer, were tested for exercise tolerance after $1/2$ hour and 1 hour and then hourly up to 6 hours. In patients taking molsidomine, an increase of maximum Watt-minute product from $\bar{x} = 308.3$ ($s_{\bar{x}} = 45.4$) to $\bar{x} = 744.4$ ($s_{\bar{x}} = 138.7$) was found after 1 hour, with effectiveness over 5 hours. During molsidomine administration, S-T lowering was decreased from $\bar{x}$ 2.5 mm ($s_{\bar{x}} = 0.3$) to a minimum of $\bar{x} = 0.7$ mm ($s_{\bar{x}}$

(3–10) Dtsch. Med. Wochenschr. 105:1216–1219, Aug. 29, 1980. (Ger.)

= 0.28) during identical work load. Action on the S-T segment lasted for 3 hours.

Molsidomine decreased blood pressure and increased heart frequency without reaching statistical significance. Blood plasma levels of molsidomine correlated with the drug action with a maximum after 1 hour and a half-life of 2.03 hours. One patient complained of light pressure in the head. There were no other side effects.

The study showed that, after 2 mg sublingual molsidomine, the exercise tolerance (Watt-minute product) increased by 144% and that the ischemic S-T lowering was decreased by 71% during identical work load. These findings point to improvement of myocardial oxygen balance during exercise. From studies of other authors, it can be determined that molsidomine brings about lowering of myocardial oxygen consumption and improvement of blood supply to the subendocardial myocardium.

Molsidomine is easily tolerated. The mechanism for increased work tolerance and prophylaxis for angina pectoris in patients with coronary heart disease is similar to that of the nitro group of compounds. With sublingual application, effectiveness is noted within the first 30 minutes; it reaches a maximum in 1 hour and lasts 5 hours. Therefore a dose of 2 mg three to four times daily is recommended. Because a linear relation exists between the effect and the blood plasma level, it is assumed that an increase of the individual dose produces a stronger effect. Therefore, further study is desirable.

▶ [Exercise-induced angina is a distressing condition, and there is always interest in potential new remedies. This compound has undergone trials since 1970 and was authorized for use in West Germany in 1978. Like the nitro compounds, it acts mainly on the venous reservoirs, reducing the preloading of the left ventricle and thus myocardial oxygen consumption. The effect is said to persist for 3 hours, with a substantial gain of symptom-limited effort tolerance.—R.J.S.] ◀

3–11 **Combined Neurogenic and Vascular Claudication.** Many patients who experience pain or discomfort in the legs during exercise and find relief in rest are automatically labeled as having intermittent claudication due to peripheral vascular insufficiency. However, this condition is often imitated by the radiculopathy associated with a narrow lumbar spinal canal. J. C. De Villiers (Univ. of Cape Town) considers problems involved in differentiating the neurogenic and vascular components in such cases.

Of 102 patients treated for cauda equina compression due to narrow lumbar spinal canal of various causes, 8 (7.7%) had evidence of severe peripheral vascular disease. Seven had arteriographic evidence of severe atheromatous vascular occlusive disease; the eighth had severe peripheral vascular disease. All 8 patients with combined disease were initially thought to have vascular claudication, leading to considerable delay before the correct diagnosis was established and appropriate treatment begun.

The symptoms and signs in vascular and spinal claudication are compared in the table. Plain roentgenograms are unhelpful in differ-

(3–11) S. Afr. Med. J. 57:650–654, Apr. 19, 1980.

COMPARISON OF SYMPTOMS AND SIGNS IN VASCULAR AND SPINAL CLAUDICATION

	Vascular claudication	Cauda equina claudication
Backache	Uncommon, can occur in aorto-iliac occlusion	Common, but need not be present
Leg symptoms	Quantitatively related to effort	May be brought on by effort; directly related to posture of extension of spine
Quality	Cramp-like, tight feeling; intense fatigue; discomfort; pain may be absent	Numbness, cramp-like, burning, paraesthetic; sensation of cold or swelling; pain may be absent
Relief	Rest of affected muscle group	Rest not enough; postural alteration of spine to allow flexion is necessary in most
Onset	Simultaneous onset in all parts affected	Characteristic march up or down legs
Urinary incontinence	Does not occur	Very rare
Impotence	Common in aorto-iliac (A1) disease (failure to sustain erection)	Very rare (? failure to achieve erection)
Wasting of legs	Global in AI disease	Cauda equina distribution in severe cases
Trophic changes	May be present; absent in AI disease	Absent, but may be present in combined disease
Sensory loss	Absent	Not uncommon; common after exercise
Ankle jerks	Often absent in patients over 60	Common, particularly after exercise
Straight leg raising	Full	Often full

entiating these conditions. Calcification of the aorta is common and not necessary significant. Clinical findings and provocative testing should indicate the next line of investigation. If symptoms are predominantly of a vascular type and operation is clinically indicated, aortography is required. Myelography can reveal the typical features of canal narrowing and impingement on the cauda equina. In patients with combined disease, diagnosis is less a matter of differentiating two conditions as of evaluating the relative importance of groups of symptoms and signs so as to assign to the particular pathologic process its place as primary or secondary in the production of the patient's symptoms.

The patient with combined disease is a particular challenge to the surgeon. The patient with associated vascular disease may be at greater risk if there has been any further compression or undue manipulation of the already compressed cauda equina nerve roots at laminectomy. The patient with combined disease who undergoes the vascular operation first also needs special attention during positioning on the operating table.

▶ [Leg discomfort arising during exercise and relieved by rest is perhaps too readily diagnosed as intermittent claudication. This article provides a useful discussion of differential diagnosis, with particular reference to the possibility of cauda equina compression arising from a narrowing of the lumbar spinal canal. It is stressed that this syndrome can coexist with peripheral vascular disease, and management in such a situation is discussed.—R.J.S.] ◀

3–12 **Physical Conditioning Augments the Fibrinolytic Response to Venous Occlusion in Healthy Adults.** R. Sanders Williams, Everett E. Logue, James L. Lewis, Thomas Barton, Nancy W. Stead, Andrew G. Wallace, and Salvatore V. Pizzo (Duke Univ.) examined the effects of physical conditioning on fibrinolysis at rest and after local venous occlusion in healthy adults at risk of cardiovascular disease. Eighty-two subjects who registered for a 10-week fitness program participated in an assessment of treadmill performance and fibrinolytic activity at the start and end of the program. Complete data on fibrinolysis were available for 69 subjects. Fibrinolytic activity was measured indirectly as hydrolysis of ^{3}H-casein by plasmin generated after activation of purified human plasminogen by plasminogen activators present in the euglobulin fraction of the subject's plasma. Subjects exercised under supervision three times weekly for 10 weeks. Sessions consisted of 10 minutes of stretching exercises followed by 30 to 45 minutes of continuous walking or jogging at an exercise intensity sufficient to elevate the heart rate to 70% to 85% of the maximum achieved on each person's initial treadmill test.

The exercise program produced a distinct aerobic conditioning effect, defined as a reduction in heart rate at submaximal treadmill work loads. Significant changes in plasma fibrinolytic activity also occurred. The increment in fibrinolytic activity stimulated by venous occlusion was highly significant (Fig 3–1). The decrease in fibrinolysis was highly significant. The exercise program did not alter factor VIII procoagulant activity significantly. The augmentation in stimulated fibrinolysis after the conditioning program was greater in women than in men and greater in persons who initially had lower levels of aerobic fitness, as assessed by treadmill performance, than in persons who were initially more fit.

The data were derived from a population free from overt cardiovascular disease, but it appears that moderate physical activity can enhance the fibrinolytic response stimulated by venous occlusion, pre-

(3–12) N. Engl. J. Med. 302:987–991, May 1, 1980.

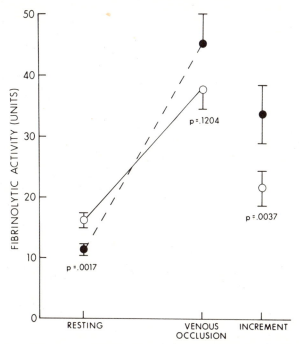

Fig 3–1.—Mean fibrinolytic activity at rest and after venous occlusion. Increment induced by venous occlusion (stimulated fibrinolysis) was measured at entry *(open circles)* and after 10 weeks of physical conditioning *(solid circles)*. Probability values refer to statistical analysis by Student's t test for paired samples (two tailed). Vertical lines represent SEM. (Courtesy of Williams, R. S., et al.: N. Engl. J. Med. 302:987–991, May 1, 1980.)

sumably through enhanced vascular endothelial release of plasminogen activators. Enhanced fibrinolysis in response to thrombotic stimuli could be an important mechanism in the beneficial effect of habitual physical activity on the risk of cardiovascular disease.

▶ [A subnormal fibrinolytic response to venous occlusion seems to be a characteristic of patients with coronary artery disease, diabetic retinopathy, and venous thromboembolism. It is encouraging to find that 10 weeks of moderate physical activity is sufficient to enhance the venous occlusion response of unfit but otherwise normal adults; the same type of experiment should now be repeated in patients with cardiovascular disease.—R.J.S.] ◀

3–13 **Exertional Heat Stroke: The Runner's Nemesis.** Lawrence E. Hart, Brian P. Egier, Arthur G. Shimizu, P. Janet Tandan, and John R. Sutton report heat stroke in an experienced runner who participated in a race conducted under extreme environmental conditions. Casualties from heat stroke are more common in novices who exceed their training efforts when racing and in well-trained competitors who strive for improved performances by suddenly increasing their pace midway through a long-distance race.

Man, 41, collapsed after 9 km of a 10-km race. He had been physically active since adolescence and had been jogging consistently for the previous 9

(3–13) Can. Med. Assoc. J. 122:1144–1150, May 24, 1980.

years. The race began when the temperature was 31.6 C, the relative humidity 80%, and the humidex 40.5 C. The patient drank 250 ml of water just before the race and 300 ml at the halfway mark. He reported no premonitory symptoms.

At admission, the patient was comatose, unresponsive to painful stimuli, and sweating profusely. The pulse rate was 180 beats per minute with regular rhythm, blood pressure was 140/90 mm Hg, and respiratory rate was 36 per minute. Serum potassium and chloride and blood glucose concentrations were elevated. Intravenous administration of Ringer's lactate was started. The patient was placed on a cooling blanket and given oxygen by mask. He required intravenous administration of diazepam to control early signs of convulsion and decerebrate posturing of one arm. After 6 hours he became conscious and had no neurologic deficit. Heat-induced acute renal failure, rhabdomyolysis, disseminated intravascular coagulation and hepatic necrosis were diagnosed. The patient underwent peritoneal dialysis on alternate days. Renal function was slow to recover. The first indication of a diuretic phase occurred 3 weeks after admission; peritoneal dialysis was then discontinued.

Body temperature invariably rises above 38 C during a marathon run, and if the runner is dehydrated the rectal temperature may rise above 40 C. The dividing line between such elevated temperatures and overt heat stroke is tenuous and may depend on personal differences in thermoregulation and the predisposition to heat stroke. Early recognition is essential for effective management of heat stroke. The cornerstones include prompt cooling, appropriate rehydration, and correction of circulatory collapse. Even under ideal circumstances of diagnosis and management, the prognosis in moderate to severe heat stroke is guarded. Atypical features, as in this case, can easily complicate the course and outcome of this potentially fatal condition. Full recovery from heat stroke is no reason for complacency, as heat intolerance in former heat stroke patients has been reported, and recurrences in susceptible persons are therefore possible.

▶ [Heat stroke is an all-too-frequent accompaniment of "fun runs" in the North American summer, and there is need for a much more effective campaign of public and medical education. It is disappointing that the present article does not direct more attention to this aspect of the reported case. Why was the race held at 1:45 P.M. in mid-June? Why was the race permitted to proceed when ambient temperatures were above the standards described in any textbook of sports medicine? A phone call to the organizers before a race is worth many hours of subsequent sophisticated medical care!—R.J.S.] ◀

3-14 **Heat Stroke: Report of 3 Fatal Cases With Emphasis on Findings in Skeletal Muscle.** R. C. Kim, George H. Collins, Chaidong Cho, Keiji Ichikawa, and Harry Givelber (SUNY, Upstate Med. Center) report 3 fatal cases of heat stroke encountered in the central New York area during 2 months. All 3 patients had a body temperature above 41 C, altered level of consciousness, hot dry skin, and one or more predisposing factors. Patient 1, a woman, aged 23, in the 39th week of pregnancy, had incessant choreiform activity which made it difficult for her to eat, drink, or sleep, and her dehydrated, hyperkinetic state led to development of heat stroke. Patients 2 and 3, men

(3–14) Arch. Pathol. Lab. Med. 104:345–349, July 1980.

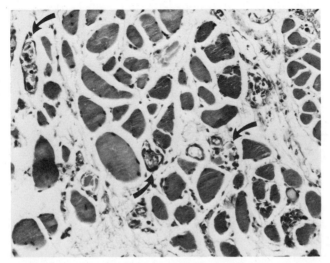

Fig 3–2.—Case 3, man, aged 79. Transverse section of muscle dissected from tissue surrounding thyroid gland, showing presence of many fibers undergoing fragmentation of sarcoplasm (e.g., *arrows*). Hematoxylin-eosin; original magnification × 152. (Courtesy of Kim, R. C., et al.: Arch. Pathol. Lab. Med. 104:345–349, July 1980; copyright 1980, American Medical Association.)

in their 70s, were dehydrated and had cardiovascular disease, but in neither case was heat stroke associated with overexertion.

In addition to laboratory and postmortem findings indicative of dysfunction of many organ systems, including acute renal failure, there was morphological evidence of widespread damage to skeletal muscle. Affected fibers showed striking swelling and irregularity of configuration with sharply defined zones of pallor or staining and loss of striations within the sarcoplasm. A number of fibers, singly and in clusters, showed either coagulative necrosis or fragmentation and disintegration of the sarcoplasm (Fig 3–2). These changes resemble those reported in cases of rhabdomyolysis associated with extreme exertion, influenza, idiopathic childhood rhabdomyolysis, idiopathic paroxysmal myoglobinuria, and malignant hyperthermia.

The mechanism by which muscle necrosis occurs is not known, but the prevailing view is that of direct thermal injury to cells.

3–15 **Physiologic Body-Cooling Unit for Treatment of Heat Stroke.** The classic treatment for heat stroke is to immerse the patient in ice water or to sponge with ice water and fan the patient. However, the rapid and extensive cutaneous vasoconstriction that occurs when the skin temperature is lowered is physiologically undesirable; the heat production of a heat stroke patient is 2–3 times greater than normal, and the shivering induced by a rapidly lowered skin temperature aggravates this effect. Also, conscious patients find ice water immersion extremely uncomfortable.

J. S. Weiner and M. Khogali (London School of Hygiene and Trop-

(3–15) Lancet 1:507–509, Mar. 8, 1980.

ical Medicine) describe a system for rapid evaporative cooling from a warm skin. Finely atomized water under pressure is sprayed over the whole body surface. The water leaves the nozzles at 15 C, but the spray is combined with warm air (45 C) blown from a height of 50 cm over the body at about 0.5 m/second^{-1}. This keeps the wet skin at about 32–33 C.

Artificial hyperpyrexia was induced in 6 volunteers, aged 24–35 years, by having them wear impermeable plastic suits and hoods while exercising on a bicycle at 1.5–2.0 kp in a room at 48 C dry bulb (db) and 30 C wet bulb (wb) until a tympanic temperature of 39.5 C was reached (about 20–25 minutes). Seven different cooling procedures were then tested in a room at a temperature of 20–22 C (db) or 17–19 C (wb): (1) The subject lay on a net suspended over a tub without any cooling treatment. (2) The subject lay on a water-filled mattress at 20 C. (3) The subject was immersed in a water bath kept at 15 C. (4) The subject lay on the suspended net, and atomized water at 15 C was sprayed continually from above and below while air at room temperature was blown over the subject to evaporate the wet surface. (5) The subject on the net was sprayed as in (4), but warm air at 35 C at the outlets which reached the subject at 25 C was used and air movement was about 0.4 m/second^{-1}. (6) The subject was treated as in (5) except the air was warmer, 40 C at the outlets and 30 C at the body surface. (7) The subject was treated as in (5) except the air was 45 C at the outlets and 32–33 C at the body surface and air movement was increased to about 0.5 m/second^{-1}.

Mean time, in minutes, to achieve a drop in core temperature of 2

Fig 3–3.—Time taken to cool from 39.5 to 37.5 C. Numerals in brackets indicate number of experiments. (Courtesy of Weiner, J. S., and Khogali, M.: Lancet 1:507–509, Mar. 8, 1980.)

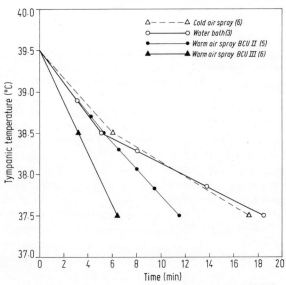

C was 33.7 for the control procedure, 19.3 for the water mattress, 18.4 for the water bath, 17.2 for cold air spray, 15.5 for warm air spray at 35 C, 11.4 for warm air spray at 40 C, and 6.5 for warm air spray at 45 C (Fig 3–3).

The warm air spray method, in which there is good air circulation and air temperature at the body surface is 30–35 C during spraying, cools hyperpyrexial patients more rapidly and comfortably than other methods. It permits efficient and hygienic administration of ancillary treatment. Preliminary clinical findings confirm its effectiveness.

3–16 **Metabolic and Respiratory Alterations of Heat Stroke.** Charles L. Sprung, Carlos J. Portocarrero (Miami, Fla.), Antoine V. Fernaine, and Peter F. Weinberg (New York) studied metabolic and respiratory variables in 12 women and 9 men, aged 20–95 years (mean, 65), admitted consecutively with heat stroke. No patient ingested alcohol before admission and only 1 had exertion-induced heat stroke. Seven patients had diabetes mellitus and 10 had psychiatric illnesses (8 of these were receiving medication known to predispose to heat stroke development). Mean rectal temperature was 41.6 C. Fourteen patients were hypotensive on admission or soon thereafter; none had septicemia.

Seven patients had metabolic acidosis (mean pH, 7.20 ± 0.04; PCO_2, 32 ± 2 mm Hg; bicarbonate level, 12 ± 1 mEq/L), 7 had combined metabolic acidosis and respiratory alkalosis (mean pH, 7.39 ± 0.01; PCO_2, 25 ± 1 mm Hg; bicarbonate level, 15 ± 1 mEq/L), 4 had respiratory alkalosis (mean pH, 7.45 ± 0.01; PCO_2, 30 ± 1 mm Hg; bicarbonate level, 20 ± 1 mEq/L), 1 had metabolic and respiratory acidosis (pH, 7.13; PCO_2, 52 mm Hg; bicarbonate level, 17 mEq/L), and 1 had respiratory acidosis (pH, 7.30; PCO_2, 56 mm Hg; bicarbonate level, 27 mEq/L). The 15 patients with metabolic acidosis had a mean pH of 7.28 ± 0.03, PCO_2 of 30 ± 2 mm Hg, bicarbonate level of 14 ± 1 mEq/L, lactate concentration of 6.5 ± 1.0 mEq/L, and an anion gap of 26 ± 4 mEq/L. Nine patients were hypocalcemic (mean calcium value, 7.8 ± 0.3 mg/dl), 5 were hypophosphatemic (mean phosphorus value, 2.0 ± 0.2 mg/dl), and 9 had rhabdomyolysis.

Of the 21 patients, 9 (43%) died, including 8 (57%) of the 14 who were hypotensive and 1 (14%) of 7 who were normotensive. Metabolic acidosis and increased admission lactate concentrations did not correlate with mortality or hypotension. The time interval between onset of symptoms and treatment did not correlate with mortality.

The predominant metabolic change in heat stroke is metabolic acidosis secondary to increased lactate content or respiratory alkalosis, or both. Hypocalcemia is common and hypophosphatemia is not infrequent. Temperature correction of arterial blood gases is important for accurate assessment of the metabolic and respiratory alterations of heat stroke. Changes in metabolic and respiratory measurements because of temperature conversions can lead to alterations in diagnostic and therapeutic decisions. Temperature correction of PO_2 may prevent

(3–16) Arch. Intern. Med. 140:665–669, May 1980.

needless intubation of patients incorrectly judged to be severely hypoxic.

Heat-induced illness should be anticipated whenever high environmental temperatures persist for more than 48 hours. Patients with predisposing factors should be told to avoid heat stress. Air conditioners or fans should be used whenever possible. Patients with prodromal symptoms of heat stroke should rapidly receive medical attention.

3–17 **Heat Injuries Among Recreational Runners.** Recommendations for preventing heat injuries in athletes are often based on studies of Olympic-caliber competitors. Richard C. Rose III, R. David Hughes, Dabney R. Yarbrough III, and Steven P. Dewees attempted to define the population at risk and make suggestions for preventing heat injuries in recreational runners, whose numbers are increasing rapidly.

Of 36 runners who required impatient or outpatient treatment at a hospital for heat stroke, heat exhaustion, or heat cramps after 4 races 8–21 km in length held on hot, humid days in Georgia or South Carolina during 1978, 27 completed questionnaires concerning life-style, health status, training, and experiences during the race. Controls were randomly selected from uninjured runners matched for age, sex, and event. The incidence of heat injuries in the 4 races was 0.2%–0.3%.

The patients were less well trained than the controls and had been jogging for an average of 22.7 months, jogged 31.2 km/week, and averaged 6.5 km on each training run; respective values for controls were 40.6 months, 49.9 km/week, and 9.5 km/run. Only half the runners in either group deliberately attempted to acclimate to heat by running in midafternoon. Most runners in both groups drank fluids within 4 hours of the start of the race but fewer than half in either group drank anything during the race. After the race 74% of the patients, but only 11% of the controls, said they felt they had run harder during the race that ever before. Fifteen patients (75% of those who believed they had run harder than ever before) cited psychologic factors as the cause. Variables such as height, weight, general health, medications taken regularly, smoking, and alcohol consumption before the race were similar in the two groups. The 14 injured patients who finished the race trained at an average velocity of 4.92 minutes/km and completed their race at an average velocity of 4.76 minutes/km. The controls averaged 5.17 minutes/km in training and 4.73 minutes/km during the races. Before the race, patients estimated velocities that were not significantly different from their training pace, whereas controls estimated velocities that were significantly faster than their training pace.

Training is important in the prevention of heat injury among recreational runners. The roles of acclimation to heat and of fluid ingestion are less clear. Races should not be held when temperatures are above 28 C. Because reward is clearly a factor in "race fever," souve-

(3–17)   South. Med. J. 73:1038–1040, August 1980.

nir T-shirts could be given to all registrants to eliminate the need to "finish at all costs."

▶ [The article by Kim et al. (3–14) earlier in this chapter discusses the pathology that may be operative in severe heat stroke, with a diffuse rhabdomyolysis common to various conditions including malignant hyperthermia and certainly febrile diseases. The article by Weiner and Khogali (3–15) presents a newer modality for therapy and the principle behind it. The practical use of this treatment remains to be documented by multiple-center testing, but it has theoretical appeal. The preceding article by Sprung et al. points out an important point for therapy, that the predominant metabolic change in heat stroke is metabolic acidosis secondary to increased lactate content and/or respiratory alkalosis in which hypocalcemia is common and hypophosphatemia is fairly common.

This article from Georgia and South Carolina, where a combination of increased heat and humidity may be operative to a greater extent than in some parts of the world, concerns the practical implications of heat injury and the population that is exposed. It is important in its reiteration that training appears to be significant in defining those who will be less prone to heat injury as a consequence of the training process. Circumstances under which a marathon or any long-distance run is permitted are again discussed and the importance of these factors is stressed. I don't think the ending comment concerning reward is too practical. I rather doubt that it will be easy to persuade people who start a prolonged run to avoid "finishing at all costs." It is likely that this personality factor is built into those who make the initial psychologic commitment.—L.J.K.] ◀

3–18 **Stress Hematuria: Athletic Pseudonephritis in Marathoners.** Stress hematuria is frequently described but poorly understood. Michel Boileau, Eugene Fuchs, John M. Barry, and Clarence V. Hodges (Univ. of Oregon) reviewed the findings in 383 marathoners, aged 14 to 54 years, who were assessed for hematuria and proteinuria after a 26-mile run. Sixty-four runners (17%) had urine specimens that contained hemoglobin after the race. Of 204 runners tested for protein, 30% had positive tests. Albumin but not myoglobin was identified; immunoglobulins were present in 88% of cases. Abnormalities reappeared after a repeat marathon in fewer than 40% of subjects tested after more than one race. No urologic abnormalities were documented in 38 runners who have been evaluated, but none of them had hematuria at the time of study. Sixteen had previously had hematuria. Of 10 male runners with postrace hematuria who were restudied after another marathon a year later, half showed hematuria again.

More athletes exhibit proteinuria than red blood cells in the urine after heavy exertion. It has been suggested that the protein leak indicates early glomerular membrane changes, and that the leak increases with progressive stress to permit the passage of red blood cells. Previous studies suggest that athletic pseudonephritis may occur in 60% to 80% of athletes after heavy exercise, but this study indicates a much lower incidence. The condition does not always reappear after subsequent heavy exertion. Most subjects with athletic pseudonephritis have no urologic symptoms. Any urinary abnormality should be proved at repeat urinalysis, and the patient should be reevaluated after 48 to 72 hours. Subjects should be questioned re-

(3–18) Urology 15:471–474, May 1980.

garding trauma, pain, other urinary symptoms, and previous renal parenchymal disease. Subjects with persistent urinary abnormalities or a suggestive history should be evaluated further.

▶ [Hematuria and proteinuria are common in athletes after heavy exercise, with hematuria in 17% and proteinuria in 30% of 383 marathon runners. The problem is how to destinguish significant organic disease from what is usually transient and benign as a condition. The authors recommend the following: (1) Prove the urinary abnormality by repeat urinalysis. (2) Reevaluate the patient and a urine specimen after a rest of 48 to 72 hours. (3) Obtain a history of any possible trauma or a history of significant acute pharyngitis. (4) Rule out a history of prior renal parenchymal disease. (5) Only then proceed to the urologic and medical workup in those patients with persistent urinary abnormality and an abnormal history.—L.J.K.] ◀

3–19 **Exercise-Induced Acute Renal Failure in an Athlete.** T. M. Bach and D. B. Clement describe an active, vigorously training athlete in whom renal failure followed two strenuous sprint races. Myoglobinuria was suspected but never proved.

Man, 24, a 400-m runner, was hospitalized with acute renal failure after a 3-day history of severe back pain, nausea, and vomiting. Three days earlier he had competed in an indoor track meet. He had been training 90 minutes per day, 5 or 6 days per week. On the morning of the races he had only a small glass of orange juice and may have entered the races in a slightly dehydrated state. He raced in the 600- and 300-m events, about 1 hour apart. After the second race he was exceptionally thirsty and drank considerable amounts of water and juice. Within an hour he began to have a sharp, knife-like pain in the low back area, followed shortly by nausea and vomiting. On admission his tongue was dry, blood pressure was 160/100 mm Hg, and pulse was 44 beats per minute. Urine production reached the lowest value 2 days after admission, 400 cc in 24 hours. Myoglobin could not be demonstrated at any time, including examination after a provocative exercise stress test undertaken 12 days after admission. The presumptive diagnosis was myoglobinuria causing acute tubular necrosis and acute renal failure secondary to exercise-induced dehydration and metabolic acidosis. Since tests for myoglobin were not done in the first 3 days of the illness, total proof of the diagnosis was impossible.

Numerous physiologic factors were present in this case that mimic predisposing factors in experimental models. A state of dehydration is probable, considering the patient's intense thirst, alcohol consumption the previous evening, and low fluid intake the day of the race. The intense arousal state associated with sprint competition would have resulted in a large sympathetic discharge before and during the race.

This case of exercise-induced acute renal failure in a well-trained athlete emphasizes the need to avoid the convergence of dehydration, acidosis, and the sympathetic discharge of competition with the possibility of rhabdomyolysis and myoglobinemia. Preventive measures include a gradually progressive training program plus adequate fluid intake before and between races.

▶ [Renal damage resulting from marathon racing under warm conditions is a problem well recognized by the sports physician. However, this is the first report of possible visceral harm from two brief, sprint-type events (300 m and 600 m). The authors sug-

(3–19) Can. Fam. Physician 26:591–595, April 1980.

gest that renal blood flow was greatly reduced by sympathetic discharge, and it may be that the discharge was perpetuated by the knowledge of a second race to be undertaken within one hour. A second unusual feature of this case was preliminary dehydration associated with overindulgence in alcohol the previous night.

It would possibly be worth testing renal function in a group of typical track competitors before and after competition.—R.J.S.] ◄

3–20 **Extracellular Hyperosmolality and Body Temperature During Physical Exercise in Dogs.** Intravenous infusions of isotonic cerebrospinal fluid containing excessive concentrations of sodium and calcium lead to body temperature increases and decreases, respectively, suggesting that sodium and calcium ions have a specific action on the thermoregulatory centers. S. Kozlowski, J. E. Greenleaf, E. Turlejska, and K. Nazar conducted exercise experiments on 8 dogs after intravenous infusions of hypertonic sodium chloride and mannitol to learn if thermoregulation during exercise could be affected by extracellular fluid hyperosmolality without alteration of the plasma Na^+ concentration. Rectal temperature responses to exercise after preexercise infusions of hypertonic sodium chloride and mannitol were compared in dogs running at moderate intensity for 60 minutes on a treadmill.

Sodium chloride infusion increased plasma Na^+ by 12 mEq/L ($P<.05$), whereas mannitol decreased plasma Na^+ by 9 mEq/L ($P<.05$). Plasma hyperosmolality was increased by 15 mOsm/kg after each infusion ($P<.05$). After both sodium chloride and mannitol infusions, rectal temperature increased by 1.9 degree C; this was 0.5 degree higher than the increase observed after noninfusion exercise ($P<.05$). Mannitol and sodium chloride infusions reduced hematocrit and plasma protein concentration, though the difference between control and infusion values was significant only for hematocrit at the beginning of exercise.

The most significant finding was that sodium- and mannitol-induced hyperosmolality caused an excessive increase in exercise-induced rectal temperature in dogs. The increase in the osmotic concentration of extracellular fluid may play a major role in the impairment of thermoregulation during exercise. An excessive increase in exercise-induced rectal temperature can be caused by extracellular hyperosmolality per se, with no increase in the sodium concentration of extracellular fluid.

► [Previous authors have not tested the possibility that the supposed effects of sodium and calcium ions on thermoregulation really arise from changes in osmotic pressure of the extracellular fluid, and thus intracellular dehydration. The results presented in this article support this hypothesis, because during exercise, rectal temperature is augmented whether plasma osmolality is increased by sodium ions or by mannitol.—R.J.S.] ◄

3–21 **Intra-Abdominal Pressure Rise During Weight Lifting as Objective Measure of Low Back Pain.** The abdominal cavity is important in providing support for the lumbar spine. Jeremy C. T. Fairbank, John Patrick O'Brien, and Peter R. Davis (Oswestry, England)

(3–20) Am. J. Physiol. 239:R180–R183, July 1980.
(3–21) Spine 5:179–184, Mar.–Apr. 1980.

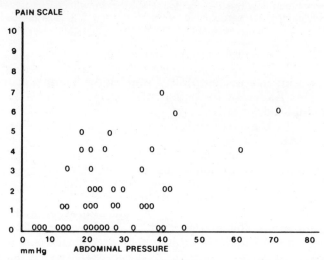

Fig 3–4.—Pressure rise in individual patients plotted against pain experienced during weight lifting. (Courtesy of Fairbank, J. C. T., et al.: Spine 5:179–184, Mar.–Apr. 1980.)

examined the relation of intra-abdominal pressure changes during weight lifting with increased pain in men with chronic, nonspecific, low back pain. None of the patients had spinal surgery or had an obvious major psychologic component. Twenty-three patients with back pain, mean age 39.1 years, and 11 controls of similar age were studied. A series of weight lifts was performed with a pressure transducer in the stomach.

The patients, who had back pain for a mean of over 7 years, all reported pain at the time of study. All but 1 had increased pain with at least 1 lift, and 3 had additional pain with all lifts. Increases in intra-abdominal pressure were greater in the patient group, and those with additional pain had greater pressure responses than the others on weight lifting. Abdominal pressure is related to pain in Figure 3–4. In patients with different pressures on both sides with lateral lifts, the pressure rise was greater on the side of pain.

Painful weight lifting is significantly related to increased intra-abdominal pressure in patients with chronic nonspecific low back pain. This maneuver may be of value both in differential diagnosis and in monitoring progress with treatment. The pressure response appears to be a reflex beyond the patient's normal conscious control. Variations in this response may be a factor in individual differences in degree of low back pain. The findings explain the high incidence of hernias noted in patients with low back pain.

▶ [An interesting set of observations is presented here that suggest that low back pain may be related to increased abdominal pressure and this in turn may be mediated via an abdominal pressure response that is a reflex function not under normal conscious control. This has considerable individual variation as it is measured. Whether this relates to the high incidence of hernia in patients with low back pain can only be conjectural at this point and was the subject of original discussion by Davis in 1959 (*Lancet*

2:155–157, 1959). These data would support the sense of having weight lifters use abdominal compression via a weight belt or binder when lifting or in the setting of low back pain itself to reduce intradiscal pressure and to reduce abdominal pressure.— L.J.K.] ◄

3–22 **Aquatic Pathogens: Sources of Disease** are discussed by Michael Rolnick, Thomas Stair, and Eric Silfen (Georgetown Univ.). Millions of persons are exposed to aquatic pathogens and microorganisms from other persons when swimming in pools, lakes, or the ocean. An inadequately chlorinated pool allows the spread of pharyngoconjunctival fever caused by adenovirus. Hepatitis virus, poliovirus, and ECHO, Coxsackie, and parainfluenza viruses also have been isolated from swimming pools and can be controlled by adequate chlorination. *Pseudomonas aeruginosa* can be found in pools, freshwater lakes and ponds, and whirlpool baths. It is the primary pathogen in "swimmer's ear." In a wound it can produce exotoxins that cause inflammation, edema, and hemorrhage. *Aeromonas hydrophila* is a freshwater bacterium that causes cellulitis. *Mycobacterium marinum,* found in both fresh and salt water, causes "swimming pool granuloma." Rashes may be caused by *Pseudomonas*. Dysentery has resulted from ingestion of *Shigella* by river swimmers. Amebas also may be ingested, causing dysentery. Sinusitis can be caused by an ameba, *Naegleria fowleri,* found in fresh water and in swimming pools.

Infections occur when the local concentration of organisms in the water is high. Rapid mixing of water by currents and a high salt concentration limit infectious epidemics in ocean swimmers, but swimming pools contain a limited volume of water that is continually recharged with flora from swimmers. Contamination can be reduced by requiring swimmers to shower and by prohibiting swimmers with respiratory infections, skin eruptions, conjunctivitis, diarrhea, etc. The reflex to urinate on entering the water is reduced by heating the pool to 75 F or more. Filtered, chlorinated, recirculated pool water is less effective in suppressing growth of organisms than water in which a certain volume is drained and replaced with fresh water by the "overflow-refill" method. A free chlorine level of 2 ppm and a pH close to 7.8 should be present for several hours.

▶ [This excellent paper is as practical as any to be found for treating that population who may present with dermatitis, enteritis, or major disease related to swimming exposure. It will make you think twice before jumping into the typical motel swimming pool; indeed, any chlorinated pool is suspect unless testing is meticulous and the value of free chlorine level is known to be above 2 ppm. The presence of *Staphylococcus* and *Pseudomonas* in the home hot tub has been well publicized and needs no further comment. The following points are worth reiteration for practical knowledge.

1. In saltwater exposure, the pathogens will be *Vibrio* species usually presenting as cellulitis, otitis, or sepsis and responsive to empiric doxycycline until culture reports are returned; or the local presence on skin of the so-called swimming pool granuloma which is due to *Mycobacterium marinum*, which may take weeks to months to clear and, if antibiotics are needed, may require drugs of the antituberculous family, such as ethambutol and rifampin.

2. Swimmer's itch secondary to the *Pseudomonas* species of the Great Lakes basin

(3–22) Consultant, p. 34, July 1980.

and the salt water of Rhode Island, Florida, and Hawaii fortunately is self-limited and may respond to topical corticosteroids or antihistamine alone.

3. Dysentery can be due to either the ingestion of *Shigella* organisms or *Entamoeba histolytica.* Increasing interest has been present in *Campylobacter,* which must also add to the differential and which should be cultured for routinely. Any enteritis deserves the full-blown workup of culture and parasite study, and it remains true that very few laboratories handle parasite evaluation well. Treatment will be so varied, depending on etiology, that it should be reserved for the precise definition of cause.

4. Progressive necrotizing frontal sinusitis should cause the appropriate concern that would warrant the exclusion of an ameba *(Naegleria fowleri).* This is not common, but may progress to fatal meningoencephalitis and, if recognized, can respond to intrathecal amphotericin. This is a freshwater and swimming pool exposure.

5. Lastly, it is clear that the ocean is a far safer place in which to swim because of the built-in protective factors of admixture by current, high saline concentration that inhibits growth of organisms other than those mentioned, and a large volume of distribution. Nevertheless, even here, and dependent on one's level of paranoia, certain preventive measures may pertain. For example, I feel strongly that scuba diving anywhere near significant human habitation or the flushing of a boat's head is a sport that is reasonably covered by γ-globulin prophylaxis to any level of exposure because of the ubiquity of the hepatitis virus, which is not inhibited by saline. This would be especially true in the Caribbean or Pacific tropics.—L.J.K.] ◄

3–23 **Sudden Drowning Syndrome.** D. S. Smith (St. Louis) reports that cold water, alcohol, and nonswimming sportsmen are the primary elements of the sudden drowning syndrome.

Wearing a personal flotation device (PFD) and rolling into a ball or fetal position and huddling with others are effective defenses against hypothermia. Swimming, treading water, bobbing in the water, and removing clothing are questionable practices in most cold water situations. Although most boating and swimming activity occurs during July and August, only 50% of drownings occur during this period. This is because the water is used mostly by fishermen, hunters, and canoeists in the fall and spring, and these sportsmen rarely tell people where they are going or when they will return. Also, most game fish are found in unpopulated areas in cold water.

Alcohol increases heat production and loss and interferes with balance. Thus, the outdoorsman who drinks is a prime target for hypothermia and a deadly plunge into cold water. As many as 52% of all water victims may be legally intoxicated at the time of death. After 3 hours of exposure to wind, sun, glare, vibration, noise, and alcohol in a normal boating situation, a boat operator becomes fatigued to the point that reaction time may double.

Drowning is usually a relatively rapid, yet almost unperceived event to incidental observers. The average drowning occurs in 20–60 seconds, with a mean of 40 seconds, after the nonswimming victim either sinks from a collapsing, air-filled plastic float, or steps, falls, or is shoved into deep water. The three nearly universal signs of drowning are involuntary rapid above-water breaststroke motions of the arms, an open but not vocalizing mouth, and a rolled-back head.

Being able to swim and feel confident and relaxed in the water is the best defense against the sudden drowning syndrome. Nonswim-

(3–23) Physician Sportsmed. 8:76–83, June 1980.

mers must wear PFDs; unfortunately, many otherwise reasonable adults refuse to admit they cannot swim and believe that PFDs are hot, uncomfortable, and not macho. Defenses against cold water involve wearing PFDs, keeping the head out of the water, and minimizing heat loss. Contrary to common belief, the last thing a person suddenly immersed in cold water should do is remove clothing, because air trapped in clothing and boots can support and insulate him if he does not struggle. A clothed person who falls into the water should roll onto his back and slowly hand scull to safety. If wearing a PFD, he should assume the fetal position.

The mammalian diving reflex permits mammals such as whales to voluntarily restrict the flow of warm oxygenated blood to the extremities and thus to remain under water for long periods. Human beings apparently have the same ability, although it is generally involuntary. In cold water drownings, the need for oxygen is reduced dramatically and blood flow is redistributed to the heart, lungs, and brain. Because a person in the diving reflex looks, feels, and acts dead, efforts to resuscitate him should continue until the internal temperature has been elevated to normal. Young persons submerged in cold water as long as an hour may be resuscitated. Middle-aged persons have survived without brain damage even after 15–20 minutes in warmer water. Properly rewarming the heart with warm, moist, oxygen inhalation-resuscitation has been increasingly successful. The primary barrier to this therapy is a belief, especially in rescue personnel, that the brain dies after 4 minutes presumably without oxygen. Another problem is that even after being successfully revived, a hypothermia victim may die within 24–48 hours from pulmonary complications. More research and better distribution of information are needed in these areas.

▶ [This review of the problem of drowning serves as no more than a general and superficial overview. It is worth reiterating the classic visual triad of the drowning person, one which is not commonly appreciated and which accounts for many drowning accidents in the country club pool, city natatorium, or otherwise supervised facility and gives very little time for recognition and lifesaving. These three signs are the involuntary rapid above-water breaststroke arm motions, the open and nonvocalizing mouth, and the rolled-back head.—L.J.K.] ◀

3-24 **Principles and Problems of Underwater Diving.** Albert B. Craig, Jr., (Univ. of Rochester) has reviewed the physics and physiology of diving, a sport which has a small margin of safety. The modern self-contained underwater breathing apparatus (scuba) includes air in pressurized tanks and a regulator to reduce the pressure from the tanks to the pressure of the water surrounding the diver. The airflow starts when the diver inhales and shuts off when he exhales. The expired gas escapes into the water and rises to the surface.

Most diving accidents are related to hydrostatic pressure. From the surface to a depth of 10 m, the water pressure doubles to two atmospheres. In both breath-holding and scuba diving, damage often results if pressure differences develop in the body. For pressure to

(3–24) Physician Sportsmed. 8:72–82, March 1980.

equalize in the inner ear sinuses, air must flow from the conducting airway into these pockets via Valsalva's maneuver or swallowing. If the pressure in the inner ear is not equalized, the pressure difference across the tympanic membrane may cause it to rupture, intracapillary pressure may cause the capillaries to rupture, or blood may seep into the inner ear to equalize the pressure and provide a good culture medium for development of ear infection. Pressure differences may also develop between the skin surface and pockets of air in the diving suit and cause petechiae that coalesce to form bruises.

Pressure differences can also develop on ascent. For breath-holding divers this seldom occurs because air flows out of the inner ear and sinuses more easily than it flows into these regions. However, if scuba divers ascend from even shallow depths while holding their breath, the pressure inside the lungs increases and an arterial air embolus may form or the lung can rupture and lead to pneumothorax. For suspected air embolism, the diver is immediately placed in a recompression chamber where the pressure is increased to a level somewhat greater than that at the bottom (to reduce bubble size) and given 100% oxygen to breathe (to speed absorption of gases from the bubble).

Both scuba and breath-holding divers are exposed to decompression illness, or "the bends." As divers descend, the partial pressure of nitrogen or helium increases and the gas is absorbed into the blood, transported, and absorbed by the tissues. The amount of gas absorbed is related to the time spent at a given depth. During ascent the gas flows in the opposite direction, but if it does not leave an area rapidly enough, a bubble will form the way bubbles form when the cover is removed from a carbonated beverage. Ascending divers must consider decompression and make stops to allow for transport of gas. For instance, a diver who has been at 100 ft for 60 minutes must stop at 20 ft for about 10 minutes and again at 10 ft for 30 minutes. If ascent is too rapid bubbles in the skin may cause itching and bubbles in joints can cause pain. Decompression illness in the pulmonary system is characterized by dyspnea, coughing, and painful breathing. Central nervous system involvement may cause bizarre symptoms such as numbness, weakness, and paralysis anywhere in the body. If central nervous system involvement is suspected, recompression should be undertaken by experienced personnel. The United States Air Force maintains 24-hour telephone advice on diving problems and the availability of recompression chambers (512/536-3278). During transport to a recompression facility, the patient should breathe 100% oxygen. If a trip must be made by unpressurized plane, the lowest feasible altitude should be chosen.

A scuba diver who runs out of air can share an air supply with a partner while going to the surface if both divers remain calm. It is also possible to make a free ascent from depths as low as 650 ft. Breath-holding divers can also run out of air and die of hypoxia because the hyperventilation which precedes breath-holding decreases the partial pressure and stores of carbon dioxide, the buildup of which is the major signal that tells a diver to surface. In the meantime, the oxygen decreases and the diver loses consciousness, makes an inspiratory gasp, and drowns.

▶ [There are very few sports, in my view, that can be as delightful and as safe as underwater diving under controlled conditions and yet have such a small margin of mechanical safety if there is equipment failure and, in particular, if there is human failure. Significant mistakes in judgment or technique are often fraught with tragedy. The practical face of this is that, in reality, far too many people are certified to do their thing before they are truly able in the setting of ocean dives and the unexpected conditions of current, temperature, adverse visibility, or equipment failure. A strong case can be made for the obligatory presence of a dive master for the first 50 to 100 hours after certification, but it is unlikely that this idea will sell in a sport where the numbers of divers certified relate to the amount of equipment sold. The comment is made in this paper that a free ascent can be made from as deep as 650 feet. Don't try it, and recognize that this presumes a submarine accident.—L.J.K.] ◀

3–25 **Dysbarism in Paradise.** Kenneth W. Kizer has analyzed the preliminary findings in 157 cases of dysbarism treated by the U.S. Navy Undersea Medical Service at Pearl Harbor from 1977 to mid-1979. This includes almost all cases occurring in Hawaii. Of the patients, 73% were civilians, 22% were active-duty military personnel, and 5% were military dependents or retirees; 94% were men or boys. Five percent of the patients were aged 10–19 years, 81% were aged 20–39, and 14% were older than age 40.

About 14% of the cases occurred in untrained persons, such as commercial fishermen and coral divers. Several patients were diving instructors who apparently felt they did not have to adhere to safe diving principles. Many sport divers who had had formal training had little knowledge of the decompression tables or of fundamental safe diving principles. Although experience should teach respect for safe diving practices, 12% of the patients had been diving less than 1 year, 27% had been diving 1–5 years, 26% had been diving 5–10 years, and 35% had been diving more than 10 years. It is estimated that more than 70% of the total case population were working divers, both commercial and military, with the largest single group being diving fishermen.

About 10% of all patients had cerebral air embolism, which usually occurred after they ran out of air at depth. Of all cases of decompression sickness, 41% were "pain-only bends"; 59% involved serious symptoms. The fact that pain-only bends reportedly constitute 70%–90% of all decompression sickness occurring in divers suggests that in Hawaii many cases of decompression sickness are not treated. More than one third of all cases and 62% of serious cases presented with lumbar spinal cord involvement: numbness, tingling, and weakness of one or both legs were the most common symptoms. Strenuous exertion at depth, believed to predispose one to decompression sickness, was reported by 32% of the patients.

One fourth of the patients reported not missing any required decompression time, but many were not truthful in their reporting because of fear of appearing naive or because they did not know their

(3–25) Hawaii Med. J. 39:109–116, May 1980.

real depth. A third of the patients missed up to one-half hour of decompression, a third missed one-half to 4 hours, and 6% missed more than 4 hours. The severity of presenting symptoms did not always correlate with the amount of missed decompression. Several fishermen who missed more than 2 hours had pain-only bends, but some of the worst neurologic cases were seen in sport divers who missed less than 10 minutes. One half of the patients noted symptoms less than 10 minutes after surfacing; 77% had symptoms within 1 hour. Time interval between symptom onset and beginning of treatment was less than 1 hour in 7% of the cases, 1–6 hours in 49%, 6–24 hours in 35%, and more than 24 hours in 9%. Much of the delay was due to reluctance of afflicted divers to seek treatment.

Recompression treatment gave complete relief of symptoms in 58% of the patients, substantial relief in 25%, and moderate or minimal relief in 17%. Because patients with paraplegia and similar neurologic damage resulting from decompression sickness do much better in the long term than those with similar neurologic injuries due to trauma or stroke, very aggressive treatment, including hyperbaric oxygen therapy in the initial stages, is indicated for these cases. Although U.S. Navy Treatment Table 5 may be used to treat pain-only bends when depth and bottom time are known, Treatment Table 6 is needed to treat those with a large decompression debt, long delay in seeking treatment, and with uncertainty about their reported diving profile.

Patients who have had an air embolism or serious decompression sickness with permanent residual damage should never dive again. In cases where all symptoms resolve after treatment, a 6-month period of no diving is recommended. A patient treated for pain-only bends should not dive for at least 4 weeks.

▶ [This nice summary of experience with the Naval hyperbaric decompression chamber at Pearl Harbor for treatment over the 2-year interval 1977–1979 includes an impressive number of cases, 157, of either decompression sickness or air embolism. It is distressing that over 85% of these accidents involved experienced people diving longer than 1 year. A high percentage, over two-thirds, involved working divers, the largest group of which were the diving fishermen. Recompression therapy is very effective and, if available, a great resource. Even when paraplegia or similar neurologic damage occurs, divers with these patterns of neurologic symptom distress and apparently the pathologic lesion do much better in the long-term than those with similar neurologic injuries due to trauma or stroke. Clearly, not enough attention is paid to the U.S. Navy decompression tables, which still stand as the general standard. As indicated in prior YEAR BOOK discussion, even these may be too liberal, as data were collected on a young and healthy age group. The author states that patients who have had air embolism or serious decompression sickness with any residua should never dive again. It is hard to argue with that position. He would contend that in cases where all symptoms resolve after treatment, a 6-month period of no-diving is recommended.—L.J.K.] ◀

3–26 **Adverse Effects of Contact Lens Wear During Decompression.** David R. Simon and Mark E. Bradley (Naval Med. Res. Inst., Bethesda, Md.) investigated the effects of corneal contact lens wear during and after exposure to hyperbaric and hypobaric conditions in 2 men, both Navy divers. The volunteers wore either soft (membrane)

(3–26) J.A.M.A. 244:1213–1214, Sept. 12, 1980.

lenses or fenestrated (0.4-mm hole in center) or nonfenestrated hard (polymethylmethacrylate) lenses while being subjected to pressures equivalent to an underwater depth of 45.5 m (150 ft) for 30 minutes and an altitude of 11,277 m (37,000 ft) for 15 minutes.

During and after decompression, the divers experienced soreness of the eyes and decreased visual acuity, and they saw halos when viewing lights when wearing nonfenestrated hard contact lenses. These effects were attributed to the formation and trapping of nitrogen bubbles in the precorneal tear film. The bubbles disappeared after 30 minutes at sea level, but nummular patches of corneal epithelial edema were apparent in the areas overlaid by the bubbles. The corneal stroma was uninvolved. During the altitude studies, only a few bubbles appeared under the hard nonfenestrated lenses and these disappeared within 10 minutes without symptoms.

It is hypothesized that the accumulation of nitrogen bubbles underneath the nonfenestrated polymethylmethacrylate lens is related to the lack of permeability of the polymer to nitrogen and to inadequate tear exchange.

▶ [Hard contact lenses are a problem for divers, apparently with corneal edema the most serious deleterious effect during decompression. Other secondary risks relate to the possibility of corneal infection if corneal epithelium is compromised and, at the symptomatic level, simple pain and transient visual impairment. The answer is straightforward. Divers should wear fenestrated hard lenses, membrane contact lenses (soft), or, preferably, as a first choice, spectacles. Although not mentioned in the article, it would seem to me that the risk of flooding a mask and losing a contact lens would add an economic incentive to leaving such lenses behind.—L.J.K.] ◀

3–27 **A Repetitive Dive Syndrome: Stress at Depth.** K. Jerome Diercks (Univ. of Texas, Austin) describes a predictable, reproducible diving stress syndrome manifest during and after the second of two standard, 25-minute dives at 30 m made 24 hours apart. Severe dorsocranial headache, nausea, and mild dyspnea occurred. The headache and nausea developed during the second dive at depth and became worse after surfacing. The nausea resolved within 10 to 15 minutes after the dive. The headache persisted for up to 6 hours. A period of nondiving preceding the first dive was necessary to elicit the stress response. The divers ascended and descended at nominal rates of 60 feet per minute. Air consumption was nominally 19 L per minute. Water temperature varied. Subjects sometimes vomited.

This syndrome was not observed when up to five dives were made daily with a maximum interexposure interval of only 5 days, but it appeared when a 3-week nondiving interval was imposed because of acclimatization to a rather intense compression-decompression regimen. The syndrome was not observed when similar dives were made subsequently. The phenomenon may be amenable to study with an animal model. It is disconcerting to divers to expect possible stress after a "safe" compression-decompression exposure.

▶ [This article describes a heretofore unreported syndrome of headache, nausea, and dyspnea associated with uneventful diving to nondecompression limits followed by a significant interval of no diving (21 days), with this particular syndrome then develop-

---

ing after repetitive diving again to nondecompression depths. A larger study group is clearly indicated to validate the repetitive pattern of symptom distress. If this is accepted as true, the next question raised would be whether decompression is, indeed, appropriate for subclinical bubble formation at what has heretofore been assumed as nondecompression-limit diving. It is important that this not be accepted as a true syndrome without additional data to exclude chance, environmental, or psychologic factors that may be relative to the isolated study.—L.J.K.] ◄

3–28 **Effects of Diving on Pregnancy.** Marthe B. Kent reports the results of a workshop held to determine the limits of safe diving for pregnant women and whether female divers are at greater risk than male divers because of physiologic changes peculiar to the female or because of oral contraception. Fife et al., in 1978, subjected pregnant sheep to simulated air dives and obtained evidence suggesting that the fetus of this animal, which has placental microcirculatory dynamics similar to those of human beings, might be at greater risk of decompression sickness than the mother. A dive considered to be safe for human beings produced air bubbles in the umbilical artery but not in the maternal jugular vein.

Little information is available on which to base a comparison of male and female susceptibility to decompression sickness. Definitive studies of susceptibility have not been made in pregnant women. Heavy exercise and stress are known to reduce uterine artery blood flow temporarily. Flow is also reduced by high partial oxygen pressures and certain drugs. Diving may produce circulatory changes similar to those seen in eclampsia. Uterine artery blood flow may be reduced by the diving reflex. The well-being of the healthy pregnant woman is probably not compromised by nonstrenuous diving to depths less than 4 atmospheres absolute. Fetal oxygen poisoning is not expected from compressed-air scuba diving. The effects of a moderately increased maternal inspired Po_2 on the fetus are unknown. Serious intrauterine hypoxia or asphyxia might have catastrophic consequences. Bolton reported an increased frequency of congenital anomalies in the offspring of women who dived while pregnant in a questionnaire survey.

Diving is not contraindicated for the normal, healthy, nonpregnant female; however, the fetus may be at greater risk than the diving mother, and no profiles have been established for diving that is definitely safe for the fetus. Until more knowledge in this area is available, it is recommended that women who are or may be pregnant not dive.

▶ [This is the major workshop on the effects of diving on pregnancy, a subject that has been debated pro and con for some years. The conclusions are clear that the pregnant woman should not dive because of the risk of pressure phenomena on the fetus. Having said that, it is rather like the conundrum of x-ray exposure in pregnancy. How do you always know when you are pregnant in the first trimester? Perhaps this interdiction should apply to those planning pregnancy as well.—L.J.K.] ◄

3–29 **Getting High: The Pathophysiology of High Altitude** is described by Charles H. Scoggin, York Miller, and Robert Tate. Many persons today are journeying to areas situated at high altitude, gen-

(3–28) Undersea Med. Soc., Bethesda, Md., 1980.
(3–29) Top. Emerg. Med. 2:53–61, October 1980.

erally defined as above 2,000 m, or 7,200 ft. The most obvious effect of high altitude on normal persons is a reduction in work capacity, i.e., more time or effort is required to achieve a given objective. A reduction in available oxygen necessitates a series of acute and chronic physiologic responses, both advantageous and disadvantageous. Initial stimulation of breathing leads to arterial hypoxemia and respiratory alkalosis. Long-time living at high altitude leads to a decreased ventilatory drive to breathe, especially in response to hypoxemia. A bicarbonated diuresis compensates for the respiratory alkalosis and coincides with improved oxygenation and decreased symptoms caused by high altitude. Pulmonary diffusion and pulmonary blood flow improve on chronic adaptation to high altitude, and the red blood cell mass increases. Heart rate also increases at high altitude, but cardiac output is unchanged; there is a fall in stroke volume.

Acute mountain sickness usually occurs within 24 hours of rapid ascent to high altitude. Retinal hemorrhage, cerebral edema, or coma may develop, although symptoms usually abate over 24–48 hours. The use of diuretics or steroids is controversial, although acetazolamide appears to improve oxygenation at high altitude. Sedative-hypnotic agents should be used cautiously in this setting. High-altitude pulmonary edema occurs both in lowland sojourners to high altitude and highland residents who return after a visit to low altitude. The best management is improved oxygenation and rapid evacuation to low altitude. There appears to be a tendency for the condition to recur in susceptible persons. Chronic mountain sickness typically occurs in highland persons, usually men, and is manifested as lethargy, headache, and a hematocrit over 60%. Pulmonary hypertension may be present. Treatment traditionally has been by periodic phlebotomy. The disorder is secondary to chronic hypoventilation and subsequent chronic hypoxia, especially during sleep. Medroxyprogesterone, a respiratory stimulant, increases oxygenation and improves symptoms.

▶ [The reader should refer to the extensive discussions on this topic in the 1980 YEAR BOOK OF SPORTS MEDICINE, pages 194–197. This paper is a general summary of the present view of the problems. The one change worthy of comment is that most knowledgeable people might now recommend that persons who become symptomatic with acute mountain sickness should now take acetazolamide (Diamox), 250 mg three times a day for 3 days prior to ascent and through a period of initial exposure. This can be very effective for the acute symptoms, including insomnia.

The authors are particularly firm in their view that sedatives and hypnotics should be used with great circumspection for insomnia because of possible depression of respiration and potentiation of hypoxemia. This principle is valid. It is a narrow line that will be tempting to cross if symptoms still persist; the drugs that might be those of choice for sedation and hypnotic effect, in my view, would be low-dose azepam drugs such as lorazepam (Ativan) in minimal dosage. Barbiturates are contraindicated, as are the stronger hypnotic drugs. I feel that lorazepam is preferable to the commonly used flurazepam (Dalmane) because of the cumulative blood levels that may occur with the latter.—L.J.K.] ◀

3–30 **High-Altitude Pulmonary Edema in Persons Without the Right Pulmonary Artery.** Peter H. Hackett, C. Edward Creagh,

(3–30) N. Engl. J. Med. 302:1070–1073, May 8, 1980.

Robert F. Grover, Benjamin Honigman, Charles S. Houston, John T. Reeves, Aris M. Sophocles, and Mechteld Van Hardenbroek have presented reports of 3 men (1 described below) and 1 woman, aged 21– 56 years, without a right pulmonary artery who had high-altitude pulmonary edema at moderate altitudes (2,000–3,000 m). These conditions are so uncommon that their association by chance is highly unlikely.

Man, 26, traveled from Wisconsin to Winter Park, Colorado (altitude, 2,750 m), and skied at altitudes of up to 3,300 m for 2 days despite increasing headache, nausea, and dyspnea. He received ampicillin and an expectorant for presumed bronchitis but became progressively more dyspneic. Four days after arrival he was found on the floor, comatose, febrile (38.8 C), cyanotic, and incontinent of urine. He was given oxygen (10 L/minute) and flown to the hospital. His condition improved rapidly on descent into Denver (altitude, 1,600 m). On admission he was lethargic, confused, ataxic, and dehydrated. Respirations were 32 per minute, blood pressure was 150/90 mm Hg, urinary specific gravity was 1.030, and rales were present over the entire left side of the chest. An arterial blood sample with the patient breathing oxygen through a nonrebreathing reservoir mask showed that the partial pressure of oxygen (Pa_{O_2}) was 45 mm Hg, partial pressure of carbon dioxide (Pa_{CO_2}) was 29 mm Hg, and pH was 7.43. Normal values during air breathing at 1,600 m are Pa_{O_2} 65–70 mm Hg, Pa_{CO_2} 34–38 mm Hg, and pH 7.38–7.42. At lumbar puncture, performed because of marked meningismus, the opening pressure was 220 mm Hg. An x-ray film of the chest (Fig 3–5) showed extensive infil-

Fig 3–5.—Admission x-ray film for skier shows infiltrates in left side of chest, small hemithorax on right, shift of mediastinum to right, and asymmetric vascular markings. (Courtesy of Hackett, P. H., et al.: N. Engl. J. Med. 302:1070–1073, May 8, 1980.)

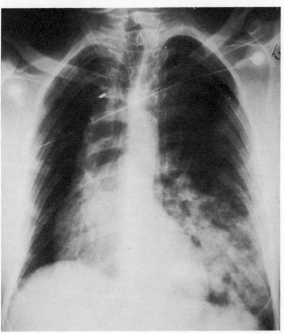

trate in the left lower lobe, no infiltrate on the right, a shift of the mediastinum to the right, and a small hemithorax and no pulmonary artery shadow on the right. On treatment with high-flow oxygen and antibiotics, the neurologic and pulmonary symptoms cleared in 3 days. Perfusion lung scans showed perfusion of the left but not the right lung. On the seventh hospital day a sample of arterial blood drawn with the patient breathing air showed Pa_{O_2} of 72 mm Hg, Pa_{CO_2} of 30 mm Hg, and pH of 7.45.

In 3 patients the time sequence of symptoms after arrival at moderate altitude, rapid resolution with descent and oxygen, x-ray films of the chest, and abnormalities in arterial blood gas all confirmed the diagnosis of high-altitude pulmonary edema. In the fourth patient, who had similar symptoms, pulmonary edema was confirmed at autopsy. Absence of the right pulmonary artery was established in 1 patient at autopsy, in 2 with pulmonary angiography, and in 1 with perfusion lung scanning. All had roentgenographic evidence that the right main pulmonary artery was absent. All had edema in the left lung, which received the entire right ventricular output, suggesting that the hemodynamic alterations of high pressure and flow in the pulmonary artery are important in the pathogenesis of high-altitude pulmonary edema.

Absence of a pulmonary artery can be diagnosed with an x-ray film of the chest. High altitude can be very hazardous for persons with this anomaly. Any severe form of high-altitude illness at only moderate altitude should raise the suspicion that there is a predisposing factor.

▶ [High-altitude pulmonary edema presenting at elevations of 3,000 m or lower should alert one to the possibility of absence of the right pulmonary artery, which certainly poses an acute threat to life in such persons even at modest altitude. Further, this article suggests that the hemodynamic alterations of high pressure and flow in the pulmonary artery are important in the pathogenesis of high-altitude pulmonary edema. In this uncommon situation, the pulmonary edema develops in the left lung, which receives the entire right ventricular output.—L.J.K.] ◀

3–31 **Intravascular Hemolysis in Acute Mountain Sickness.** The cause of acute mountain sickness is unclear. Raymond E. Lovlin, S. Rowlands, George R. Kinnear, and Eric Rast (Univ. of Calgary) report a case suggesting that red blood cell hemolysis may be contributory.

Man, 20, in excellent health and active in sports and mountaineering, climbed to 3,300 m, after 2 days at 2,500 m in Mexico, and noticed restlessness and thirst. Next day he climbed to 4,200 m and later developed headache and mild nausea. Cheyne-Stokes breathing occurred during sleep. Severe headache and anorexia ensued, with cyanosis and listlessness. The subject became difficult to arouse and reported double vision. Speech was somewhat slurred. There were no signs of pulmonary edema. Ataxia was profound during descent. Improvement was rapid on descent, and the subsequent course was uneventful except for traveller's diarrhea. Intravascular hemolysis was observed when finger-prick samples were obtained as part of a study of the effects of exercise on the red blood cells.

This subject exhibited most symptoms and signs of acute mountain

(3–31) Aviat. Space Environ. Med. 51:271–272, 1980.

sickness. It is hoped that others will seek evidence of hemolysis in subjects with acute mountain sickness. The authors have also documented headache, nausea, and hemoglobinemia in a young man subjected to a simulated altitude of 4,200 m in a hypobaric chamber for 48 hours.

▶ [The complication of intravascular hemolysis in acute mountain sickness has not been reported previously, to my knowledge. In experiments in the rat, this hematologic abnormality has been shown with exposure to high altitude, but only for extended intervals (10 to 40 days). This would be something to consider in the differential diagnosis of acute mountain sickness that proved refractory or uncommonly severe. It would be appropriate in this patient to question a possible relationship of the disorder to Darvon and barbiturates, which were taken during the climb, and possibly to administration of other drugs not reported during the Mexican experience. The workings of chance and idiosyncratic disease expression are operative in mountaineers as well as the ordinary patient.—L.J.K.] ◀

3–32 **Treatment of Accidental Hypothermia: Prospective Clinical Study.** Accidental hypothermia to below a central temperature of 35 C may occur with exposure of otherwise healthy persons to cold or wet conditions, or in the very young or elderly, or in the general population from drugs and alcohol. I. McA. Ledingham and J. G. Mone (Glasgow) carried out a prospective, 15-year study of patients in an urban environment with accidental hypothermia. A total of 44 cases were seen between 1963 and 1978. Most patients were rewarmed with use of a radiant heat cradle over the torso. Two patients had thoracotomy and mediastinal irrigation with warmed fluids. Warmed intravenous fluids and oxygen also were used. Patients were followed for a month after the episode of hypothermia. Another 89 hypothermic patients were treated by less aggressive measures during this period, and 77 cases were available for analysis.

Mean age of the study group was 44 years. Most patients had a lowest core temperature below 32.3 C. Poisoning was the precipitating factor in 25 cases, with drugs in 18. Nineteen patients had various illnesses. No consistent relation was found between blood pressure and temperature, and heart rates were not as low as might have been expected. About 40% of patients had obvious respiratory impairment; 9 were apneic. Hemoconcentration, thrombocytopenia, and leukocytosis were common. Rewarming was achieved at a mean rate of 1.13 degrees C per hour; mean duration of rewarming was 8 hours. Twenty-one patients had intermittent positive-pressure ventilation with warmed, humidified gas. One third of patients had a systolic pressure below 70 mm Hg during rewarming, and 7 received drugs. Mortality was 27%; only 2 patients died during rewarming. Nonsurvivors were older than the survivors, but no significant difference in admission temperature was found. Mortality in the retrospective series was 60%. Mortality was 32% in 19 patients who were hypothermic as a result of drug or alcohol abuse.

More aggressive management of accidental hypothermia, including rewarming, results in a shorter period of close monitoring and more

(3–32) Br. Med. J. 280:1102–1105, Apr. 6, 1980.

rapid diagnosis of the underlying condition. Few patients in this prospective series died of factors related to hypothermia. Many in the retrospective group died while they were still hypothermic and before a definite diagnosis was made.

3–33 **Accidental Hypothermia Treated Without Mortality.** Even though slow rewarming after accidental hypothermia ends in death for 45%–100% of patients revived in this manner, rapid rewarming for resuscitation has been slow to gain acceptance because of early failures and the shock and vascular collapse attributed to it. David H. Frank (Univ. of California, San Diego) and Martin C. Robson (Univ. of Chicago) conducted a prospective study of 10 patients with accidental hypothermia treated by rapid rewarming in a Hubbard tank and aggressive fluid resuscitation. All the patients had rectal temperatures below 34 C (mean, 30.4 C). When the core temperature reached 37 C, the patient was transferred to the intensive care section of the burn unit and monitored for 24–48 hours. Seven patients had a significant, concurrent medical problem that was treated as necessary.

All the patients survived. Sodium bicarbonate was required in each case, even though only 1 patient was severely acidotic at admission. All patients had elevated levels of serum creatine phosphokinase. Rapid infusion of Ringer's lactate was required by most to establish and maintain normal blood pressure. Four patients were hypoglycemic at admission. Frostbite that required additional treatment was present in 5 patients. Concomitant medical problems that were treated included alcoholism, stroke, myxedema, tuberculosis, and paraplegia.

It is concluded that the victim of accidental hypothermia is best treated by returning the metabolism to a normal temperature as rapidly as possible while controlling fluid volume and acidosis.

3–34 **Accidental Hypothermia: Management Approach.** There is much controversy regarding the best management of victims of accidental hypothermia. William J. Mills, Jr., reviewed 50 Alaskan cases. Many patients had temperature recordings of 34.9 C because low-reading core temperature thermometers were lacking at many hospitals. The patients were warmed by several methods. There were 4 deaths. Most patients were dehydrated, had mild to severe acidosis, and showed evidence of hyperkalemia during or after warming. Cerebration was present at much lower temperatures than was previously thought to be likely. More time was available for patient care when slower, spontaneous warming methods were used, and less was available when rapid rewarming methods were used. Patients with freezing injury appeared to obtain better extremity results when rapid warming and thawing methods were used.

Accidental hypothermia is characterized by decreasing function of metabolic systems, dehydration, loss of caloric reserve, enzyme system dysfunction, and tissue hypoxia. Metabolic acidosis, renal dys-

(3–33) Surg. Gynecol. Obstet. 151:379–381, September 1980.
(3–34) Alaska Med. 22:9–11, Jan.–Feb., 1980.

function, and increasing loss of neuroregulation are other problems. The core temperature should be elevated in a controlled manner. Fluid-electrolyte imbalance should be corrected, as should dehydration and acid-base imbalance, and renal function should be restored. Correction of hypovolemia with glucose-water or physiologic saline solution is important. Warming may be spontaneous or may employ such methods as rapid external rewarming, peritoneal dialysis, extracorporeal circulation, use of warm inspired air, or thoracotomy with lavage. Inhalation of warm, moist air helps prevent a further drop in core temperature. A planned approach is essential. Rewarming should be done only with total patient control.

▶ [There is considerable controversy regarding the best management of accidental hypothermia, with the main argument centering about the rapidity of rewarming as well as the given technique. Frank and Robson, in the preceding article, are firm in their view that rapid rewarming is the treatment of choice and that slow rewarming has a significant risk. On the other hand, this article by Mills and supplemental writings make a strong case for control of the environment of the patient as soon as retrieval is accomplished and then warming by any method that is familiar and effective, which includes spontaneous slow rewarming or rapid mechanical rewarming. His points seem well taken, as 14 patients had warming more or less slowly and 17 had rapid rewarming, including 10 with associated severe frostbite. The significant point is that these simple methods are available in even the smallest of our outlying hospitals.

The argument that a minimum of cardiologic resuscitative measures be undertaken is also impressive, as it recognizes that the cold heart is not responsive to defibrillation procedures and electroshock and this is a very different situation than the true cardiac arrest of normothermia. Cardiopulmonary resuscitation in this situation is indicated, therefore, only with the totally unresponsive patient with no signs of life; defibrillation is not advised at a temperature below 85 F. The Mills' data are hard to dispute.— L.J.K.] ◀

3–35 **Early Sympathetic Blockade for Frostbite: Is It of Value?** The concept of altering the natural course of frostbite injury by regulating the circulatory state during or just after rewarming evolved during World War II and the Korean conflict. David L. Bouwman, Sydelle Morrison, Charles E. Lucas, and Anna M. Ledgerwood (Wayne State Univ.) attempted to determine whether sympathetic blockade, implemented acutely after exposure, improves healing of frostbite injury. Sixty male and 6 female patients with an average age of 34 years were seen with frostbite during 1976–1978. Alcoholic inebriation was a factor in 50 patients. None had isolated first-degree frostbite. Thirty-three had second-degree frostbite at admission, and 33 had estimated deep injury from which tissue loss was anticipated. Twenty-two of the latter patients were seen within 48 hours after injury. Four patients seen during 1976–1977 received dextran intravenously, but this practice was later discontinued. Of 18 patients with bilaterally symmetric injuries, 3 had operative sympathectomy within 20 hours of admission and 15 received ipsilateral intra-arterial infusion of 0.25–0.50 mg of reserpine within 1 hour of admission and were operated on after an average of 3 days. Eight patients had lumbar and 10 had dorsal sympathectomy.

All patients with second-degree frostbite responded to local care;

(3–35) J. Trauma 20:744–749, September 1980.

none had late tissue loss. All those admitted with late deep frostbite underwent late debridement and had tissue loss. Six patients with recent deep frostbite had third-degree skin losses with small wounds that healed primarily. Nine required amputation; 3 had more subtle tissue loss. Unilateral dorsal sympathectomy did not appear to influence tissue loss, and lumbar sympathectomy did not lead to early improvement on the side operated on. No patient requested contralateral sympathectomy.

The theoretical advantages of sympathetic denervation require empirical confirmation in controlled clinical studies. The present results showed both early operative sympathectomy and intra-arterial reserpine infusion with later operative sympathectomy to be ineffective in limiting tissue loss after acute frostbite injury. Contrasting findings have, however, been reported. Sympathectomy does appear to provide protection against subsequent cold exposure, and this may be important in persons who are exposed occupationally, such as professional skiers with cold sensitivity.

▶ [There is still a school of thought that advocates sympathectomy in acute frostbite, but this is becoming the minority view. This study lends strong evidence for the lack of benefit from sympathectomy even when achieved early with intra-arterially administered reserpine. The possible benefit of late protection against subsequent cold injury would not seem sufficient argument to carry out this surgical blockade other than in extreme occupational exposure.—L.J.K.] ◀

3–36 **Controlled Trial of Supervised Exercise Training in Chronic Bronchitis.** Simple unsupervised exercise produces small but significant improvements in the 12-minute walking distance in patients with severe chronic bronchitis. D. J. M. Sinclair and C. G. Ingram hypothesized that a supervised training program would produce greater improvement in such patients.

After recovering from an acute exacerbation of chronic bronchitis, 33 patients, aged 46–83 years (mean, about 65 years), performed a daily 12-minute walking distance test and stair-climbing exercise (stepping up and down on two 24-cm steps for 1.5–2 minutes twice daily) supervised by a nurse. After hospital discharge, 17 patients who lived near the hospital continued these exercises at home and were seen weekly by the nurse. The exercise schedule was increased when possible. The 16 patients who lived outside the city did not continue with daily exercise and were not reviewed by the nurse. Patients were assessed at 6 and at 10–12 months.

Apart from a significant improvement in mean forced vital capacity in the exercise group, ventilatory function, lung volumes, and diffusion were unchanged at the 6-month and final assessments. Right quadriceps strength was reduced in controls. There was no change in thigh circumference, body weight, minute ventilation, or heart rate in either group. There was a highly significant improvement in mean 12-minute walking distance at 6 and at 10–12 months in the exercise group; all patients improved, the range being 12.3%–83% (mean, 23.4%) at the final assessment. The number of steps fell significantly,

(3–36) Br. Med. J. 1:519–521, Feb. 23, 1980.

indicating an increase in length of stride. The improvement was gradual, reaching a maximum at 8 months. There was no significant change in the control group. Electrocardiograms showed no change over the study period. Chest radiographs showed emphysematous changes in 11 patients in each group. Dyspnea, general well-being, and daily activity were significantly improved in the exercise group.

In patients with severe airway obstruction and emphysema, daily physical exercise improves exercise capacity, well-being, and ability to perform daily tasks. These improvements do not depend on changes in pulmonary or cardiac function or muscle power. They probably depend on the patients becoming more tolerant of dyspnea and adapting to their physical incapacity. With motivation and perseverence, surprising improvement can be expected even in the severely disabled.

▶ [In 33 patients with severe chronic bronchitis, the controlled exercise group showed a 24% maximal increase after the relatively prolonged period of 8 to 12 months and the control group did not improve. These are impressive data. What is of interest is that this did not relate to change in ventilation, heart rate, or muscle strength. Nonspecific factors of conditioning may be implicated, and possibly the increase in forced vital capacity relates to reduced air trapping. However elusive the precise physiology, the benefits noted seem so clear and the type of program so amenable to home supervision that it is to be strongly recommended at this time as a therapy. While the discontinuance of smoking would be desirable, of course, this was excluded as a factor of significance in this study, as were factors of antibiotic use.—L.J.K.] ◀

3-37 **Exercise-Induced Asthma** is discussed by Harvey Gerhard and E. Neil Schachter. Exercise-induced asthma may occur in patients with mild or severe asthma, as well as in those who have had no

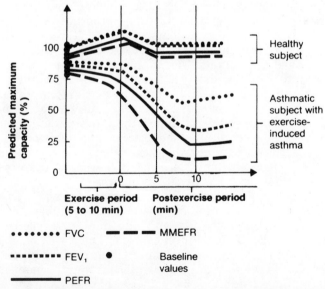

Fig 3-6.—Typical spirometric measurements after exercise in healthy person and in patient with exercise-induced asthma. *FVC*, forced vital capacity; *FEV₁*, forced expiratory volume in 1 second; *PEFR*, peak expiratory flow rate; *MMEFR*, midmaximal expiratory flow rate. (Courtesy of Gerhard, H., and Schacter, E. N.: Postgrad. Med. 67:91–102, March 1980.)

(3-37) Postgrad. Med. 67:91–102, March 1980.

PHARMACOLOGIC AGENTS IN TREATMENT OF EXERCISE-INDUCED ASTHMA

Drug	Effectiveness	Comment
Theophylline	+	Attack may occur despite adequate blood level. Can be used prophylactically
Beta-agonists (eg, isoproterenol, metaproterenol, terbutaline)	+	Act rapidly. May be used prophylactically and following onset of attack
Cromolyn sodium	+	Useful only prophylactically. Additional dose may be taken prior to exercise.
Anticholinergic agents (atropine, ipratropium bromide*)	±	Not currently approved for use in asthma but may be effective in some patients.
Corticosteroids	–	Generally not effective by either oral or inhaled route

*Not commercially available in the United States.

symptoms for years. The condition may also develop in persons not having a clinical history of asthma. In some individuals these episodes may be severe. Children and adolescents are most likely to experience exercise-induced asthma because of their greater activity levels. The typical pattern of obstruction in susceptible persons is shown in Figure 3–6. The attack becomes increasingly severe with continued exertion. The stimulus that initiates exercise-induced asthma is not well defined, but many workers believe that it is related to exchange of heat and water across the airways. All asthmatic patients are thought to become bronchospastic when subjected to vigorous exercise. Treadmill testing appears to precipitate bronchospasm more reliably than does cycle ergometer testing.

Drugs used to treat exercise-induced asthma are listed in the table. Theophylline preparations have an important role, but these drugs may not assure control of the condition despite strict adherence to a prescribed asthmatic regimen. Certain drugs, e.g., β-adrenergic agents, may be of great value in inhibiting exercise-induced asthma, and cromolyn sodium is useful in the treatment of exercise-induced attacks. Anticholinergic agents are not recommended for the treatment of asthma at present. Steroids provide little benefit in the management of exercise-induced asthma. Any regimen must be individualized, because exercise tolerance varies greatly among susceptible persons. A warm-up period before undertaking athletic activity may be of particular value to those susceptible to exercise-induced asthma. Athletic activities differ widely in their potential for inducing asthma. If a patient has persistent problems with a particular sport, the physician may recommend alternatives that are less likely to initiate an attack, e.g., baseball or golf, which require only intermittent brief bursts, rather than prolonged periods, of activity. Swimming is the optimal exercise, presumably because the warm, moist air at the water surface prevents bronchospasm.

▶ [This is a sound background article identifying the dimensions of the problem. It is pointed out that exercise-induced asthma may be relatively independent of the ordinary mild or severe expression of the disease and that it may occur in patients who have been symptom free for many years. It is also seen in patients who have no history of prior asthma. Many agents have been found effective and they are appropriately listed in the table. What the table does not include and what is important to recognize in terms of its addition to the therapeutic armamentarium is the now approved British drug albuterol (Ventolin), a very effective antasthmatic on a twice-daily basis that may reasonably be expected to be beneficial in this situation. Those data are not yet available. I should also disagree with the comment in the table that corticosteroids are generally ineffective, either oral or inhaled, in the sense that Vanceril (beclomethasone dipropionate) may have very significant beneficial effect in a given person.—L.J.K.] ◄

3–38   **Oral and Inhaled Salbutamol in Prevention of Exercise-Induced Bronchospasm.** Paul W. J. Francis, Inese R. B. Krastins, and Henry Levison (Hosp. for Sick Children, Toronto) compared the effectiveness of oral salbutamol (0.15 mg/kg body weight) and salbutamol aerosol (0.2 mg total dose) in promoting bronchodilation and in preventing exercise-induced bronchospasm (EIB) in a single-blind crossover study of 16 asthmatic children. The subjects were exercised 40 minutes after administration of the aerosol and 120 minutes after taking the oral preparation. Pulmonary function was assessed by measurement of peak expiratory flow (PEF), forced vital capacity (FVC), forced expiratory volume in 1 second (FEV_1), forced expiratory flow during the middle half of the FBC ($FEF_{25\%-75\%}$), and maximum expiratory flow after 75% of the FVC had been expired (V_{25}).

Based on changes in all parameters of pulmonary function, oral salbutamol and salbutamol aerosol were equally effective in promoting bronchodilation. Changes in PEF and FEV_1 indicated that both forms of treatment were equally effective in preventing EIB after treadmill exercising. However, based on postexercise changes in $FEF_{25\%-75\%}$ and V_{25}, the aerosol was slightly, but significantly ($P < .01$), more effective than oral salbutamol in preventing EIB. Oral salbutamol was clinically effective in preventing EIB for 4.9 hours with respect to changes in FEV_1 and for 5.8 hours as reflected by changes in PEF.

The results show that salbutamol aerosol has a faster onset of action and fewer side effects and offers greater protection against EIB in asthmatic patients. However, oral salbutamol is a useful substitute for patients who are unable to use a metered aerosol.

► [The greater effectiveness and fewer side effects of salbutamol aerosol compared to oral salbutamol are not particularly surprising. However, the fact that the oral preparation works so well is encouraging news for those who cannot administer an aerosol correctly.—R.J.S.] ◄

3–39   **Effects of Cromolyn Sodium on Airway Response to Hyperpnea and Cold Air in Asthma.** Pretreatment with cromolyn sodium can reduce the severity of airway obstruction after physical exertion in asthmatics in the laboratory, but it is not clear whether the effect is obtained in severe ambient conditions, e.g., outdoor winter sports. Cromolyn has a marked affinity for water and can freely exchange it as a function of the relative humidity of its surroundings. Frank J. Breslin, E. R. McFadden, Jr., and R. H. Ingram, Jr. (Boston) exposed

(3–38)   Pediatrics 66:103–108, July 1980.
(3–39)   Am. Rev. Respir. Dis. 122:11–16, July 1980.

8 asymptomatic asthmatic patients to cold air during exercise-induced hyperpnea, with and without cromolyn pretreatment. The 4 men and 4 women had a mean age of 26.3 years. Drugs were withheld for at least 12 hours before study. Subfreezing air was breathed from a heat exchanger as the patients hyperventilated. On study days, 40 mg of cromolyn sodium was inhaled into the lungs or sprayed into the oropharynx.

Hyperventilation of cold air resulted in marked changes in lung function, including a 45% reduction in forced expiratory volume in 1 second and a 54% fall in specific conductance. Cromolyn pretreatment significantly modified this response without affecting prechallenge lung function. The drug was much less effective when placed in the mouth than when inhaled into the lungs. Respiratory heat loss and the retrotracheal esophageal temperature were unchanged by inhaled cromolyn during eucapnic hyperpnea.

Pretreatment with cromolyn sodium is as effective in blunting the bronchoconstrictor response to simulated exercise in winter conditions as it is in reducing the obstructive consequences of physical exertion in more temperate environments. Cromolyn may act as a heat exchanger in series with the mucosa, augmenting its ability to provide water on inspiration and recover it on expiration. In contrast, atropine, presumably through its ability to limit the availability of mucosal surface water, can interfere with heat exchange within the airways and increase heat loss.

▶ [This study demonstrated that pretreatment with cromolyn was as efficient in blunting bronchoconstrictor response to simulated exercise in frigid conditions as it was in diminishing the obstructive consequences of such exertion in a more temperate environment. Unlike anticholinergic agents, cromolyn therefore remains an effective form of therapy for exercise-induced asthma even with the additional factor of severe thermal burdens being placed on the airways. The effect seems clear. The mode of action remains for precise definition, with the hypotheses including mass cell membrane stabilization and some form of direct action on smooth muscle mediated by cyclic adenosine monophosphate or phosphodiesterase inhibition.—L.J.K.] ◀

3–40 **Breathing Dry or Humid Air and Exercise-Induced Asthma During Swimming.** Omri Inbar, Raffy Dotan, Ronald A. Dlin, Ittai Neuman, and Oded Bar-Or hypothesized that the humidity of the air breathed by the swimmer could be an important, uninvestigated factor in explaining the protective effect of swimming against exercise-induced asthma (EIA). Twenty-two children, aged 9 to 15 years, whose symptoms met the American Thoracic Society definition of asthma, were studied. Each came twice, a week apart, to an outdoor swimming pool and performed a tethered swimming test. The protocols of the two sessions were identical, except that in one the relative humidity (RH) of inspired air was 80% to 90% (humid) and in the other, 25% to 35% (dry).

Although a trend toward lower values for pulmonary function was apparent in the dry swimming condition, none of the differences between the dry and humid swimming conditions was statistically sig-

(3–40) Eur. J. Appl. Physiol. 44:43–50, June 1980.

nificant. None of the pulmonary functions measured 5 and 10 minutes after either condition was reduced by more than 12% at either of the postexercise stages. Forced vital capacity, 1-second forced expiratory volume, and maximal breathing capacity were reduced by less than 7%, a reduction well within the exercise response of healthy persons. None of the differences was significant.

Air dried to 25% to 35% RH did not induce bronchoconstriction in the swimming asthmatic. It may be argued that the intensity and duration of the swimming task were insufficient to provoke EIA. However, running at similar metabolic and ventilatory rates and in comparable air dryness levels did produce bronchoconstriction in the same children.

▶ [Subjects with exercise-induced bronchospasm find swimming is one form of physical activity that they can undertake, and this is usually attributed to the relatively moist air found in the pool environment. The present report apparently casts some doubt on this hypothesis. The humidity used for treadmill running was established in a climatic chamber and is thus above suspicion. For swimming, there was dry air stored in a Douglas bag, with wet and dry bulb temperature readings just proximal to the mouthpiece. The authors suggest several other hypotheses to explain why dry air may have less effect in the pool: Because heat is lost into the water, the temperature gradient between inspired air and the respiratory tract is lessened, reducing cooling of the airway. Alternatively, an increase of central blood volume may help to maintain airway temperature. Finally, hydrostatic pressure may facilitate the expiratory phase of ventilation.—R.J.S.] ◀

3–41 **Reassessment of Effects of Oropharyngeal Anesthesia in Exercise-Induced Asthma.** The critical variables initiating an obstructive response to exercise in asthmatics are the temperature and water content of the inspired air and the amount of ventilation achieved. The role of cholinergic efferent activity in the postexertional bronchial obstructive response is unclear. An afferent pathway involving "irritant-like" receptors in the oropharynx has been proposed. Christopher H. Fanta, R. H. Ingram, Jr., and E. R. McFadden, Jr. (Boston), with the technical assistance of David Stearns and Diane Saunders, assessed the potential role of oropharyngeal receptors under conditions of constant inspired air temperature, water content, and minute ventilation in 10 atopic patients with asthma, all of whom were asymptomatic at the time of study. Airway resistance and thoracic gas volume were measured by plethysmography. The oropharynx was sprayed with either 2% lidocaine hydrochloride or water, 5–10 times, to deliver 1–1.5 ml.

Neither lidocaine nor water produced significant changes in pulmonary mechanics (Fig 3–7). No significant differences were found between the effects of lidocaine and water in hyperventilation studies in which the minute ventilation averaged 88 L/minute with water and 89 L/minute with lidocaine. Eucapnic hyperventilation was followed by a significant reduction in pulmonary mechanics with both lidocaine and water nebulization.

Pharyngeal anesthesia did not alter bronchoconstrictor consequences of a hyperventilatory stimulus in asthmatics in this study in

(3–41) Am. Rev. Respir. Dis. 122:381–386, September 1980.

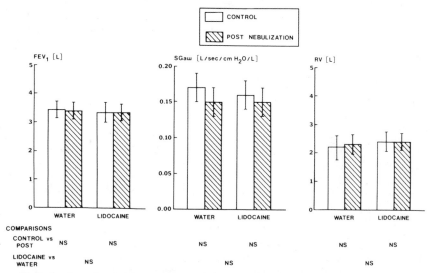

Fig 3–7.—Lung function before and after spraying the oropharynx. Heights of bars represent mean values; brackets indicate 1 standard error. The first set of bars in each graph shows the effects of water and the second, the effects of lidocaine. *FEV*₁, forced expiratory volume in 1 second; *SGaw,* specific conductance; *RV,* residual volume; NS, not significant. (Courtesy of Fanta, C. H., et al.: Am. Rev. Respir. Dis. 122:381–386, September 1980.)

which the variables that influence the obstructive response to airway cooling were precisely controlled. The findings do not support the existence of "irritant-like" receptors as essential elements in the pathogenetic results of airway cooling in the posterior pharynx. Thermally activated reflexes do exist in both normal persons and patients with obstructive airways disease, but their effects should not be confused with the thermal events that occur with hyperpnea.

▶ [Oropharyngeal anesthesia could be expected to block "irritant-like" receptors in the posterior pharynx, if present. Such receptors are excluded as etiologic factors. The syndrome of exercise-induced asthma remains real.—L.J.K.] ◀

3–42 **Life-Threatening Cold and Exercise-Induced Asthma Potentiated by Administration of Propranolol.** β-Adrenergic blockers may precipitate severe bronchospasm in patients with asthma, but they are considered safe in patients with chronic obstructive pulmonary disease without a history of reversible airway obstruction. Susan Schwartz, Scott Davies, and John A. Juers present reports of 2 patients without previously recognized bronchospastic disease and in whom acute life-threatening respiratory failure was provoked by exercise in extremely cold air. Both were receiving propranolol for hypertension.

CASE 1.—Man, 63, who smoked and had been taking 40 mg of propranolol 3 times a day for 5 months because of essential hypertension, became acutely dyspneic while walking briskly uphill on a cold (−20 C) day. On admission to St. Paul-Ramsey Medical Center, he was conscious but too short of breath

(3–42) Chest 78:100–101, July 1980.

of speak. Respiratory rate was 40, pulse was 96, and blood pressure was 220/110 mm Hg. He was cyanotic and diaphoretic. No breath sounds could be heard. He responded quickly to therapy with intravenous aminophylline and oxygen. He had no history of asthma but in retrospect did recognize a gradual increase in dyspnea on exertion during the time he was receiving propranolol. Pulmonary function tests after cessation of propranolol showed moderate airway obstruction with no response to bronchodilators. He has had no further episodes of dyspnea in the 6 months of follow-up.

CASE 2.—Man, 47, who had done strenuous work in a meat cooler (4 C) for several years and had been taking 40 mg of propranolol twice a day for 3 months because of essential hypertension, became acutely dyspneic while at work. On admission, respiration rate was 48, pulse rate was 96, and blood pressure was 164/96 mm Hg. He was cyanotic and had markedly decreased breath sounds. He improved rapidly with administration of oxygen and intravenous aminophylline. Spirometry after cessation of propranolol showed mild airway obstruction with modest bronchodilator response. The patient had stopped smoking 5 years earlier but continued to have a chronic cough. In retrospect, he was aware of other self-limited episodes of dyspnea provoked by working in the cold during the time he was receiving propranolol. He had had no episodes of shortness of breath prior to taking propranolol. After cessation of propranolol he exercised maximally on a treadmill without development of bronchospasm. He returned to work in the meat cooler and has been well for 6 months.

Patients with chronic bronchitis who are started on propranolol should be asked specifically whether they are having episodes of shortness of breath precipitated by exercise. If so, the drug should be stopped.

▶ [β-Adrenergic blockers are widely used now in the therapy of hypertension and angina pectoris. Most people respect the history of asthma, if present, as a relative contraindication. Chronic obstructive pulmonary disease without a history of asthma has not been considered a contraindication to the use of these agents. This study documents life-threatening asthma induced by exercise and cold in the clinical setting of propranolol use. It is of clear importance that the risks of exercise exposure, cold exposure, and, in particular, the combination be discussed as potential hazards in any patient in whom this family of drugs is used.—L.J.K.] ◀

3–43   **Bronchospasms Induced by Acetylcholine and by Free Running Exercise: Comparison in 50 Asthmatic Children.** P. Rufin, M. R. Benoist, R. Jean, P. Scheinmann, and J. Paupe (Paris) tested 50 asthmatic children for cholinergic bronchial sensitivity and occurrence of bronchospasm; 92% of them showed hypersensitivity to acetylcholine challenge, and exercise-induced bronchospasm occurred in 80%. On pooling, 98% had a positive response to at least one of the tests. The incidence of positive responses with the 2 tests showed the superiority of the acetylcholine test. Moreover, in 3 of 4 subjects with a negative response to the test of bronchial cholinergic sensitivity, bronchospasm was induced by exercise.

On the whole, there was a qualitative correlation between exercise-induced bronchospasm and bronchial sensitivity to acetylcholine in 38 of the 50 children, although no correlation could be demonstrated between severity of the exercise-induced bronchospasm and the

(3–43) Nouv. Presse Med. 9:1357–1360, Apr. 26, 1980. (Fre.)

threshold dose of acetylcholine. This phenomenon is explained by the differing nonimmunologic spasmogenic mechanisms involved in the two tests.

From a diagnostic standpoint, the advantage of testing for bronchial cholinergic sensitivity is certain. The physical stress test has essentially an orientational value in terms of the athletic potential of the asthmatic patient. Nevertheless, in a number of cases, the occurrence of bronchospasm after exercise will permit confirmation of a diagnosis of asthma even in the absence of bronchial hypersensitivity to acetylcholine.

▶ [There has been considerable discussion as to whether the bronchospasm brought about by physical activity is the same as that induced by pharmacologic "provocation" tests. Possible points of differentiation have included the time course of the reaction and the relative proportions of large and small airway spasm. This article supports the view that there are differences in the two types of spasm. Despite use of one of the more provocative forms of physical activity (free running, 5 minutes at maximum speed), the acetylcholine test provides a more consistent basis for the diagnosis of asthma.—R.J.S.] ◀

3–44 **Aplastic Anemia Associated With Rubber Cement Used by a Marathon Runner.** Marathon runners are subject to many unique physical problems, especially blistering of the feet. Once this occurs, some runners use rubber cement, which contains benzene as an impurity, to keep adhesive tape in place over the denuded areas while running. G. David Roodman, Eugene P. Reese, Jr., and Joseph M. Cardamone (Univ. of Minnesota) describe a runner who used rubber cement in this way for more than a year and in whom aplastic anemia developed.

Man, 26, noted leg cramping and marked fatigue while running in a marathon in October 1977. During a marathon in April 1978, he noted muscle cramping, arm heaviness, and spontaneous bruising. During the next 6–9 months, he experienced decreased exercise tolerance, petechiae, spontaneous bruising, and episodic hematochezia and melena. His only medication exposure was in April and May 1977, when he was treated with 300 mg of phenylbutazone daily for 2 days and with 200 mg of indomethacin daily for 6 weeks for a torn right Achilles tendon. In July 1978, when he was examined because of a "chronic cold" for the previous 6 months, petechiae were noted on the arms and legs, and pancytopenia was found with a hemoglobin level of 10.8 gm/dl, a white blood cell count of 3,300/cu mm, and a platelet count of 18,000/cu mm.

The patient had been using rubber cement on foot blisters for about 12 months to attach adhesive tape during daily 2- to 3-hour runs and during marathons. The rubber cement was placed on the denuded area of the feet, with adhesive tape placed over the rubber cement. The patient had palatal and buccal petechiae, a mobile, firm, nontender left axillary node measuring 0.5×0.5 cm, and scattered ecchymoses and petechiae on the chest, back, and extremities. Bone marrow aspirates and biopsy specimens showed a very hypocellular marrow. Results of laboratory studies were negative for mononucleosis, paroxysmal nocturnal hemoglobinuria, hepatitis A or B, or viral infection. Vitamin B_{12} levels, serum and red blood cell folate levels, and complement levels were normal. Therapy with 150 mg of oxymetholone daily,

(3–44) Arch. Intern. Med. 140:703, May 1980.

begun in August 1978, brought no improvement in the pancytopenia. The patient does not have an HLA-compatible donor suitable for bone marrow transplant. No in vitro evidence for suppressor T cell activity as a cause of the aplasia was found.

Aplastic anemia has been reported after exposure to many drugs and toxins, including phenylbutazone, indomethacin, and benzene, and the patient was exposed to all three of these. Because exposure to phenylbutazone and indomethacin was brief and occurred at least 6 months prior to development of symptoms, the aplastic anemia was probably due to a solvent containing benzene, to which the patient was exposed chronically up to the time of initial presentation.

▶ [Aplastic anemia has been reported after exposure to many drugs and toxins. This patient is of particular interest because he may have used a therapy in vogue among some runners for blistering of the feet, namely, applying rubber cement directly to the denuded skin and then attaching adhesive tape to permit continued running despite the blisters. In this instance, there was a chronic exposure to this agent of 2 hours daily for 12 months. Rubber cement has benzene as an impurity of the hexane used in its preparation. Benzene has a long and checkered history in the etiology of aplastic anemia. This is not a good custom for the therapy of blisters. Hopefully, the word will spread.—L.J.K.] ◀

3–45 **Olympic Drug Testing: Improvements Without Progress.** Since antidoping controls were introduced at the 1968 Winter Olympic Games in Grenoble, France, policy makers in amateur sports have disagreed on whether such controls protect the athlete or whether they are a waste of time and money. Lan Barnes has reviewed the development of drug control efforts in international sports competition.

At the 1968 winter Olympics, certain categories of drugs—sympathomimetic amines, CNS stimulants, narcotic analgesics, antidepressants, and major tranquilizers—were banned for the first time. Alcohol also was prohibited for athletes taking part in fencing and shooting events. All 86 tests at Grenoble and 667 of 668 tests at the summer games in Mexico City (1968) were negative. By the time of the 1976 games at Innsbruck, Austria, and Montreal, drug testing of Olympic athletes had become a multimillion dollar effort. The regulations had expanded to include types of banned drugs, specifically banned drugs, specifically permitted drugs, and specifically permitted uses of banned drugs. A major development at Montreal was the introduction of anabolic steroid testing. Positive results were found in 8 competitors, 3 of them medal winners. However, there were no positive drug tests at the 1980 Winter Olympics at Lake Placid, New York. A test for detecting reinfusion of an athlete's stored red blood cells has been proposed, but verifying positive results will prove difficult. Femininity testing is regarded as an expensive overreaction to a virtually nonexistent problem. It is claimed that variations in athletic performance are greater than the advantages supposedly conferred by the use of banned drugs. It is feared that the emphasis on drug testing may perpetuate drug use by Olympic athletes.

(3–45) Physician Sportsmed. 8:21–24, June 1980.

▶ [This article is a provocative peice on the growth of a multimillion-dollar screening process that some consider a waste of time and money. There may be two sides to the case, but the arguments against testing have rarely been expressed as lucidly. Certainly, there is tremendous inconsistency at this time not only in those drugs that are permitted, such as phenothiazine to treat jet lag and the use of local anesthetic injections, but the fact that some things still cannot be tested for effectively, such as blood doping and, indeed, in the area of anabolic steroids, testosterone itself—if one is inclined to the ultimate anabolic steroid. There is a certain appeal to the belief that were testing to stop, a certain glamour would leave the use of drugs. If it is true that the drugs do not make a difference in performance, the problem might very well move into insignificance. The point that the $2 or $3 million saved at each Olympics could do wonders for the Olympic movement is worth pondering. There certainly is much hypocrisy afoot when one is asked to believe that ephedrine, presently banned and having cost an American swimmer a gold medal in 1976, could conceivably affect athletic achievement, whereas caffeine is totally acceptable and has been unequivocally shown to be able to affect performance.—L.J.K.] ◀

3–46 **Insect Allergy and the Sportsman.** Thousands of Americans who enjoy outdoor activities are allergic to insect stings, especially Hymenoptera (bees, wasps, hornets, and ants). Many of these persons are unaware of this hypersensitivity, and each year at least 50–100 of them die. Claude A. Frazier (Asheville, N.C.) discusses ways to minimize the chances of being stung and steps to take if stung. Generalized systemic reactions to insect stings vary from slight to severe (Table 1). A severe generalized systemic reaction can intensify to fatal anaphylactic shock within 5–30 minutes of a sting.

Insect sting kits containing premeasured doses of epinephrine (1:1,000) with sterile syringes are available by prescription. Persons hypersensitive to insect stings should keep 1 in the home, 1 in the car, and 1 on the person whenever insects may be encountered. Patients must inject the epinephrine subcutaneously at the first sign of even a mild allergic reaction and seek medical aid immediately. Patients with severe local reactions should be assessed by skin tests or radioallergosorbent to protect against the possibility of systemic reactions if they are restung.

Immunotherapy should be initiated as soon as possible and the patient brought to a maintenance dose as rapidly as tolerated. Each of the two types of therapy available, whole body extracts and venom extracts, has its advantages and disadvantages. Patients allergic to insect stings should wear a medical warning tag stating that fact.

Steps the allergic person can take to minimize the odds of being restung are listed in Table 2. People responsible for public safety, such as nurses, forest rangers, and scout leaders, should be trained to recognize symptoms of allergic reactions and to administer premeasured injectable epinephrine when necessary. They should carry premeasured doses of epinephrine (1:1,000) with their regular first aid supplies.

▶ [This is a measured pitch for the use, or at least the potential use, and the carrying of insect sting kits, such as Ana-Kit, in the hope that they will decrease the severity of reactions and the considerable toll of 50–100 deaths per year from hypersensitivity to Hymenoptera. This is certainly to be recommended. The question of which patients

(3–46) Physician Sportsmed. 8:124–127, March 1980.

TABLE 1.—MUELLER'S CLASSIFICATION OF GENERALIZED REACTIONS

Slight general reaction

Generalized urticaria, itching, malaise, anxiety

General reaction

Any of the above plus any two or more of the following: generalized edema, constricted feeling in chest, wheezing, abdominal pain, nausea, and/or vomiting, dizziness

Severe general reaction

Any of the above plus two or more of the following: dyspnea, dysphagia, hoarseness or thickened speech, marked weakness, confusion, feeling of impending disaster

Shock reaction

Any of the above plus two or more of the following: cyanosis, fall in blood pressure, collapse, incontinence, and unconsciousness

TABLE 2.—PRACTICAL MEASURES TO AVOID BEING STUNG

1. Have some nonallergic person destroy Hymenoptera nests periodically during warm summer months as they appear around the home and yard.
2. Do not go barefoot or wear sandals outdoors.
3. Do not wear brightly colored clothing or use perfumed lotions, aftershaves, shampoos, and so on, since they attract Hymenoptera.
4. Be wary of eating outdoors, especially sugary foods or drinks, and avoid areas with garbage cans or dumps and fruit trees where fruit is rotting on the ground.
5. Do not mow lawns, clip hedges, or pick flowers.
6. Wear gloves, long pants, and long-sleeved shirts when outdoors.
7. Do not wear bright metal jewelry, belt buckles, and so on, since they attract Hymenoptera.
8. If Hymenoptera are encountered, do not swat or run, since such moves are likely to infuriate them and increase the risk of a sting. Retreat slowly, but if retreat is impossible, lie face down and cover the head with arms.

should then proceed to immunotherapy is a separate one to be handled on an individualized basis. It is a fact of life that most medical kits do not have injectable epinephrine available unless the person carries it himself or unless a physician with this equipment happens to be immediately available.—L.J.K.] ◀

3–47 **Inability of Iodination Method to Destroy Completely *Giardia* Cysts in Cold Water.** Use of a stock solution of saturated iodine is a simple method by which travelers and hikers can disinfect small quantities of water in the wilderness (Kahn and Visscher, 1975). Its efficacy against *Giardia* cysts was not known because of lack of a sensitive technique for determining *Giardia* cyst viability. Edward L. Jarroll, Jr., Alan K. Bingham, and Ernest A. Meyer (Univ. of Oregon) used a recently described method of inducing *Giardia* excystation in

(3–47) West. J. Med. 132:567–569, June 1980.

EFFECT OF SATURATED IODINE TREATMENT ON *GIARDIA* CYSTS IN CLEAR AND CLOUDY WATER

Clear Water

	3°C (26 ml of stock iodine solution)			
	Control	*15 min.*	*30 min.*	*40 min.*
RI*	0	6.87	6.87	6.87
Percent cyst mortality	0	56.5	93.3	95.9
Final pH	7.1 (range, 7.0-7.1)			

Cloudy Water

	3°C (26 ml of stock iodine solution)			
	Control	*15 min.*	*30 min.*	*40 min.*
RI	0	4.58	4.58	4.58
Percent cyst mortality	0	37.2	57.5	81.5
Final pH	7.3 (range, 7.0-7.3)			

	20°C (13 ml of stock iodine solution)			
	Control	*15 min.*	*30 min.*	*40 min.*
	0	3.29	3.29	3.29
	0	>99.8	>99.8	>99.8
	7.1 (range, 7.0-7.1)			

	20°C (26 ml of stock iodine solution)			
	Control	*15 min.*	*30 min.*	*40 min.*
	0	3.01	3.01	3.01
	0	>99.8	>99.8	>99.8
	7.3 (range, 7.0-7.3)			

*Residual iodine in parts per million.

vitro (Bingham and Meyer, 1979) as the criterion of cyst viability to test the iodination method of water disinfection.

As shown in the table, even after 40 minutes of contact time, complete destruction of *Giardia* cysts did not occur at 3 C, regardless of water quality. The data suggest, however, that if the contact time or the iodine residual was increased sufficiently, the efficacy of this method of cold water disinfection could prove satisfactory. At 20 C, iodination destroyed more than 99.8% of *Giardia* cysts in both clear and cloudy water after 15 minutes.

This and other small-quantity water disinfection methods are ineffective in the combined presence of low water temperature and increased iodine demand because survival of *Giardia* cysts is prolonged in cold water. Furthermore, no water in the wilderness can be more iodine demand-free than the clear water used in this study. Thus, while 95.9% of the cysts in cold, clear water were destroyed, a lower level of destruction can be expected in actual use.

A modified method of using a saturated iodine solution that will insure *Giardia* cyst destruction in cold water could not be formulated from the data. However, two other small-quantity water disinfection methods have effectively destroyed *Giardia* cysts at 3 C (Jarroll et al., 1980). Furthermore, bringing water to a boil destroys *Giardia* cysts instantly, so that a method of killing these organisms is available even when chemical water treatment methods are not.

▶ [The risk of *Giardia lamblia* infestation from high mountain lakes and streams heretofore thought to be immaculately pure is very real and appears to be increasing. Further bad news for the backpacker and climber is that in clear cold water the classic 1 drop of saturated iodine for 10 minutes is no longer sufficient to guarantee cyst destruction. The practical solution would seem to be to extend the time interval to perhaps 15 or 20 minutes or, better still, to bring water to a boil if there is any question as to its purity—it seems that there is a question as to the purity of all water these days. On the other hand, the use of Lugol's solution, 1 drop per glass for 10 minutes, is 99.8% effective for the traveler in the tropics and is strongly recommended not only for wilderness backpacking, but for brushing one's teeth in Mexico City.—L.J.K.] ◀

EXERCISE TESTING

3–48 **Small-Animal Ergometer** was devised by J. C. Russell, P. D. Campagna, and H. A. Wenger (Univ. of Alberta) to simulate human exercise of an intensive nature previously impossible with small animals. Even under the most demanding conditions, no injuries to the animal occur.

The ergometer consists of an endless, downward-moving vertical ladder. Some mechanism is required to motivate animals to climb rather than rest at the base of the enclosure. A nose cone assembly permits determination of respiratory gas exchange in the exercising animals.

Rats were placed in the ergometer at age 6 weeks and trained to climb and maintain position at the top of the ladder without difficulty. They were subjected to exercise sessions 4 days a week and worked at gradually increasing speeds. They were forced to climb for 1 to 5 minutes or more; duration was based on clinically apparent signs of fatigue. Heart rate was monitored and increased on exercising. Figure 3–8 shows the relation between oxygen uptake and power output for single rats from a group that was exercise conditioned.

(3–48) J. Appl. Physiol. 48:394–398, February 1980.

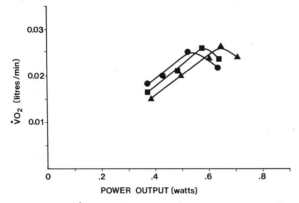

Fig 3–8.—Oxygen uptake $(\dot{V}O_2)$ as function of external power output. Different data points represent specific observations on single Woodlyn rats, aged 14 weeks, that had been subjected to 7-week program of physical conditioning. (Courtesy of Russell, J. C., et al.: J. Appl. Physiol. 48:394–398, February 1980.)

Each showed a linear increase in oxygen uptake with increasing power output with a drop after a maximum.

The vertical ladder ergometer provides a method for imposing high levels of defined work or exercise on small animals.

▶ [The regular exercising of rats is finding increased application in laboratory sports medicine. Severe controlled training experiments can be undertaken, aging studies are completed within 1–2 years, and a variety of organs can be subjected to detailed biochemical scrutiny. Unfortunately, many rats run poorly on the usual treadmill, while swimming tests may confound exercise and hypothermia. This article describes a new type of laddermill, which seems well adapted to normal rat behavior patterns. It permits the measurement of oxygen consumption, and the authors' graphs of lower output against $\dot{V}O_2$ show some quite pretty plateaus.—R.J.S.] ◀

3–49 **Linear Relationship Between the Distribution of Thallium-201 and Blood Flow in Ischemic and Nonischemic Myocardium During Exercise.** Anton P. Nielsen, Kenneth G. Morris, Robert Murdock, Frederick P. Bruno, and Frederick R. Cobb (VA Med. Center, Durham, N.C.) compared the myocardial distribution of thalium-201 and regional myocardial blood flow during pneumatic cuff ischemia and the stress of exercise in 6 dogs. Each animal received catheter implants in the atrium and aorta and a snare on the circumflex coronary artery distal to the first marginal branch. Seven to 10 μ of radioisotope-labeled microspheres were used to measure regional myocardial blood flow during quiet, resting conditions. After 1 minute of exercise on a treadmill, the circumflex coronary artery was occluded and thallium-201 and a second label of microspheres were injected; exercise was resumed for 5 minutes. The animals were killed and the left ventricle was sectioned. Approximately 80 samples of 1–2 gm each were obtained and analyzed for thallium-201 activity and regional myocardial blood flow.

(3–49) Circulation 61:791–801, April 1980.

The maximum increase in blood flow during exercise was 3.3–7.2 times resting control values. Myocardial samples in which blood flow was reduced to less than 0.10 ml/minute/gm were obtained from each dog. In each animal, linear regression analyses demonstrated a correlation coefficient of 0.98 or greater between thallium-201 distribution and direct measurements of regional myocardial blood flow (Fig 3–9).

The results show that during physiologic exercise sufficient to in-

Fig 3–9.—The relationship between thallium-201 activity and myocardial blood flow (ml/minute/gm) in six dogs during exercise and ischemia; n, number of samples analyzed. (Courtesy of Nielsen, A. P., et al.: Circulation 61:797–801, April 1980; by permission of the American Heart Association, Inc.)

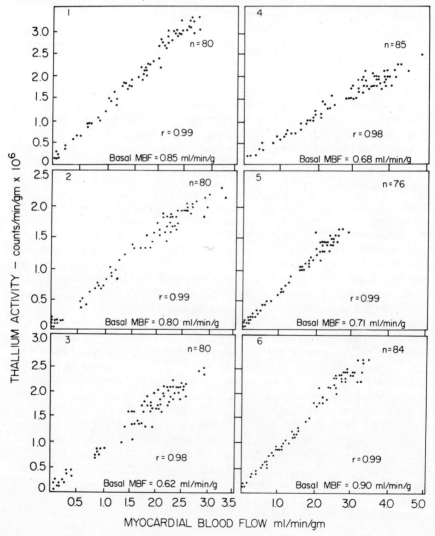

crease coronary blood flow 3–7 times control values, the myocardial distribution of thallium activity is linearly related to regional myocardial blood flow in both ischemic and nonischemic regions.

▶ [It is possible to make a relatively objective assessment of capillary blood flow in the dog by injection of microspheres of an appropriate size. Use of 7- to 10-μ microspheres demonstrates a maximum flow of about 5 times the resting value; because the resting oxygen extraction is fairly complete in the coronary circulation, myocardial ischemia is likely if the cardiac work rate is increased more than fivefold. The experiments also show a nice correlation between the regional coronery flow indicated by microspheres and by thallium-201.—R.J.S.] ◀

3–50 **Exercise Efficiency: Validity of Baseline Subtractions.** Wendell N. Stainsby, L. Bruce Gladden, Jack K. Barclay, and Brian A. Wilson reviewed the literature and considered the validity of using baseline subtractions in evaluating the efficiency of the muscles in performing external work.

Although baselines have been criticized, they have been widely used without analysis of the implications. From data in the literature for isolated muscles, calculation showed that baseline subtraction gives unreasonably high efficiencies, suggesting that baselines are invalid. For a baseline subtraction to be valid, the baseline must remain unchanged during changes in the work rate and alterations in the exercising conditions. However, baselines do change with an increasing work rate. Various metabolic and physiologic processes contribute to changes in the baseline. Calculation of exercise efficiencies is complicated by variations in the use of elastic energy storage in some types of exercise. Although baseline subtractions may be useful for obtaining information on changes in energy expenditure, they should not be construed to indicate the efficiency of contracting muscle.

Because baselines do not isolate energy expended specifically for the performance of external work, none of the exercise efficiencies (gross, net, work, apparent, delta, and instantaneous) accurately reflects the efficiency of the muscles in performing external work. Future studies of exercise metabolism should be more concerned with describing and quantifying the determinants of energy expenditure than with attempting to refine baselines.

▶ [Whether efficiency is calculated for an isolated muscle or for the body as a whole, it is necessary to make some allowance for the initial (resting) matabolism. The resting value may be subtracted, the slope of oxygen consumption against added work can be viewed, or an attempt can be made to provide a stable baseline of light work. With any of these three expedients, there is the theoretical objection that activity may (for example, through a rise of temperature) change resting metabolism. In maximum effort (12–14 times basal), small changes in the baseline do not lead to large errors. However, the problem is more serious in moderate work.

During running, mechanical efficiency exceeds the biochemically possible! This is because energy used in raising the center of gravity is stored in stretched tendons during descent and can be recovered at the next pace.—R.J.S.] ◀

3–51 **Elicitation of Maximal Oxygen Uptake From Standing Bicycle Ergometry.** John M. Kelly, Robert C. Serfass, and G. Alan Stull

(3–50) J. Appl. Physiol. 48:518–522, March 1980.
(3–51) Res. Q. Exerc. Sport 51:315–322, May 1980.

investigated whether higher maximal oxygen consumption ($\dot{V}O_{2\,max}$) values could be obtained from a continuous standing bicycle ergometer test than from a continuous sitting test. They also compared the sitting and standing bicycle test values with those obtained during continuous graded treadmill running. Twelve male students were tested twice on each of three continuous $\dot{V}O_{2\,max}$ protocols for treadmill running, pedaling on a bicycle ergometer while seated, and pedaling on a bicycle ergometer while standing. Mean age was 22.42 years and mean body weight was 75.64 kg. Expiratory volumes were measured during the last 30 seconds of each minute of exercise and heart rates were monitored continuously.

Results showed no differences among protocols for pulmonary ventilation. For $\dot{V}O_{2\,max}$, all differences were significant. The value was highest with treadmill running, intermediate with cycling in the standing position, and lowest with cycling while seated (Fig 3–10). Maximum heart rate was significantly lower on both bicycle tests than on the treadmill. There was no difference between the maximum heart rates recorded on the sitting and standing bicycle tests. The respiratory exchange ratio was higher on the sitting bicycle task than on the standing bicycle task. No other differences among protocols were significant.

The demonstration of an 8% difference of attained $\dot{V}O_{2\,max}$ favoring graded treadmill running over sitting bicycle ergometry closely agreed with findings of other research. The principal finding of this study was that standing bicycle ergometry resulted in a 4% higher $\dot{V}O_{2\,max}$ than a sitting bicycle test that used the same work increments. The standing protocol elicited 96% of the $\dot{V}O_{2\,max}$ attained during graded treadmill running. The large standard error of prediction associated with the bicycle tests, however, limits their value for esti-

Fig 3–10.—Means of $\dot{V}O_{2\,max}$ for treadmill and standing and sitting bicycle tests with percentages of treadmill values. (Courtesy of Kelly, J. M., et al.: Res. Q. Exerc. Sport 51:315–322, May 1980.)

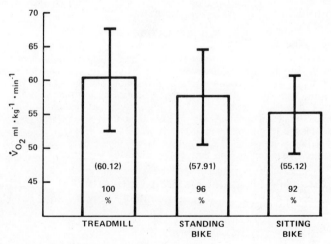

mating maximum cardiorespiratory responses that would be expected from treadmill running. Because of the higher $\dot{V}O_{2\,max}$ obtained from a standing bicycle protocol, this protocol should be considered when cardiorespiratory response to maximal work is to be measured.

▶ [It has been recognized for some years that the usual bicycle (or more correctly, cycle) ergometer test yields a lower $\dot{V}O_{2\,max}$ than the treadmill. The usual explanation is that during cycling, a high proportion of the total work load is sustained by a single muscle group (the quadriceps). The test is therefore halted by local fatigue, rather than central cardiorespiratory exhaustion. Uphill treadmill running, in contrast, involves most of the body muscles. Because the purpose of a $\dot{V}O_{2\,max}$ measurement is to assess cardiorespiratory performance, the treadmill data are more valid than those obtained on the cycle. It has previously been suggested that the use of pedal traps will enable a "central" $\dot{V}O_{2\,max}$ to be reached. However, such a tactic is not particularly suited to clinical testing. The present authors suggest that half of the error can be avoided by the expedient of standing on the pedals. Again, this may not be too suitable a procedure for older people. It must also be stressed that where the quadriceps is weakened by inactivity or disease, the errors associated with a cycle ergometer test may be much larger than 8%.—R.J.S.] ◀

3–52 **Criteria for Maximum Oxygen Uptake in Progressive Bicycle Tests.** K. Niemelä, I. Palatsi, M. Linnaluoto, and J. Takkunen (Univ. Central Hosp., Oulu, Finland) studied the different criteria for $\dot{V}O_{2\,max}$ on a simple progressive bicycle test to see if objective evidence for $\dot{V}O_{2\,max}$ in general is achieved using this test protocol.

TECHNIQUE.—The test-retest repeatability (reliability) and validity of the protocol was studied on 16 healthy men, aged 25–35 years (the "control" group). In addition, 55 men and 44 women, aged 35–62 years, all of them healthy volunteers accustomed to moderately heavy work, pedalled the progressive test once (the "normal" group). The cycle ergometer was electrically braked. Expiratory gases were collected through an open low-resistance mouthpiece; $\dot{V}O_2$, carbon dioxide production, respiratory quotient (R), tidal (V_T) and minute ventilation ($\dot{V}_E$), respiratory rate (f), and heart rate were measured every minute throughout the exercise with a computer-based system. The different criteria were evaluated as follows: (1) a plateau in $\dot{V}O_2$, (2) adequacy of a subjective criterion for establishing the end point, (3) respiratory quotient over 1.15, and (4) an increase in heart rate to maximum values estimated for age ± SD, that is, ±10 beats per minute.

No significant differences were found for the average submaximal values of $\dot{V}O_2$, V_E, R, or heart rate in two repeated progressive tests, and the average difference of $\dot{V}O_2$ at the submaximal level was $-4.1\% \pm 6.9\%$ (-110 ± 170 ml/minute). The $\dot{V}O_2$ against work load was lower in the progressive than in the constant-load test. Three types of $\dot{V}O_2$ response against work load were noticed; they were: a linear increase, an unexpectedly high increase, and a plateau; the last two only appeared when $\dot{V}O_{2\,max}$ was achieved. The last three $\dot{V}O_2$ values at least were required to define the plateau. Most commonly, subjective exhaustion was achieved, R was greater than 1.15, and maximal heart rate reached the estimated level for age, though $\dot{V}O_{2\,max}$ was not achieved. No significant differences were found between "peak $\dot{V}O_2$" in the first progressive test, the second progressive test, or the constant-load test. In the progressive test performed

(3–52) Eur. J. Appl. Physiol. 44:51–59, June 1980.

once on 55 men and 44 women, subjective exhaustion was achieved by most of the subjects, but the plateau in $\dot{V}O_2$ was shown only in 17 subjects, and the peak $\dot{V}O_2$ values were somewhat lower than expected. Moreover, R max did not correlate with peak $\dot{V}O_2$, and was more than 1.15 only in 9 subjects, and maximum heart rate was often below the estimated level.

The authors conclude that progressive cycle exercise seems to be convenient for testing the physical work capacity of people of different ages, but the establishment of the "true" physiologic maximum is more difficult: the uncommon plateau in $\dot{V}O_2$ appears to be the only useful criterion for $\dot{V}O_{2\,max}$. The value of other criteria and arbitrary end points is rather disappointing, especially if older and untrained subjects are tested. The unexpectedly high increase in $\dot{V}O_2$ may be one more sign of the approach of the "true" maximum. So far, the term "$\dot{V}O_{2\,max}$" seems justifiable on progressive bicycle exercise only when the plateau in $\dot{V}O_2$ is shown, or when repeated measurements are performed. Otherwise, other terms, for example, "peak $\dot{V}O_2$," should be used. A clear definition of the plateau is especially important when small increments of work load are used.

▶ [The prime criterion of centrally limited exhausting exercise is attainment of a plateau of oxygen consumption (the directly measured $\dot{V}O_{2\,max}$). Unfortunately, this criterion is not always realized on a cycle ergometer because of local fatigue in the leg muscles. In the present sample of 55 men and 44 women, a progressive test protocol yielded a clear plateau in only 17 instances. Further, the sometimes suggested subsidiary criteria of a respiratory gas exchange ratio >1.15 and attainment of the peak heart rate seemed unreliable. The lesson seems to be that if a cycle ergometer test is used on sedentary subjects, the result observed is a subjectively limited "peak" rather than a true maximum, and it should be described in these terms.—R.J.S.] ◀

3–53 **Master Two-Step Test: Present Status** is outlined by Jules Constant (SUNY at Buffalo). The relatively simple Master two-step test is still a popular office test throughout the world. It may not be important that the high maximal heart rates achieved by treadmill testing be reached for significant coronary artery disease to be detected. The double Master test requires about half the oxygen consumption measured during progressive exercise stress testing in sedentary, middle-aged men. Although the postexercise heart rate may reach only 50% to 60% of predicted maximum rate, the coronary circulation may be inadequate in the postexercise period. The double Master test is only about half as sensitive as the treadmill test in predicting future events, but it is not necessarily less specific. Risk ratios have not been found to be significantly better with a treadmill, a bicycle, or the double Master test. If a 1.5-minute test is negative, an augmented double Master test may safely be carried out. The use of postexercise ECG changes other than S-T depression as criteria will minimize false positive interpretations.

A double Master test can be used as an office screening procedure in prescribing exericse. Patients who can complete a double Master test with slight symptoms can probably meet the demands of any

(3–53) N.Y. State J. Med. 80:39–45, January 1980.

light job. The double Master test may be of use as an indicator of when to perform coronary angiography with bypass surgery in mind. For this indication and to learn whether ischemia due to coronary disease is present, there is no proof that a progressive stress test is superior to an augmented double Master two-step test. If a Master two-step test is markedly positive, coronary angiography may well be indicated. If only moderate S-T depression of 1 to 2 mm is found, a progressive exercise test and thallium scanning may be appropriate. If the augmented Master two-step test is negative despite a postexercise heart rate of at least 110 beats per minute, it is questionable whether anything more than medical management of symptoms and risk factors is necessary.

▶ [The sophisticated treadmill testing often is used simply to identify the presence or absence of significant coronary disease and to attempt some measure of prognosis for future coronary events. If this is all it is to be used for, the Master two-step test may be nearly as good, infinitely cheaper, and much easier to carry out in the office. There is something rather nice about seeing an enthusiast for the Master two-step test because it harks back to our simpler selves, if nothing else. It cannot give the sophisticated information about cardiovascular fitness, cardiac function, or arrhythmias that can be gleaned by expert observers from a progressive treadmill or bicycle stress test. Using the Master two-step test in the office does not preclude the need for the availability of a defibrillator and personnel trained in cardiopulmonary resuscitation.—L.J.K.] ◀

3–54 **Segmental Wall Motion Analysis in Right Anterior Oblique Projection: Comparison of Exercise Equilibrium Radionuclide Ventriculography and Exercise Contrast Ventriculography.** Thomas J. Brady, James H. Thrall, John W. Keyes, Jr., James F. Brymer, Joseph A. Walton, and Bertram Pitt (Univ. of Michigan) evaluated right anterior oblique (RAO) radionuclide and contrast ventriculography in visualization of regional myocardial wall motion at rest and during supine bicycle exercise in 39 patients with confirmed or suspected coronary artery disease. The five standard segments from 30-degree RAO contrast ventriculograms and the corresponding 10-degree RAO radionuclide segments were analyzed. Three independent observers evaluated radionuclide visualization of myocardial wall motion by using a 5-point scale ranging from normal ($+3$) to dyskinesis (-1).

Both techniques were used to study 161 rest and 164 exercise segments. There was complete agreement between the two techniques in 139 (86%) of the 161 rest segments and agreement within 1 wall motion grade in 97%. There was complete agreement in 128 (78%) of the 164 exercise segments and agreement within 1 wall motion grade in 96%. Among 22 patients with confirmed coronary artery disease, fewer segments showed complete agreement (rest, 78%; exercise, 56%), though agreement within 1 wall motion grade was essentially unchanged (rest, 95%; exercise, 91%). Radionuclide wall motion analysis was 97% sensitive for segments graded as showing marked hypokinesia, akinesia, or dyskinesis, but it was only 45% sensitive for segments graded as mildly hypokinetic ($2+$). Diagnostic agreement

(3–54) J. Nucl. Med. 21:617–621, July 1980.

among observers on whether a study was normal or abnormal was 90%.

Right anterior oblique radionuclide wall motion analysis compares favorably with analysis of RAO contrast ventriculogram segments at rest and during exercise. The greater resolution of contrast ventriculography for assessment of regional myocardial wall motion is a major factor accounting for its greater sensitivity.

▶ [This report shows that contrast ventriculography is a somewhat better method of classifying abnormal motion of the ventricular wall than is radionuclide ventriculography. Even if no more than a three-point semiquantitative assessment is attempted, the interobserver agreement of radionuclide tests is only about 80%.—R.J.S.] ◀

3–55 **Detection of Coronary Artery Disease: Comparison of Exercise Stress Radionuclide Angiocardiography and Thallium Stress Perfusion Scanning.** Myocardial stress perfusion scanning with ^{201}Tl fails to detect some patients with significant coronary artery disease. James A. Jengo, Ronald Freeman, Marianne Brizendine, and Ismael Mena compared ^{201}Tl stress testing with first-pass radionuclide stress angiography in 42 patients who had at least 75% obstruction of a coronary artery and 21 of whom had evidence of past myocardial infarction and in 16 subjects without more than 50% coronary obstruction. Radionuclide angiography was performed with ^{99m}Tc-diethylenetriamine penta-acetate in conjunction with maximal bicycle exercise. Stress perfusion studies were performed with 1.5 mCi of ^{201}Tl.

One control had a defect on the exercise thallium study, but all had normal resting perfusion scans. Each had a rise in ejection fraction of at least 0.1 on exercise. Segmental wall motion was normal at rest in all subjects but 1 and was uniformly increased on exercise in all subjects. Fifteen of the 16 controls had a normal ECG response to exercise stress. The resting perfusion study was abnormal in 22 of the 42 patients with significant coronary disease, and 24 patients developed a new perfusion defect during exercise. Some abnormality was detected in all but 3 patients. Ejection fraction decreased on exercise. Forty patients had a new wall motion defect on exercise or showed no improvement of a preexistent defect in the distribution of the diseased coronary artery or arteries. The ECG stress test was positive in 81% of patients. Perfusion scanning was 50% sensitive and radionuclide angiography was 81% sensitive in detecting other coronary lesions in the presence of past infarction. The respective specificities of the two methods were 94% and 100%.

▶ [In patients with preexisting infarction, both thallium scanning and radionuclide angiography are useful in detecting additional coronary artery disease and may serve complementary roles. Radionuclide angiography appears to be the more sensitive and specific indicator of the presence and location of significant associated coronary artery disease. Thallium stress testing offers no information on left ventricular function and only indirect evidence of the nature of coronary obstructive disease.—L.J.K.] ◀

3–56 **Exercise Testing for the Diagnosis of Coronary Artery Disease.** Previous studies have shown that the presence of an abnormal

(3–55) Am. J. Cardiol. 45:535–541, March 1980.
(3–56) Am. Heart J. 99:811–812, June 1980.

PRETEST RISK OF CORONARY DISEASE AND PREDICTIVE VALUE OF POSITIVE AND NEGATIVE
EXERCISE TESTS IN CORONARY ARTERY SURGERY STUDY (CASS)

				Predictive value (%)	
			Pre-test risk		
History	*Sex*	*No.*	*of coronary disease (%)*	*+ET**	*−ET***
Definite angina	Male	620	89	96	35
Definite angina	Female	98	62	73	67
Probable angina	Male	594	70	87	56
Probable angina	Female	240	40	54	78
Nonischemic pain	Male	251	22	39	86
Nonischemic pain	Female	242	5	6	95

*Predictive value of a positive exercise test (+ET) = percentage of positive results that are truly positive.
**Predictive value of a negative exercise test (−ET) = percentage of negative results that are truly negative.

S-T segment response to stress almost always predicted the presence of coronary artery disease. However, most of these patients were at high pretest risk of coronary disease. Recently, studies of patients with a low pretest risk who were subjected to exercise testing and coronary arteriography have shown an unusually high rate of false positive results. Donald A. Weiner, Carolyn H. McCabe, and Thomas J. Ryan (Boston Univ.) evaluated the predictive value of the S-T segment response to exercise by correlating clinical and exercise data with the results of coronary arteriography obtained from the National Collaborative Study on Coronary Artery Surgery. The patient population consisted of 1,465 men and 580 women. The exercise test was considered positive when the S-T segment depression or elevation was greater than or equal to 1 mm.

Depending on the sex of the patient and the intensity of chest pain, the pretest risk of coronary disease varied from 5% to 89%. A positive exercise test was highly correlated with the presence of coronary disease in patients with a high pretest risk of coronary disease (e.g., men with definite angina); a negative exercise test in this subgroup was likely to be a false negative response. In contrast, a negative exercise test in patients with a low pretest risk (e.g., women with nonischemic chest pain) was highly predictive of the absence of coronary disease; a positive exercise test in this subgroup was likely to be falsely positive.

The results indicate that the pretest risk of coronary disease must be considered before the results of exercise testing can be objectively evaluated (table). The results also support other studies that showed a rate of false positive exercise tests among asymptomatic patients as high as 65%. It appears that the S-T segment response to exercise testing provides little additional information to improve on the estimate of the probability of coronary disease beyond that provided by the classification of chest pain and sex of the patient.

▶ [In the past few years, clinicians have become sufficiently familiar with the epidemiologic concepts of test sensitivity and specificity to realize that there is little justification for stress testing of the general population in terms of the diagnosis of ischemic heart disease. This article shows that even if there is a history of chest pain, unless this is relatively typical of angina, a positive test result is of little help in diagnosis. On the other hand, a negative result can be used to reassure the patient with some confidence if symptons are atypical.—R.J.S.] ◄

3–57) **Exercise Testing After β-Blockade: Improved Specificity and Predictive Value in Detecting Coronary Heart Disease.** J. Marcomichelakis, R. Donaldson, J. Green, S. Joseph, H. B. Kelly, P. Taggart, and W. Somerville (Middlesex Hosp., London) point out that in asymptomatic subjects, exercise tests to detect coronary heart disease yield a high number of false positive results. Consequently, the specificity and predictive value of these tests are poor. To increase the reliability of exercise testing, the authors studied the effect of β-adrenergic blockade on the ECG response to exercise in 100 men. Group I contained 50 patients selected for coronary arteriography because of angina. All were between ages 32 and 64 years. Group II consisted of 50 asymptomatic male subjects, aged 17 to 57 years, referred for investigation of an abnormal resting ECG suggesting myocardial ischemia. Each subject performed maximal treadmill exercise tests before and after β-blockade with oxprenolol.

In group I, 34 of the 50 patients had abnormal resting ECGs indicating myocardial ischemia. In 8 of the 34 the changes were greater in the standing position. After β-blockade, 15 of the 34 abnormal ECGs became normal, 8 improved but did not become normal, and 11 were unchanged. In the 8 patients whose ischemic abnormalities were exaggerated by standing, the postural effect was less after β-blockade. In group II, 40 subjects had normal ECGs after β-blockade. In 8 of the other 10 the ECG improved and in 2 it was unaffected. In 15 of the 50 the changes were more prominent in the standing position,

---

TABLE 1.—GROUP I: EXERCISE TEST RESULTS* IN 50
PATIENTS WITH ANGINA

No medication	Oxprenolol
44 +ve (43 TP +1 FP)	43 +ve (43 TP +0 FP)
6 −ve (3 TN +3 FN)	7 −ve (4 TN +3 FN)

*TP, true positive; FP, false positive; TN, true negative; FN, false negative; +ve, positive; −ve, negative.

TABLE 2.—GROUP II: EXERCISE TEST RESULTS* IN 50
ASYMPTOMATIC SUBJECTS WITH ABNORMAL ECGS

No medication	Oxprenolol
20 +ve (1 TP +19 FP)	1 +ve (1 TP +0 FP)
30 −ve (29 TN + 1 FN)	49 −ve (48 TN +1 FN)

*TP, true positive; FP, false positive; TN, true negative; FN, false negative; +ve, positive; −ve, negative.

(3–57) Br. Heart J. 43:252–261, March 1980.

and this postural effect was abolished by β-blockade. Tables 1 and 2 show the exercise test results in group I and group II, respectively.

Incorporation of β-blockade into the standard exercise procedure for the ECG response improved the specificity and predictive value of this test without affecting sensitivity. Although β-blockade was unreliable in distinguishing ischemic from nonischemic resting ECGs, it eliminated all false positive ECG responses to exercise in both groups and abolished no true positive response. This procedure may be a useful further routine test in the investigation of coronary heart disease.

▶ [In the group of symptomless patients studied, β-blockade improved the specificity of an ECG stress test from 60% to 100%; however, the sensitivity in detecting 50% angiographic narrowing remained unaltered at a disappointingly low 50%. β-Blockade thus helps to make screening tests more effective, although it cannot overcome the inherent difficulty of a poor yield when the stress ECG is applied indiscriminately to the general adult population.—R.J.S.] ◀

3–58 **Identification of Patients With Left Main and Three-Vessel Coronary Disease With Clinical and Exercise Test Variables.** Donald A. Weiner, Carolyn H. McCabe, and Thomas J. Ryan (Boston Univ.) investigated which, if any, exercise test variables could serve as important predictors of left main or three-vessel coronary disease when used in conjunction with the clinical history. A consecutive series of 436 patients referred for evaluation of suspected or known coronary artery disease, who were able to undergo both exercise testing and coronary arteriography, were studied. All underwent graded treadmill exercise testing according to the standard Bruce protocol. The patients were divided into group I (35 patients), with 50% or greater narrowing of the left main coronary artery; group II (89), with three-vessel coronary disease without left main coronary artery disease; group III (188), with one- or two-vessel coronary disease including 31 with proximal left anterior descending coronary artery disease; and group IV (124), with angiograms that revealed no significant coronary artery disease. Five clinical and 11 exercise test variables were compared with the findings of coronary arteriography in the 436 patients.

Group I patients had earlier onset of S-T segment depression, which was more prolonged and appeared in a greater number of ECG leads, than did group II patients. Individual clinical or exercise test variables did not detect left main coronary disease because of their low sensitivity or predictive values. The pattern of 2 mm or more downsloping S-T segment depression that starts in stage 1, lasts at least 6 minutes into recovery, and is displayed in at least five ECG leads, was highly predictive (74%) and reasonably sensitive (49%) for detection of left main or three-vessel coronary disease. These criteria had a sensitivity of 74% and a predictive value of 32% for detection of isolated left main coronary artery disease. The table summarizes the results.

Identification of patients with left main or three-vessel coronary disease can be improved by combined analysis of several readily ob-

(3–58) Am. J. Cardiol. 46:21–27, July 1980.

COMBINATIONS* OF EXERCISE TEST VARIABLES FOR
DETECTION OF LEFT MAIN (GROUP I) AND LEFT MAIN OR
THREE-VESSEL CORONARY DISEASE (GROUPS I AND II)

	Group I (n = 35)		Group I and II (n = 124)	
	Sensi-tivity (%)	Predictive Value (%)	Sensi-tivity (%)	Predictive Value (%)
Combination I	77	24	57	69
Combination II	74	32	49	74
Combination III	57	38	36	83

*Combination I: 2 mm or more downsloping S-T segment depres-
sion with S-T depression beginning in stage 1; combination II: combination I plus S-T depression lasting 6 or more minutes and involving 5 or more leads; combination III: combination II plus exercise-
induced angina and treadmill time 6 minutes or less.

tained features of the exercise test. Analysis of the clinical features
of all 436 patients disclosed no single variable that helped distinguish
left main from three-vessel coronary disease or predict the presence
of left main coronary artery disease. Results of the study confirm that
the exercise test should be regarded semiquantitatively, rather than
in the customary qualitative format.

▶ [Many authors claim a high sensitivity and/or specificity for their method of detecting left main or three-vessel disease, or both. It is thus very helpful to have in a single
table the values for sensitivity and specificity of many of the commonly proposed criteria. Exploration of various possible combinations of criteria supports the widely held
view that the most effective group of variables are S-T depression >2 mm, beginning
early in a progressive test, lasting more than 6 minutes, and involving five or more
leads.—R.J.S.] ◀

3–59 **Superior QRS Axis of Ventricular Premature Complexes: An
Additional Criterion to Enhance the Sensitivity of Exercise
Stress Testing.** The presence or frequency of ventricular premature
complexes during exercise stress testing has shown a poor correlation
with the presence of underlying coronary artery disease. T. Joseph
Mardelli, Joel Morganroth, and Leonard S. Dreifus (Lankenau Hosp.,
Philadelphia) studied 63 patients with ventricular premature complexes and ECG or angiographic evidence of coronary heart disease,
or both, and 10 control patients with normal coronary arteriograms
to determine whether the morphological features (right or left bundle-branch block) or axis of exercise-induced ventricular premature
complexes enhance the sensitivity of exercise stress testing to underlying coronary artery disease.

Uniform ventricular premature complexes were seen in 45 of the
63 patients, while 18 had complexes with multiple axes (Fig 3–11).
Forty-eight patients (76%) showed at least one venticular premature
complex with a superior axis between − 30 and − 120 degrees, 13
(21%) had a ventricular premature complex with an axis between
− 30 and + 150 degrees, and 2 had an indeterminate axis. All 10 of

(3–59) Am. J. Cardiol. 45:236–243, February 1980.

CORONARY ARTERY DISEASE

N = 63 PATIENTS

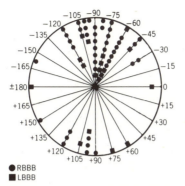

● RBBB
■ LBBB

Fig 3–11.—Distribution of the axes of exercise-induced ventricular premature complexes in 63 patients with coronary artery disease. A ventricular premature complex with a right bundle-branch block *(RBBB)* pattern is shown by a circle, and one with a left bundle-branch block *(LBBB)* pattern is shown by a square. (Courtesy of Mardelli, T. J., et al.: Am. J. Cardiol. 45:236–243, February 1980.)

the control subjects had a QRS axis of ventricular premature complexes in the normal range (between −30 and +150 degrees). A right bundle-branch block was present in 37 patients (59%), a left bundle-branch block was seen in 16 (27%), and 10 (14%) showed both right and left bundle-branch block patterns. Of 63 patients tested for coronary artery disease by the criterion of S-T segment depression, 38 had an abnormal S-T segment response of 1 mm or greater depression, while 25 had a normal or borderline test with 1 mm or less S-T segment depression. Twenty-one of these 25 patients had a ventricular premature complex with a superior axis. Thus, the sensitivity of the exercise stress test was enhanced from 60% to 94% when the S-T segment depression criterion was used in conjunction with the axis of ventricular premature complexes. Diagnostic sensitivity was not improved by the presence of a left bundle-branch block pattern.

It is suggested that the presence of ventricular premature complexes with an abnormal superior axis appears to be a specific marker for coronary artery disease and that the use of this criterion adjunctively with S-T segment depression may enhance the sensitivity of exercise stress tests in patients with a nondiagnostic response.

▶ [Previous authors have noted that "hazardous" premature ventricular contractions can be distinguished by (1) a polyfocal origin, (2) increasing frequency during exercise, and (3) occurrence early during repolarization. This article adds a fourth adverse criterion (a superior electric axis). It is suggested that when used in conjunction with S-T segmental depression, this finding increases sensitivity in the detection of angiographic coronary vascular disease.—R.J.S.] ◀

3–60 **Detecting Abnormalities in Left Ventricular Function During Exercise Before Angina and S-T Segment Depression.** Mark T.

(3–60) Circulation 62:341–349, August 1980.

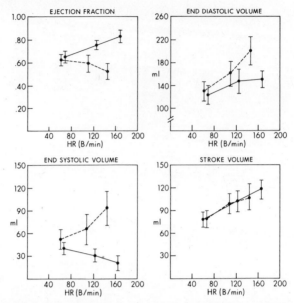

Fig 3–12.—Hemodynamic responses to exercise in 10 normal subjects *(solid lines)* and 25 patients with coronary artery disease *(broken lines)*. Means ± SD are presented at rest and for two exercise levels. *HR,* heart rate. (Courtesy of Upton, M. T., et al.: Circulation 62:341–349, August 1980; by permission of the American Heart Association, Inc.)

Upton, Stephen K. Rerych, Glenn E. Newman, Steven Port, Frederick R. Cobb, and Robert H. Jones (Duke Univ.) used radionuclide angiocardiography to determine if abnormalities in left ventricular function precede angina pectoris and ECG evidence of myocardial ischemia.

Twenty-five men, with a mean age of 51 years, who had stable coronary artery disease formed the study group. Ten had a history of myocardial infarction and 8 had pathologic Q waves on the 12-lead ECG. Ten men, with a mean age of 32 years, served as controls. After a resting radionuclide angiocardiogram was made, exercise was begun on an isokinetic cycle ergometer with the subject sitting. First-pass radionuclide angiocardiography was used to assess left ventricular performance. In the patients with coronary artery disease, the first radionuclide study during exercise was performed before and the second after the onset of S-T segment depression.

In all normal subjects, the left ventricular ejection fraction increased more than 5%, end-diastolic volume increased less than 25%, and end-systolic volume decreased from rest to two levels of exercise. Wall motion was normal at rest and increased with exercise. No patient with coronary artery disease had chest pain or S-T segment depression during the first level of exercise. The ejection fraction decreased or increased less than 5% in 18 patients, end-diastolic volume increased more than 25% in 9, end-systolic volume increased in 19, and a segmental contraction abnormality developed in 14. Hemodynamic and wall motion abnormalities occurred in all patients during the second level of exercise when S-T segment depression was present. The 25 patients with coronary artery disease and the 10 normal subjects had comparable mean heart rates and blood pressures at rest. During both levels of exercise, heart rate was significantly faster in patients than in normal subjects. Although mean stroke volume and stroke work progressively increased in both groups during exercise, 6 patients with coronary artery disease had an actual decrease in stroke volume from rest to the second level of exercise (Fig 3–12). Stroke volume and stroke work were not significantly different in the two groups at rest or during the lower level of exercise. However, the mean stroke volume was slightly higher in the normal subjects at the higher exercise level.

The significant abnormalities in left ventricular function that were detected by radionuclide angiocardiography occurred in most patients before clinical symptoms or ECG evidence of myocardial ischemia. By the time the ECG showed S-T segment depression, all patients had wall motion abnormalities and significant hemodynamic alterations. Angina pectoris and S-T segment shifts are frequently late signs of myocardial ischemia, and noninvasive radionuclide angiocardiography may be used to detect myocardial ischemia in patients suspected of having coronary artery disease.

▶ [Most investigators recognize that readily detected anginal pain is often a late manifestation of exercise-induced myocardial ischemia, not appearing until there is gross S-T segment depression. The present authors suggest that the S-T response is itself a late indicator relative to functional data obtained by radionuclide angiocardiograms. Phenomena such as a decreasing ejection fraction and increases of end-systolic and end-diastolic volumes certainly suggest that the myocardium is becoming hypoxic, but given the 20-year age difference between "coronary" and "normal" subjects, it may be rash to assume that such hypoxia is always pathologic. Another recent paper on this topic (Caldwell, J. H., et al.: *Circulation* 61:610–619, 1980) has concluded that radionuclide ventriculography has a high sensitivity but a poor specificity in detecting significant coronary vascular disease.—R.J.S.] ◀

3–61 **Automated and Nomographic Analysis of Exercise Tests.** Recently, manufacturers of exercise testing equipment have developed and marketed small computer systems that analyze exercise-induced S-T segment changes. Michael H. Sketch, Syed M. Mohiuddin, Chandra K. Nair, Aryan N. Mooss, and Vincent Runco (Creighton Univ., Omaha) evaluated a commercially available, automated exercise ECG analysis system in 107 patients referred for evaluation of chest pain and derived a nomogram to estimate the severity of coronary artery disease. The results of coronary arteriography, visual analysis of 12-lead ECGs and ECG lead V_5, and automated analysis of ECG lead V_5 were correlated.

The S-T integrals of $+5$ through -6 μV-s were definitive of a negative test. Automated analysis of V_5 after exercise had virtually the same sensitivity, specificity, and predictive value as visual analysis ($P<.05$ Fig 3–13). However, this close correlation was not observed using integrals recorded during exercise. As with visual analysis of

(3–61) J.A.M.A. 243:1052–1055, Mar. 14, 1980.

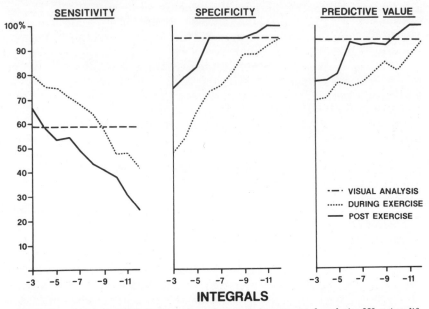

Fig 3–13.—Comparison of during-exercise and postexercise automated analysis of V_5 using different S-T integrals for cutoff of normality. Values for visual analysis were derived from postexercise V_5 ECGs. (Courtesy of Sketch, M. H., et al.: J.A.M.A. 243:1052–1055, Mar. 14, 1980; copyright 1980, American Medical Association.)

exercise-induced S-T segment changes, there was a relatively high number of false negative results with automated analysis. However, patients with false negative tests had significantly less (P<.01) severe coronary artery disease than those with true positive tests. Using multiple-regression analysis of the severity index, duration of exercise, and the most negative exercise-induced S-T integrals of ECG lead V_5, a regression formula was derived that made it possible to differentiate mild and severe disease.

Although automated analysis of the S-T integral is valid and provides useful information, it should not be assumed that automated analysis obviates the need for visual analysis of exercise tests and physician evaluation of other factors related to coronary artery disease.

▶ [By suitable adjustment of the cutoff point, the automated system has a sensitivity and a specificity almost equal to that of direct inspection of the ECG record. However, the physician must still examine the tracing to pick out such features as arrhythmias, conduction defects, S-T segment elevation, and changes in R wave amplitude.— R.J.S.] ◀

3–62 **Clinical Value of Early Exercise Testing After Myocardial Infarction.** Currently, there are few objective guidelines to identify patients at risk during convalescence after myocardial infarction. Robert A. Stein, William Walsh, Florence Frank, Antoine Fernaine, and

(3–62) Arch. Intern. Med. 140:1179–1181, September 1980.

Norman Krasnow (SUNY, Downstate Med. Center) prospectively assessed the clinical usefulness of predischarge exercise ECGs in 47 patients a mean of 17 days after myocardial infarction. Each subject was rated by the resident and attending physician as to anticipated exercise capacity, angina, and ventricular arrhythmias during moderate exercise. Anticipated discharge drug regimens and activity loads of convalescence were also listed. The graded-interval ergometric exercise protocol was terminated when the exercise protocol was completed (450 kilopondmeters per minute; approximately 5 mets, oxygen cost), 75% of the age-predicted maximum heart rate was attained, or established clinical conditions appeared. Convalescent regimens were altered on the basis of test results.

No complications were observed during evaluation. Of 31 patients who completed the exercise protocol, 25 were correctly rated by both the resident and attending physician. Because of limited exercise tolerance, 6 patients were given more restricted convalescent programs. Nine patients reported anginal pain during exercise; in 5 of these patients this was not anticipated. Severe arrhythmias were observed in 10 patients; 4 of these were already receiving antiarrhythmia medication. Of the other 6 patients with arrhythmias, 3 were anticipated by both the resident and attending physician. As a result of testing, the convalescent regimens of 22 (47%) of the patients were changed. It is noted that the patients were less anxious about exercising on a cycle ergometer than on a motor-driven treadmill.

It is concluded that predischarge exercise testing provides the clinician with relevant objective information not obtainable from history and physical examination. The routine use of predischarge exercise ECG testing, when not contraindicated, is recommended.

▶ [Exercise testing is important in identifying those predisposed to coronary artery disease. It is of obvious importance after myocardial infarction in identifying those in whom the convalescent activities have to be modified or, conversely, the subgroup that can be exercised progressively as a therapeutic modality and in the course of a return to normal physiologic function.

This study advances the concept of predischarge treadmill testing, assessing this prospectively in 47 patients approximately 2 weeks after the initial infarction. No significant complications were experienced. The testing served to limit exercise as a predictor in 6 patients. In clinical practice, this is becoming a very common phenomenon and a definite option of practical significance prior to patient discharge.—L.J.K.] ◄

3–63 **Serial Ambulatory Electrocardiography and Treadmill Exercise Testing After Uncomplicated Myocardial Infarction.** Treadmill exercise testing has been found to elicit prognostically important ventricular ectopic activity in selected patients soon after myocardial infarction. However, this testing method has been withheld from patients with clinically significant left ventricular dysfunction because of the potential risks. Robert F. DeBusk, Dennis M. Davidson, Nancy Houston, and John Fitzgerald (Stanford Univ.) compared the diagnostic and prognostic value of ambulatory electrocardiography and treadmill exercise testing in 90 men who had been treated for acute myocardial infarction. The patients, none of whom had clinically

(3–63) Am. J. Cardiol. 45:547–554, March 1980.

significant deterioration of left ventricular function, were tested at 3, 11, 26, and 52 weeks after the episode. Ambulatory electrocardiography was performed at the end of exercise testing.

The prevalence of any treadmill-induced premature ventricular complex increased significantly, from 42% at 3 weeks to 53% at 11 weeks, but it was relatively constant thereafter. The prevalence of any premature ventricular complex detected by ambulatory electrocardiography ranged from 77% to 83%; no significant changes were found in subsequent tests. The prevalence of premature ventricular complexes induced by exercise ranged from 25% to 31%, whereas the prevalence recorded by ambulatory electrocardiography ranged from 33% at 3 weeks to 53% at 11 weeks. The peak frequency of premature ventricular contractions on treadmill tests and in ambulatory electrocardiograms did not change significantly during the year after infarction. Coronary events occurring within 2 years of infarction were significantly associated with ischemic S-T segment depression of 0.2 mV or greater or a peak work load of less than four multiples of resting energy expenditure on the treadmill test at 3 weeks. However, the presence of premature ventricular complexes during exercise or ambulatory electrocardiography at any time was not predictive of coronary events.

Ambulatory electrocardiography seems to be the better technique in patients with clinical heart failure. However, in patients without clinical heart failure, treadmill testing may be preferable when performed as soon as 3 weeks after uncomplicated myocardial infarction, because it may yield prognostic information not available from ambulatory electrocardiography.

▶ [Plainly, there are advantages in distinguishing high-risk patients soon after infarction. Such persons can progress more cautiously in exercise programs and receive closer monitoring of drug dosages and early consideration for surgical treatment if their condition is deteriorating. Unfortunately, many of the patients suspected to be at high risk are not good candidates for stress testing, and it has thus been suggested that ambulatory monitoring be used as an alternative. These authors were unable to deduce prognostically valuable information from the ambulatory record of premature ventricular contractions, pointing out the need to accept the risks of stress testing.— R.J.S.] ◀

3-64 **Electrocardiographic Exercise Testing and Ambulatory Monitoring to Identify Patients With Ischemic Heart Disease at High Risk of Sudden Death.** Ambulatory ECG monitoring and exercise testing provide different information regarding the electrophysiologic state of the myocardium. The finding of ventricular extrasystoles may have different implications regarding the degree to which the patient with ischemic heart disease is at risk of sudden death depending on which technique has been used. Ljudmila A. Ivanova, Nikolai A. Mazur, Tatiana M. Smirnova, Alexander B. Sumarokov, Vladimir A. Nazarenko, and Elena A. Svet (USSR Acad. of Med. Sciences, Moscow) assessed the prognostic value of ambulatory ECG monitoring (Holter monitoring) and exercise testing in 144 men with

(3–64)   Am. J. Cardiol. 45:1132–1138, June 1980.

PROGNOSTIC SIGNIFICANCE OF BIVARIATES FOR SUDDEN DEATH WITHIN
TWO YEARS OF FOLLOW-UP STUDY

Bivariate	2×2 Matrix (number of patients)		Predictive Accuracy (%)	Risk Ratio	Sensitivity (%)	Specificity (%)	Chi Square
HR & ST	6	13	32	10	60	90	16.40*
	4	121					
HR & ET$_2$	4	5	44	10	40	96	15.16*
	6	129					
ET$_2$ V PM$_4$	8	32	20	10	80	76	11.94*
	2	102					
ET$_2$ & ST	3	5	38	7	30	96	7.74†
	7	129					
ET$_2$ V PM$_5$	5	17	23	5	50	87	7.33†
	5	117					
HR & PM$_3$	6	26	19	5	60	75	6.68†
	4	108					
ST & PM$_3$	5	19	21	5	50	86	6.21‡
	5	115					
HR & PM$_4$	3	8	27	5	30	94	4.59§
	7	126					
PM$_3$ V PM$_4$	9	67	13	8	90	50	4.48§
	1	67					
ST V PM$_5$	7	45	13	4	70	66	3.89§
	3	89					

*$P < .001$.
†$P < .01$.
‡$P < .02$.
§$P < .05$.
Note: PM$_5$ indicates grade 5 ventricular extrasystoles during prolonged monitoring; V, symbol of inclusive disjunction; &, symbol of conjunction; HR, maximal exercise heart rate not greater than 115 beats/minute; ET$_2$, grade 2 ventricular extrasystoles during exercise test; PM$_4$, grade 4 ventricular extrasystoles during prolonged monitoring; ST, depression of S-T segment during exercise test; PM$_3$, grade 3 ventricular extrasystoles during prolonged monitoring.

established ischemic heart disease. All monitoring and exercise variables were analyzed by prognostic stratification in which all univariates were used to establish all the possible bivariates and trivariates.

During a 2-year follow-up period, 12 deaths were reported, 10 of which occurred suddenly. Univariates strongly associated with sudden death were reduced maximal exercise heart rate, frequent exercise-induced ventricular arrhythmias, exercise-induced S-T segment depression, and grades 3 and 4 ventricular extrasystoles revealed by 24-hour Holter monitoring. Conjunction and inclusive disjunction of these variables were used to identify groups of patients at very high and very low risk of sudden death. Bivariates associated with a 10-fold increase in sudden death were grade 2 ventricular extrasystoles induced by exercise terminated at a heart rate of 115 beats per minute or less and S-T segment depression during exercise testing terminated at a heart rate of 115 beats per minute or less ($P < .001$; table). The best prognostic stratification was found using inclusive disjunction of exercise-induced grade 2 ventricular extrasystoles and grade 4 extrasystoles detected by Holter monitoring in conjunction with reduced maximal exercise heart rate ($P < .001$). A reduced maximal exercise heart rate by itself did not constitute an independent risk factor for sudden death. However, in 3 patients with reduced maximal exercise heart rate and frequent ventricular extrasystoles and S-T segment depression induced by exercise, the death rate was 100%. Patients at very high risk were identified by combinations of exercise variables, while those at very low risk tended to have combinations of monitoring variables.

The results indicate that ambulatory ECG monitoring and exercise testing provide different prognostic information that may be complementary in identifying patients at high risk of sudden cardiac death.

▶ [This report is interesting in showing the similarity of concerns of cardiologists in the United States and the Soviet Union. The authors adopted a multivariate approach. Using this technique, they found that Holter monitoring added to the prognostic information provided by stress testing alone. (This stands in contrast to the view of DeBusk et al. in the preceding article.) Unlike some American reports, the best combination of variables (exercise premature ventricular contractions, Holter premature ventricular contractions and low maximum heart rate) did not include S-T segmental depression.—R.J.S.] ◀

3-65 **Exercise Testing in the Geriatric Patient** is discussed by Lawrence J. Laslett, Ezra A. Amsterdam, and Dean T. Mason. Exercise stress testing in geriatric patients has been somewhat controversial because of possible risks, but all patients should be evaluated as individuals, and there is no evidence that age alone increases the risk of stress testing. The most common indication is the possibility of ischemic heart disease. Many geriatric patients with valvular disease deserve a consideration of surgical correction, as do those with aortic stenosis. Exercise testing is of importance in establishing the level of activity that is safe relative to provocation of arrhythmias. The stress test is the key to prescribing training programs in the rehabilitation of patients with coronary disease. Exercise testing in patients with peripheral vascular disease can determine the degree of functional limitation.

Older patients may not be comfortable with standard treadmill protocols. A protocol starting at a lower work load and increased more gradually, such as that of Chung, may be more useful than the Bruce protocol. The Patterson protocol is even easier. Some flexibility in the use of these protocols is permissible without jeopardizing the standardization of results in terms of work load achieved. A cycle ergometer may provide an alternative to some elderly patients who fear the treadmill or are unsteady. Early fatigue and light-headedness due to deconditioning and vasoregulatory inefficiency must be kept in

(3–65) IM, pp. 53–61, September 1980.

mind in testing elderly subjects. Significant calcific aortic stenosis may prevent an appropriate systolic pressure rise with exercise.

Geriatric patients should be considered for exercise stress testing on the basis of the same criteria as those used in any other age group, but particular attention should be given with regard to the flexible use of exercise protocols, coaching and reassurance, and maintenance of alertness for any difficulties. In this way, safe and informative stress testing can be performed on most elderly patients.

▶ [There was an initial concern that exercise stress testing in the geriatric patient might be associated with an increased frequency of complications. This has been shown not to be the case if common sense, modified protocols, and a certain flexibility are applied. It should be pointed out that this is a very positive and necessary use of stress testing because this group of patients often has coronary artery disease, and it has exactly the same implications in terms of diagnosis and prognosis for recovery from coronary artery events. I think it may be even more important to identify the subtleties of activity that may be permitted the elderly. It should be noted that a cycle ergometer can be a sturdier platform for some elderly people than a treadmill, especially in the setting of unstable back, knee, or hip disease.—L.J.K.] ◀

EXERCISE THERAPY

3-66 **Walking for Fitness: Slow but Sure.** A regular, vigorous program of walking has been shown to exert a training effect. Paul Schultz has reviewed the literature on health benefits of walking.

Walking can be of significant aerobic value. It has been shown to increase maximum oxygen uptake, decrease heart rates and resting blood pressure, and decrease body weight and percent of body fat. It is estimated that one has to walk for 1 hour at a rate of 3.5 mph to improve fitness. At a rate of more than 3.7 mph, the energy required for walking increases exponentially. Since there is an apparent tendency to break into a jog because of the biomechanics of walking at 4–4.5 mph, a walk-jog regimen may be helpful for some persons. Variations in grade, terrain, and weight carried can affect the amount of energy expended.

Guidelines of the American College of Sports Medicine and the American Heart Association for prescribing walking as an exercise are briefly reviewed.

▶ ↓ The following study by Schoenfeld et al. not only has a precise group of controlled subjects, but used differential backpack loading. Doubling the load during the fourth week for a study group improved aerobic capacity almost twofold. It is of marked significance, I think, that this study demonstrates that participants with a lower initial level of physical fitness are going to have more improvement in $Vo_{2\,max}$ than subjects who start with a higher level of fitness. Walking has the salutary benefit of being much kinder to aging joints and is much more readily accepted by the nonathlete and by those not naturally attuned to running. Face it. Running is not easy. It is basically for the lean and those with sturdy joints. Most others tend to be early dropouts from any long-range program. Add to these facts our knowledge that it is not what you do but how long you do it that really counts in terms of exercise benefits and even caloric expenditure. Walking has much to recommend it.—L.J.K. ◀

3-67 **Walking: Method for Rapid Improvement of Physical Fitness.** Physical fitness programs have not induced most people to be physi-

---

(3–66) Physician Sportsmed. 8:24–27, September 1980.
(3–67) J.A.M.A. 243:2062–2063, May 23/30, 1980.

cally active. Some activities, such as jogging, are unsuitable for many people and harmful for some. Yehuda Shoenfeld, Gad Keren, Tuvia Shimoni, Chaim Birnfeld, and Ezra Sohar (Tel-Aviv Univ.) examined the efficacy of walking with a backpack load as a method for improving physical fitness.

Forty-four sedentary men with a mean age of 19 years (range, 18–23 years), mean height of 178 cm, and mean weight of 76 kg walked at a speed of 5 km/hour with a 3-kg backpack load for 30 minutes a day, 5 days a week, for 3 weeks. At this time, 32 (group A) terminated the experiment and 12 continued to march for another week: 6 (group B) had the same backpack load and 6 (group C) had a load of 6 kg.

By the end of the 3- to 4-week experiment, predicted aerobic work capacity had increased by 15% in the 32 men in group A, by 18% in the 6 men in group B, and by 32% in the 6 men in group C. An improvement in predicted aerobic work capacity of more than 20% occurred in 34% of the men in group A, 50% of those in group B, and 67% of those in group C. A comparison of results for 7 men from group A with low initial physical fitness and for 7 with high initial fitness showed an increase in predicted aerobic work capacity of 30.4% in the former group and of only 2.7% in the latter group. An increase in work capacity of more than 20% was noted in 4 of 7 men with low initial fitness and in none of the 7 with high initial fitness.

It is possible to substantially improve aerobic physical fitness in just 3 weeks by walking daily with a light backpack load. This program is most useful for people who have low initial aerobic work capacity. Walking is relatively safe. It can easily become a way of life and be recommended as a popular method of physical activity, even for elderly people. The main determinant of the rapid increase in aerobic work capacity is apparently the increase of the weight of the backpack load, rather than speed or duration of walking.

▶ [Backpacks are becoming a more acceptable feature of urban life-style, particularly among the young. The executive who walks to the station in the morning gets valuable exercise, but carrying his books and papers in an attaché case places an asymmetric load on the spine. A backpack would be a much more physiologic approach to the morning "constitutional."—R.J.S.] ◀

3–68 **Losing Weight Through Exercise.** Barry A. Franklin and Melvyn Rubenfire (Wayne State Univ.) discuss exercise myths and misconceptions, along with gimmicks, gadgets, and fads promoted as "miracle" agents to reduce body weight.

To discount that exercise requires relatively little caloric expenditure, it can be noted that laborers, soldiers, and endurance athletes can consume about 6,000 calories (kcal) daily, yet remain thin. To discount that "a pound of fat can be worked off by splitting wood for 7 hours," it is noted that the calorie-expending effects of exercise are cumulative, and if the 7 hours of chopping are divided into 20 minutes daily, 0.45 kg of fat could be lost in just 21 days (or 7.65 kg in 1 year).

(3–68) J.A.M.A. 244:377–379, July 25, 1980.

Another misconception is that exercise stimulates the appetite, making food intake equal to or greater in energy value than the energy cost of the exercise. However, rats exercised for 1 hour daily show lower than normal food intake and body weight. Research with human subjects shows similar exercise-induced appetite suppression.

Walking, running, and bicycling are popular. Unless a person walks very slowly or runs very fast, the caloric cost per distance is relatively independent of speed. For a given distance, bicycling uses one half and one third of the kilocalories used for walking and running, respectively (Fig 3–14).

Passive exercise devices that "do the work for you" are promoted as effortless methods to reduce body weight. However, studies show that 307 periods of vibration of 15 minutes each are needed to lose 0.45 kg of fat. Special weight-reducing clothing and inflatable outfits rely chiefly on dehydration, localized pressure, or constriction of tissue.

Advocates of spot reduction believe that by exercising a specific body area, the fat in that area will be reduced. However, in accomplished tennis players, the arm circumferences in the playing (active) arm are greater than in the nonplaying arm, but there are no differences in fat deposits as assessed by subcutaneous skinfolds.

Exercise with or without caloric restriction offers advantages over dieting alone. It improves the function of the cardiorespiratory and muscular systems. It can be an enjoyable leisure time activity. Finally, weight loss through exercise consists primarily of fat as opposed to the water loss or loss of vital lean tissue that can occur with "fad" diets.

Exercise therapy for obesity should be of long duration, use large muscle groups, be maintained continuously, and be rhythmic and aerobic in nature. Stored carbohydrates provide almost all of the energy needed for short periods of high-intensity exercise, but after 30 minutes of exercise, stored fat provides most of the energy; thus the "long slow distance" concept is important when fat is the energy substrate of choice. The minimal threshold of exercise for fat loss includes continuous exercise lasting at least 20–30 minutes with an intensity sufficient to expend 300 kcal or more per session and carried

Fig 3–14.—Gross energy requirement for 1.6 km. (Courtesy of Franklin, B. A., and Rubenfire, M.: J.A.M.A. 244:377–379, July 25, 1980; copyright 1980, American Medical Association.)

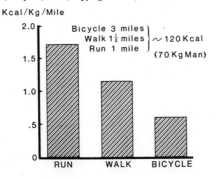

out at least 3 days per week. Exercise programs performed twice a week are relatively ineffective in reducing fat regardless of intensity or duration. Incorporating a regular exercise program into an otherwise hypokinetic life-style is not enough. Patients should increase physical activity in everyday living, for example by parking the car farther away from stores, using manual rather than power tools, using stairs instead of elevators, eliminating home extension telephones, and making other energy-requiring substitutions.

▶ [I like this paper because, while not profound, it deals with many of the misconceptions that come up relative to exercise, caloric intake, and weight loss. It lays many common misconceptions to rest and would be nice to have in pamphlet form for broad distribution. Perhaps a single point that I should reiterate is that if one decreases an exercise program to 2 days or less a week, it is going to be relatively ineffective in reducing body weight and fat stores. It is also important to recognize that the incorporation of a regular exercise program into an otherwise sedentary life-style is not enough and that changes in attitude and behavior are important. If one is really serious and exercises vigorously, there is a built-in dividend that I think is more effective than usually is appreciated in terms of an automatic decrease of appetite and intake. This may be why exercise is effective for weight loss if it is carried out methodically and at a realistic level of intensity.—L.J.K.] ◀

▶ [I have had occasion to investigate certain types of weight-reducing clothing for the Canadian Ministry of Consumer Affairs, pending the laying of legal charges for false advertising. The garments were flimsy pieces of plastic that very quickly disintegrated, and the decrease of body dimensions claimed could not have been produced even by adding together decreases in circumferences at a multiplicity of measuring sites. The companies concerned tend to operate out of "box offices" and are difficult to bring to prosecution.—R.J.S.] ◀

3-69 **Importance of Sport and Physical Training in Preventive Cardiology** is discussed by W. Hollmann, R. Rost, and H. Liesen.

Coordination, or the standard of functioning of the central nervous system and of the skeletal muscles during a given movement, can be improved by training. This will improve the performance of patients with peripheral arterial diseases or coronary insufficiency by lowering the oxygen requirement of the muscles for a given submaximal performance.

Flexibility, or the maximum amount of movement voluntarily attainable in joints, can be increased through appropriate exercise. In this way, patients with degenerative joint changes can regain greater flexibility and the elderly can maintain sufficient flexibility to cope with everyday life.

Strength is the muscle tension that can be voluntarily developed against a fixed resistance in a given position. Static and dynamic strength can be increased by training. This may prevent posture anomalies from developing, reduce the effects of existing degenerative joint changes, and enable even the elderly to maintain muscle efficiency. Strength training does not stimulate the cardiopulmonary system.

Speed refers to the degree of quickness in any cyclic movement. Speed training has no significant effect on the cardiopulmonary system. In the elderly or in persons with organic lesions, speed training may be hazardous.

(3–69) J. Sports Med. Phys. Fitness 20:5–12, March 1980.

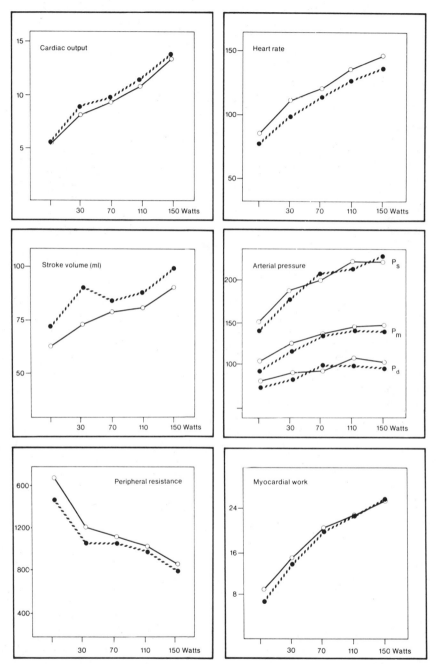

Fig 3–15.—Behavior of hemodynamics before and after 10-week endurance training of elderly men. (Cardio-Green method). (Courtesy of Hollmann, W., et al.: J. Sports Med. Phys. Fitness 20: 5–12, March 1980.)

Endurance is the ability to maintain a given level of work for a long time. Of its eight different forms, general aerobic endurance is of particular importance to health. This can be increased by carrying out dynamic work by large groups of muscles for at least 10, and preferably 30–45, uninterrupted minutes. In healthy men and women younger than age 50 years, work intensity should be high enough to produce a pulse rate of 130–150 beats per minute; in those older than age 50 years, a pulse rate during training of 180 minus the age in years should be reached. Exercise at these levels should be carried out daily or at least 3–4 times a week.

Exercise-induced improvement of general aerobic endurance comes about via an increase in cardiopulmonary and metabolic efficiency and economization of all circulatory and respiratory processes. Resting cardiac frequency is reduced. Exercised muscles show better capillarization and improved oxygen diffusion. Peripheral metabolic adaptations include increased myoglobin level, increased activity of aerobic enzymes, increased intramuscular glycogen level, and nearly unchanged cardiac output (Fig 3–15). In this way, it may be possible to obtain relative protection against the effects of existing degenerative cardiovascular changes.

▶ [Most authors believe that the *maximum* cardiac output increases roughly in proportion with the gain of maximum oxygen intake during training. It is in submaximum work that the cardiac output shows little change.—R.J.S.] ◀

3–70 **Exercise for Postcoronary Patients: Assessment of Infrequent Supervision.** There is evidence that prolonged, supervised, graded physical activity aids rehabilitation after myocardial infarction and may reduce the risk of reinfarction, but substantial personnel and facilities are needed in such efforts. Terence Kavanagh and Roy J. Shephard (Univ. of Toronto) assessed a "tapered" program in which postcoronary patients are required to sustain an exercise regimen after a year of training in a medically supervised program, with reinforcing visits to a rehabilitation center at 2-month intervals. Thirty of 49 study patients appeared to have reached a plateau of training after attending weekly exercise sessions for about a year, whereas 19 were still improving when transferred to the 2-month program. Thirty-one other patients continued regular weekly attendance in the second year of follow-up.

Most patients were thought to have made useful but not dramatic gains in aerobic power on initial rehabilitation. Ten patients were judged as noncompliant with experimental rehabilitative efforts, but their weekly mileages and pulse rates were not much poorer than those reported by the other subjects. Twenty-three other patients sustained their level of cardiorespiratory fitness, whereas 16 showed small continuing gains in aerobic power. Some subjects who regressed reported having missed the encouragement of group members and the discipline of regular observation and complained that suitable facilities were lacking in their area of residence.

(3–70) Arch. Phys. Med. Rehabil. 61:114–118, March 1980.

Infrequent supervision of postcoronary rehabilitation was safe in this study, but its therapeutic efficacy was doubtful. Gains in aerobic power were small, compared with those in patients managed in the standard supervised manner. Patients who are confident that they can exercise may be most suitable for infrequently supervised programs. Psychotherapy may be a useful preliminary to transfer of a patient to a program of infrequently supervised exercise.

▶ [This is an important study, I think, pointing out that human nature, predictably, will out. As a patient group leaves the discipline of close supervision, the discipline may well be lost, the effectiveness and significant statistical gains of a program may suffer accordingly, and one gets the feeling that the whole sense of mission may be defused. In this study of 49 patients where follow-up became deliberately intermittent, with personal activity prescription and physician supervision once every 8 weeks, 20% demonstrated a deterioration of cardiorespiratory fitness over the ensuing year and the therapeutic effectiveness was doubtful in some of the other patients in terms of gains of aerobic power and some objective evidence of deterioration of exercise cardiogram. The similarity to what is observed in weight-losing groups or alcohol-abstinence groups is obvious. The possible conclusion that can be drawn is that the highly motivated persons, as in any area, are defined by their own self-sufficiency. For the rest, who are more prone to herd instinct patterns of behavior and deviance, ongoing closer supervision may be the unfortunate necessity, with all that it implies in terms of expense and compliance.—L.J.K.] ◀

3–71 **Long-Term Effects of Physical Training Program on Risk Factors for Coronary Heart Disease in Otherwise Sedentary Men.** Although favorable associations between physical fitness and risk factors for coronary disease have been reported, the protective effect of physical activity in itself has yet to be elucidated. Anthony W. Sedgwick, John R. Brotherhood, Ann Harris-Davidson, Roger E. Taplin, and David W. Thomas (Adelaide, Australia) evaluated the effects of a physical fitness intervention program on "classic" risk factors for coronary heart disease in 370 sedentary men, aged 20 to 65 years, 5 years after initial intervention.

Analysis of the group as a whole and in 10-year age groups showed no significant difference in any measurement between the initial and the final examination. Nonetheless, several individual changes were observed. Twenty-eight percent of the men lost more than 2 kg, whereas 27% gained more than 2 kg. Although overall smoking was unchanged, light and moderate smokers tended to smoke less or stop altogether. Except for a slight reduction in type IV hyperlipoproteinemia, there was little overall change in serum lipid values. On the basis of a questionnaire, 339 of the men were classified as being active or inactive; 34% were active. The mean working capacity of the inactive men had fallen to preintervention values, but it was 17% higher in the active group. There were no significant changes in physical risk factors and smoking habits between the two groups. Regression analysis showed that the percentage of risk factor variance accounted for by the change in fitness was close to zero for systolic and diastolic blood pressure, serum cholesterol concentration, and Quetelet's index and was 1.06 for serum triglyceride concentration.

(3–71) Br. Med. J. 2:7–10, July 5, 1980.

The results do not support the view that risk factors for coronary heart disease in healthy men are improved by taking up regular aerobic exercise, though physical fitness may be increased. Since no direct observations of heart disease were made, the possibility that physical activity protects against heart disease cannot be dismissed.

▶ [Several authors have recently indicated a disappointing long-term response to fitness programs. The present study was conducted with a relatively receptive group (volunteers, 95% of whom had "white-collar" or administrative occupations). After a 12-week fitness program, they were encouraged to exercise on their own. The 34% who were initially active sustained a 17% increase of physical working capacity over a 5-year period, but the remainder showed no change. Neither active nor inactive subjects showed any consistent long-term change in cardiovascular risk factors. Plainly, there is a need for much stronger reinforcement programs or changes of societal attitudes before patients can be expected to continue a healthy life-style introduced to them at a 3-month fitness class.—R.J.S.] ◀

3–72 **Vigorous Exercise in Leisure-Time: Protection Against Coronary Heart Disease.** J. N. Morris, M. G. Everitt, R. Pollard, S. P. W. Chave, and A. M. Semmence (London) examined the incidence of coronary heart disease (CHD) in relation to vigorous leisure-time exercise in a population of sedentary workers. A total of 1,138 first clinical episodes of CHD occurred in 17,944 middle-aged male office workers in Britain between 1968 and 1970. These men, white-collar workers of executive grade, represented 86% of those eligible for study. Average follow-up was $8^{1}/_{2}$ years. Vigorous exercise was defined as activities likely to produce peaks of energy expenditure of 7.5 kcal/minute, a threshold equivalent to heavy industrial work.

Vigorously exercising individuals had lower rates of fatal and nonfatal primary CHD events (table). At ages 40–65 years, fatal first heart attacks occurred less than half as frequently in active men. The rise in mortality with increasing age was small in active men, an

VIGOROUS EXERCISE (VE) AND INCIDENCE OF CORONARY HEART
DISEASE (CHD) IN MALE EXECUTIVE-GRADE CIVIL SERVANTS*
First attacks CHD 1968–78

	All men		Reporting VE sports		Reporting no VE	
Clinical presentation	Cases	Rate %	Cases	Rate %	Cases	Rate %
Total incidence†	1138	6·3	66	3·1	981	6·9
Fatal first attacks:						
40–49*	138	1·6	9	0·8	115	1·7
50–54	129	2·7	8	1·3	109	2·9
55–65	208	4·5	7	1·5	187	5·0
40–65†	475	2·6	24	1·1	411	2·9
Non-fatal first attacks						
40–49	243	2·9	22	2·0	195	3·0
50–54	192	4·0	12	1·9	167	4·4
55–65	228	5·0	8	1·7	208	5·6
40–65†	663	3·7	42	2·0	570	4·0

*Ages of men and report of exercise at survey, 1968 to 1970.
†Rates standardized for age by conventional indirect method.

(3–72) Lancet 2:1207–1210, Dec. 6, 1980.

effect that continued into early old age. The effect of vigorous exercise was independent of a family history of premature cardiovascular mortality, physique, and cigarette smoking habits. There was no indication that the "effect" of vigorous exercise was the result of active men being younger or taller, or being nonsmokers.

Adequate exercise may be postulated to be one of the body's defenses. "Adequate" exercise connotes dynamic aerobic activity involving the free movement of large muscle groups above the intensity required for a training effect. Central and peripheral cardiovascular efficiency, and perhaps coronary flow, appear to be enhanced by vigorous activity. The evidence that ectopic beats are fewer in active men may indicate lesser myocardial sensitivity. Those men in the present population who engaged in vigorous activity and did not smoke had a rate of fatal first heart attacks about 20% of that observed in nonexercising men who smoked cigarettes.

▶ [A more enthusiastic position than in some other papers is presented in this article, which argues that vigorous exercise confers some protection in all categories—in obesity, in short stature, in those predisposed to coronary artery disease, and in smokers. The general thrust of these data may be true, but the reservations are still appropriate.—L.J.K.] ◀

3–73 **Sports for the Physically Disabled: The 1976 Olympiad (Toronto).** The first international sporting event for physically disabled persons was held in 1952 at Stoke Mandeville Hospital in England, and in 1956 the Stoke Mandeville Games were formally recognized by the International Olympic Committee. Twenty years later, the first Olympiad for the Physically Disabled was held in Toronto. Robert W. Jackson and Alix Fredrickson (Toronto Western Hosp.) report various medical aspects of the event.

The 1976 Olympiad was the first international event with full competition for blind, paralyzed, and amputee athleees. More than 1,500 athletes from 38 countries participated in wheelchair games (12 events), blind games (8 events), and amputee games (11 events). An international team of physicians carefully evaluated the degree of disability of the athletes to permit fair and equal competition. The athletes were accommodated in university housing and transported 15 miles a day to the games site. Small infirmaries were available at the residences. Also, near the games site a school was converted into a field hospital and rest areas were provided. All of the medical staff were volunteers. The field hospital was manned for two shifts daily, each staffed by at least 3 physicians, 3 nurses, 3 receptionists, and 3 physical therapists. In addition, 2 physicians, 4 or more trainers, 2 nurses, and 2 physical therapists rotated around various venues of the games site. Physicians treated 285 patients, 184 of whom were athletes, for various problems. Sixty physical therapists treated 119 athletes and 20 trainers treated 114 participants. It was apparent that the physically disabled athletes were slightly more vulnerable to stress and fatigue than able-bodied athletes.

(3–73) Am. J. Sports Med. 7:293 ·296, Sept.–Oct. 1979.

Until the 1976 Olympiad, disabled athletes faced several problems: they were not regarded as serious competitors by the press and the general public; they did not have easy access to suitable training facilities; and chances for competition were few. However, the Toronto Olympiad showed that sports for the disabled has evolved from a purely rehabilitative activity to a true sporting event.

▶ [Hopefully, the attitudes of those involved with sports medicine programs have advanced to a position of total acceptance of sports for the physically disabled. These people can become outstanding athletes and enjoy athletics as much or more than any other athlete. Athletics can be a major portion of their lives, even more so than with others who have many more options from which to choose. We should provide as much support and as many opportunities as possible for the physically disabled to become involved with athletics.—F.G.] ◀

3-74 **Physical Education: Integrating the Handicapped.** David Cushing reviews developments in the integration of the handicapped into physical education programs in the wake of the Rehabilitation Act of 1973 and the Education for All Handicapped Children Act of 1975, or Public Law 94-142 (PL 94-142), and discusses the role of the physician in these programs.

Section 504 of the Rehabilitation Act guarantees the civil rights of the handicapped, whereas PL 94-142 guarantees equal opportunities for educational services to handicapped children of school age, who are estimated to number 4 million to 8 million. Public Law 94-142 is designed to move handicapped children from special schools to public school settings under the provisions of the Individualized Education Program (IEP). The IEP provides for special education and related services, including medical and nonmedical evaluations and psychological services. Integration of handicapped individuals into normal physical education classes will rely heavily on the physicians' evaluation and advice regarding acceptance into the program and the kind and amount of physical activity in which a handicapped child can engage. Some states have interpreted the PL 94-142 regulations in such a way that the physician is involved in a broad range of services for the handicapped. Ohio State University researchers recently completed official guidelines for implementing PL 94-142 that are, in part, intended to establish an organizational protocol between physicians and educators.

However, physical education is often ignored in favor of integrating the handicapped into the classroom, and medical attention to the physical education needs of these children is occasional at best. This may be, in part, because physicians are all too willing to excuse handicapped children from physical education classes. On the other hand, because the definitions are written so broadly, almost any child exhibiting normal adolescent behavior patterns can be defined as handicapped and so become eligible for the IEP. Because so many children are potentially eligible, it is feared that meeting the needs of the handicapped will bankrupt local school districts. This has not yet proved to be the case. Nonetheless, some believe that Section 504

(3-74) Physician Sportsmed. 8:121-125, January 1980.

and Pl 94-142 are the beginning of federal regulation of all medicine because they apply comprehensively to direct and indirect recipients of federal monies. There is also the fear that the schools will become the primary vehicle of medical care for not only handicapped children, but for all children. Despite the anticipated legal obstacles, an expanded commitment to professional training and a high degree of cooperation among physicians, educators, and the handicapped themselves are necessary to meet the law's requirements.

▶ [It is very easy to recommend athletic activity for the disabled such as that described in the preceding article. Those athletes are screened carefully and compete against those with similar levels of disability. The integration of the physically handicapped into physical education programs has not gone as well. I wish I had an answer to this problem. In general terms, the solution probably will be found through education and cooperation of all those involved.—F.G.] ◀

4. Sports Injury

4–1 **The Role of Orthopedic Surgery in Sports Medicine** is discussed by John A. Ogden (Yale Univ). Orthopedists and sports physicians have a role in helping each athlete, whether professional, amateur or "casual," to minimize debilitating injury and attain maximal benefit from a physical, musculoskeletal endeavor. Too often the relation of orthopedics to sports medicine connotes only one sport, football, and one location, the knee. This leads to a misconception of the role of orthopedic medicine and surgery in the overall realm of sports and of the appropriate interaction with other physicians and allied personnel concerned with the care of athletes.

Participation in sports is increasing with more leisure time available to Americans, and an increasing part of the population is being exposed to potential musculoskeletal injury. Knowledge of the mechanisms of injuries in a given sport will help prevent accidents and resulting damage. In some sports such as swimming there is more risk of repeated microtrauma than of acute gross trauma. Most young female gymnasts have abnormal lower back findings. Dancers as well as athletes may require orthopedic attention.

Further study is needed in the area of drug effects on the musculoskeletal system. The indiscriminate use of steroid injections is unwise. Further research is needed not only in the area of women's athletics but in the entire realm of muscle physiology as well. Youth represents a large segment of the athletic population, but understanding of many of the normal and abnormal effects of intensive athletic training and competition on the developing chondro-osseous skeleton is inadequate. Changes in equipment must take into account the possible effects on the rest of the "game." The overall goal is to recognize patterns of injury and develop ways of preventing them. The aim is to reintroduce athletes into activity as soon as feasible after injury without compromising excellent medical care.

▶ [The willingness of the author, an orthopedic surgeon, to look beyond sports medicine as it related to football, the knee, and professional athletics is noteworthy. His desire to consider injury prevention as a priority matter is also unique. Will such exceptional concepts find their place?—J.S.T.] ◀

4–2 **The Reality and Acceptance of Risk.** The taking of risks is an inevitable fact of life. Bertram D. Dinman (Pittsburgh) reports the risk of death for various voluntary activities, including some sports,

(4–1)   Yale J. Biol. Med. 53:281–288, July–Aug. 1980
(4–2)   J.A.M.A. 244:1226–1228, Sept. 12, 1980.

VOLUNTARY RISKS*

	Deaths/ Person/yr, Odds
Smoking, 20 cigarettes per day	1 in 200
Drinking, 1 bottle of wine per day	1 in 13,300
Soccer, football	1 in 25,000†
Automobile racing	1 in 10,000
Automobile driving (United Kingdom)	1 in 5,900†
Motorcycling	1 in 50
Rock climbing	1 in 7,150‡
Taking contraceptive pills	1 in 50,000
Power boating	1 in 5,900†
Canoeing	1 in 100,000‡
Horse racing	1 in 740†
Amateur boxing	1 in 2 million†
Professional boxing	1 in 14,300‡
Skiing	1 in 1,430,000‡
Pregnancy (United Kingdom)	1 in 4,350§
Abortion, legal, <12 wk	1 in 50,000§
Abortion, legal, >14 wk	1 in 5,900§

*All numerical data presented as rounded-off values.
†Based on deaths per million participants per year.
‡Based on deaths per million hours per year spent in sport.
§Based on deaths per million pregnancies per year.

and natural events and discusses factors involved in the assessment and interpretation of risks.

The odds of death occurring per person per year as a result of voluntary activity range from 1 in 50 for motorcycling to 1 in 2 million for amateur boxing (table). On the basis of efforts made to reduce hazards, it appears that the boundaries of acceptable risk are between 1:1,000,000 and 1:100. Society seems to accept voluntary risks of at least one order or magnitude greater than involuntary risks.

In our society, determination of what is safe is based on an objective, empirical data-based process of risk assessment, followed by a normative, subjective social determination of risk acceptability. Although the risk assessment process is often based on incomplete information and estimates, it can lead to statements of risk probabilities or odds ratios for common life activities.

▶ [This philosophical essay recognizes, "Most often the risk assessment process is based on incomplete information and estimate." The author's conclusion is appropriate: "Even a virtuous life has its risk, as illustrated by the Chinese proverb: 'The couple that goes to bed early to save candles ends up with twins.'"—J.S.T.] ◀

4–3 **Nonresponse in Sample Surveys: The Problem and Some Solutions.** Sample surveys are becoming increasingly common in phys-

(4–3) Phys. Ther. 60:1026–1032, August 1980.

ical therapy research, yet the problem of nonresponse has not been discussed in the literature. Donna R. Brogan (Emory Univ.) discusses the bias that can result from a low response rate in sample surveys and reviews some methods to increase response rates.

A larger sample size does not avoid the bias of nonresponse. Surveys involving more personal contact (e.g., telephone or personal interviews) are believed to produce a higher response rate than mail surveys alone. Combinations of these approaches can be used to increase the response rate; follow-up contact with nonrespondents also increases the response rate. A more intensive approach to nonresponse is to select a subsample of nonrespondents for an all-out follow-up effort. By using the weighted averages of the original respondents and the subsample response, an unbiased estimate of the overall population can be obtained. However, the expense of an all-out effort may be too great to assure that the subsample response will be representative of the entire group. Formulas have been developed for the variance of the weighted average, and for the estimated variance when the initial sample size is greater than 50.

It is recommended that subsampling of nonrespondents be used in sample surveys in which a large nonresponse rate is expected.

▶ [Although this article is found in the physical therapy literature, this isn't the only group that could benefit from this contribution. The technique described is not new; as the author aptly states," Although this technique was first proposed about 30 years ago . . . the method does not appear to be well known among researchers in general." The author presents examples to demonstrate how far off one can get by treating nonresponse as simply random and thus ignorable.—J.S.T.] ◀

4–4 **Bicycle Accidents and Injuries. Random Survey of A College Population.** The circumstances surrounding the occurrence of bicycle accidents in one area were studied by a review of police reports and medical records. Diana L. Kruse and Andrew A. McBeath (Univ. of Wisconsin) investigated the incidence of and injuries occurring in bicycle-related accidents by sending a questionnaire to 1,200 randomly selected college students who represented 3.1% of all students registered at the University of Wisconsin, Madison.

There were 856 (71%) respondents, over 60% of whom were cyclists. Of the bicyclers, 29% had been involved in an accident during the previous 3 years and 13% had an accident within the immediately preceding year. Roadway conditions were most frequently reported as the major contributing factor (52%), whereas the presence of another person was cited by 41% as a causative factor. The automobile was the major contributor to the accident in only 26% of incidents. Of those involved in accidents, 62% sustained an injury and 32% of these individuals sought medical attention. Only 8% of the accidents were reported to the police. It is projected that if public monies were spent to make bicycle-safe railroad crossings, to repair rough roads, and to install sewer gratings, 29% of these accidents could possibly have been prevented.

(4–4) Am. J. Sports Med. 8:342–344, Sept.–Oct. 1980.

It would appear that studies based on police or hospital records have underestimated the hazards and morbidity of bicycling.

▶ [This excellent study demonstrates that bicycle injury data based on police or hospital records underestimate the hazards and morbidity of this activity.—J.S.T.] ◀

4–5 **Bicycle Spoke Injuries.** Bicycle spoke injury occurs when a child sitting behind a parent adducts his thighs for a stable position on the seat and catches his legs, which are long enough to reach the wheel, in the spokes. Moshe Roffman, Moshe Moshel, and David G. Mendes (Rothschild Univ., Haifa, Israel) describe the mechanism of injury, treatment, and outcome in 25 children aged $2^{1}/_{2}$–4 years who suffered a variety of bicycle spoke injuries, from mild contusion and skin laceration to hematomas and fractures, all located at and above the ankle. In soft tissue injuries, the wound was cleaned and dressed and the child was sent home with instructions for rest and leg elevation. In more serious cases or when a fracture occurred, the leg was placed in a plaster cast after reduction. Of the 25 children, 20 were released but reexamined the next morning in the outpatient clinic and followed up once a week until complete recovery. Five children needed hospitalization for periods up to 3 days. Children with only soft tissue injury were treated for 2–6 weeks; treatment of fractures required 8–10 weeks. Many parents lost time from work during the treatment period, with substantial economic loss.

A study of the mechanism of injury show that the foot is caught in a slight inversion between the spokes and pulled forward until the lateral side of the ankle reaches the vertical rod of the bicycle frame. The ankle is crushed against the rod, which results in soft tissue damage. If the wheel does not stop immediately, the foot is carried

Fig 4–1.—Rigid plastic net to prevent bicycle spoke injury. (Courtesy of Roffman, M., et al.: J. Trauma 20:325–326, April 1980.)

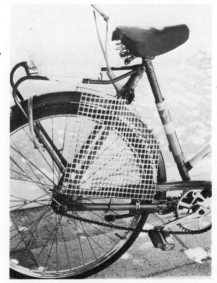

foward and the ankle is angulated into varus against the rod, resulting in fracture of the tibia and fibula. In the 3 children presenting with fracture, a short oblique fracture of the distal tibia with varus deformation was noted.

Six months after completion of treatment, hypertrophic scars and dystrophic vasomotor changes were noted in 7 cases (28%), which prevented wearing of a shoe and prolonged the disability. Skin grafts were not required in any case. Immediate treatment and close follow-up probably prevented this complication.

Ten children (40%) were injured during the first bicycle ride, and the parent was not aware of the danger from the bicycle wheel. To prevent injury in children, a stiff plastic net that fits to the bicycle frame and covers the wheel (Fig 4–1) is suggested. The device may prevent serious injury.

▶ [Of note is the fact that this series of 25 bicycle spoke injuries occurred among a population of 616 children with orthopedic problems seen during a 1-year period (June 1976, thru June 1977) in the emergency room of the Rothschild University Hospital in Haifa, Israel.—J.S.T.] ◀

4–6 **Board Surfing and Bodysurfing Injuries Requiring Hospitalization in Honolulu.** Laurette A. Chang (Univ. of Hawaii) and Clarence E. McDanal, Jr. (Univ. of Alabama) reviewed the records of board surfing and bodysurfing patients admitted to a center in Honolulu during 1973–1977. There were 26 board surfers, 21 bodysurfers, and 2 persons who were struck on the beach by bodysurfers. About half the board surfers were aged 15–20 years, whereas 76% of the bodysurfers were over age 20, chiefly 26–30 years. There were no deaths and only one incident of salt water aspiration with near-drowning.

Most board surfing injuries were due to trauma from a surfboard. Six patients had head injuries, and 2 required surgery for depressed skull fractures. One surfer had an eye enucleated. Three subjects had blunt chest and abdominal trauma; 1 required a partial hepatectomy. All patients with musculoskeletal injuries had a good outcome, except for a boy who completely transected the common peroneal nerve and had loss of motor function despite realignment. Nine bodysurfers had spinal fractures and 1 had a cervical spinal contusion. One patient with a spinal fracture had paralysis with permanent loss of function, and another had a slow return to ambulation. Two bodysurfers had head injuries; 1 had a basal skull fracture and the other, a frontal contusion. The musculoskeletal injuries included 4 knee injuries with torn ligaments, 2 with a torn medial meniscus as well; 4 lower extremity fractures; 2 acromioclavicular joint separations; and a shoulder dislocation with ulnar nerve dysfunction.

▶ [One cannot help but be impressed by the severity of the injuries incurred by these activities.—J.S.T.] ◀

4–7 **Propeller Injuries Incurred in Boating Accidents.** Ronald J. Mann (Univ. of Miami) treated 32 patients with propeller injuries

(4–6) Hawaii Med. J. 39:117, May 1980.
(4–7) Am. J. Sports Med. 8:280–284, July–Aug., 1980.

between 1963 and 1978. In the literature, waterskiing injuries are reported as most prominent, and the injuries incurred by a waterskier struck by a boat propeller are disabling and dangerous. In this author's experience, most patients with propeller injuries were thrown from a racing or speeding boat or were divers accidently run over by a boat propeller. In 1978 in the United States there were 1,761 boating injuries, of which 92 were caused by a propeller. In the author's series there were 20 deaths. Five patients had amputations inflicted by the boat propeller. Three patients had an above-knee amputation, 1 patient had bilateral above-knee amputation and survived, and 1 patient had an above-elbow amputation.

Propeller injuries are devastating and catastrophic, and basic surgical principles of wound care must be followed. The wounds can be considered to be contaminated when first seen, since seawater contains *Pseudomonas* species and lake water may be contaminated with raw or treated sewage. After debridement, all wounds should be left open and either closed or grafted later. Closure is usually preceded by debridements every 48 hours in the operating room until the wound is ready for closure or grafting. Broad-spectrum antibiotics and the usual resuscitative and supportive measures are used. Fractured limbs are initially placed in skeletal traction or immobilized in plaster.

▶ [This article calls attention to a group of serious recreational injuries with a mortality of 20%. Also, it points out the grossly contaminated nature of the propeller wounds.—J.S.T.] ◀

4–8　**The Challenge of Boxing: Bringing Safety Into the Ring** is discussed by Mike Moore. Some consider boxing a murderous and suicidal sport, but others consider it justifiable and useful if strictly controlled. Although amateur boxing is strictly controlled, legislation pertaining to professional boxing varies among the states, and in some cases the situation is chaotic. A total of 335 deaths have occurred in boxing since 1945. The circumstances of recent professional boxing deaths—particularly that of Willie Classen, who had been under indefinite medical suspension but lied to the New York State Boxing Commission about a recent bout in London—emphasize the need for federal legislation covering medical supervision in boxing and the need for international cooperation in maintaining boxing records.

Presently, the New York State Boxing Commission requires that ringside physicians and other officials must take a course in neurology. Fight officials must record the amount of punishment a fighter absorbs, and computerized axial tomography scanning is required for boxers who have sustained head injury or been knocked out. Computerization of boxing records now is under way. In other states the trend has been to do nothing until a tragedy occurs. While deaths in the ring lead to great public outcry, dementia is a less dramatic sequel. There may be individual differences in how well the brain can take blows. The nature of boxing virtually precludes the adaptation

(4–8)　Physician Sports Med. 8:101–105, November 1980.

of protective equipment to lessen damage from head blows. Short of this, the greatest challenge to professional boxing is acceptance of the physician as an integral part of the ring fraternity. Amateur boxing has profited from an association of ringside physicians.

▶ [Anecdotal and editorial in content, this article does bring into focus a major health problem in sports: boxing fatalities. The authors might well have attempted to convert the incidence of worldwide amateur and professional boxing deaths into fatalities rates.—J.S.T.] ◀

4–9 **On the Causes of Traumatic Dental Injuries With Special Reference to Sports Accidents in a Sample of Finnish Children: A Study of Clinical Patient Material.** Seppo Järvinen (Univ. of Kuopio) has investigated the causes of traumatic dental injuries in Finnish children. The series included 98 girls and 223 boys with 450 traumatically injured permanent anterior teeth recorded during 1972–1975 in school dental clinics in the city of Lahti. Slight injuries (63.3%) included crown infraction, enamel fracture, enamel-dentin fracture, and concussion; serious injuries (36.7%) included complicated crown fracture, crown-root fracture, root fracture, subluxation, luxation, and exarticulation. In girls, the most common cause of injury was falls (36.7%) and in boys, sports (33.6%). Among the sports accidents, gymnastics dominated for girls and ice hockey for boys. The proportion of severe injuries was significantly higher in ice hockey and bicycling accidents (60% and 48%, respectively), as compared with injuries in other sports activities (23.7%).

Because of the great variety of causes of traumatic dental injuries, it is difficult to prevent their happening; however, the use of mouth protectors, not only in organized sports but also in free-time games, is strongly recommended.

▶ [In view of this study including what appears to be a defined and controlled population, it is unfortunate that the author did not express the results in terms of dental injury rates. However, the recommendation that mouth protectors be used not only in organized sports but also in free-time games is sound.—J.S.T.] ◀

4–10 **High Cost of High School Football Injuries.** James W. Pritchett (Paradise Valley, Ariz.) has examined year-to-year (1965, 1976–1977) and state-to-state (6 western United States) cost variations in relation to injury site, severity, and repetition of high school football injuries. Data were collected from the files of the largest single insurer of secondary school students in these states. Analysis was made through a specially programmed Qantel 1300 computer. The average claim cost was $34.72 in 1965, $149.93 in 1976, and $177.95 in 1977. The average cost was lowest in Utah and highest in California. In the 1976–1977 season, 3,501 claims from 15,252 players were reported; 401 (2.6%) players had more than 1 claim in a season, accounting for 882 (25.2%) of all claims received. Relatively minor injuries (sprains, strains, contusions, and abrasions) accounted for 72.3% of all injuries but only 42.4% of medical costs. Lower extremity injuries accounted for one-third of the injuries and one half of the costs. Knee injuries

(4–9) Acta Odontol. Scand. 38:151–154, 1980.
(4–10) Am. J. Sports Med. 8:197–199, May–June 1980.

alone accounted for 12.7% of all injuries and 31.8% of all medical costs paid by the insurance company.

There seems to be a high probability that trainers and team physicians can contribute to cost reduction through injury prevention. Flexibility examinations before competition, followed by appropriate conditioning for stretching tight muscles or strengthening weak muscles to stabilize joints, may significantly reduce the cost and frequency of injury. Programs for trainer and coach education in recognition and treatment of football injuries are recommended. The fact that 40% of all medical expenses go for repeatedly injured players suggests that careful examination of players for fitness, agility, stamina, and psychologic factors combined with adequate rehabilitation and strict compliance with playing criteria on return to participation could substantially reduce these costs.

▶ [The article would be more appropriately titled "The Cost of High School Football Injuries." Calling it "high cost" reflects a bias that is not supported by comparative data regarding other sports or nonsporting activities. The author's use of 1965 data as a basis of comparison is also questionable; note that the average number of injuries per reporting district that year was 29, whereas the average per district in 1976 and 1977 was only 4.—J.S.T.] ◀

4–11 **Three-Year Summary of NAIRS Football Data.** Wesley Alles, John W. Powell, William E. Buckley, and Edward E. Hunt, Jr. (Penn State Univ.) report a summary of results of a 3-year study of injuries in football undertaken as part of the National Athletic Injury/Illness Reporting System (NAIRS) and recently submitted to the U.S. Consumer Product Safety Commission. The NAIRS system relies on data submitted on a voluntary basis by athletic trainers across the country. It defines a reportable injury as any injury causing cessation of an athlete's participation for at least 1 day following injury. A minor injury is a reportable injury in which the athlete could return to participation within 1 week from day of onset. A significant injury involves time loss greater than 7 days. Injuries involving time loss of 8–21 days are termed moderate and those involving time loss of longer than 21 days, major. Severe injuries are those that are permanently disabling.

Data for 1975–1977 football seasons show that a high school football team experienced about 8 reportable injuries per 1,000 athlete-exposures, or 32 reportable injuries per season. College teams record about 11 injuries/1,000 athlete-exposures, or 83.6 reportable injuries per season. However, high school teams report only 2 significant injuries/1,000 athlete-exposures, whereas college teams report 3/1,000 exposures.

Data show a low frequency of cerebral neurotrauma: 5 of 100 athletes experienced a reportable concussion, and 5 of 1,000 athletes experienced significant concussions. Because NAIRS computer programs can tabulate data in a variety of ways, it was possible to investigate whether a particular helmet was associated with neurotrauma more than expected. No such association was found.

(4–11) Athletic Training 15:98–100, Summer 1980.

To determine whether surface hardness contributes to additional injury, NAIRS analyzed injury data on concussions, using college data. Evidence did not support the belief that surface hardness adds to the risk of sustaining a significant concussion. However, significant meniscus/knee sprains and ankle sprains demonstrate slightly higher rates for both artificial surfaces (Astroturf and Tartanturf) than rates observed for these injuries on natural grass. Further analysis demonstrated that a college team could expect to sustain 1 or 2 additional significant injuries per season per team if all exposures were on either of the two artificial surfaces rather than on natural grass. A cause-effect relationship is not proved, however. Multivariate statistical tests may permit identification of other factors that may relate to the association.

It is concluded that the utility of the NAIRS data is based on year-to-year continuation of systematic data collection along with increased number of teams.

▶ [The 1979 Summer issue of *Medicine and Science in Sports* contained an article by K. S. Clarke and J. W. Powell entitled "Football Helmets and Neurotrauma: An Epidemiological Overview of Three Seasons." This was abstracted in the 1980 *Yearbook of Sports Medicine.* The current offering from *Athletic Training* is virtually an edited version of the work published in 1979.—J.S.T.] ◀

4–12 **Football Injury Update—1979 Season.** Football fatalities have decreased dramatically over the past 20 years. Frederick O. Mueller and Carl S. Blyth (Univ. of North Carolina at Chapel Hill) report findings of the *Forty-eighth Annual Survey of Football Fatalities 1931–1979* (National Collegiate Athletic Association and American Football Coaches Association) and discuss reasons for the decline.

TABLE 1.—FATALITIES DIRECTLY DUE TO PLAYING FOOTBALL

	SANDLOT	PRO AND SEMIPRO	HIGH SCHOOL	COLLEGE	TOTAL
1960	1	1	11	1	14
1961	3	0	10	6	19
1962	6	1	12	0	19
1963	1	1	12	2	16
1964	4	1	21	3	29
1965	4	0	20	1	25
1966	4	0	20	0	24
1967	5	0	16	3	24
1968	4	1	26	5	36
1969	3	1	18	1	23
1970	3	0	23	3	29
1971	2	0	15	3	20
1972	3	1	16	2	22
1973	2	0	7	0	9
1974	0	0	10	1	11
1975	1	0	13	1	15
1976	3	0	15	0	18
1977	1	0	8	1	10
1978	0	0	9	0	9
1979	0	0	3	1	4
Total	50	7	285	34	376

(4–12) Physician Sportsmed. 8:53–55, October 1980.

TABLE 2.—STATUS OF INJURED FOOTBALL PLAYERS

	1977	1978	1979	TOTAL
High School				
Permanent paralysis	6	8	3	17
Recovery	1	8	6	15
College				
Permanent paralysis	1	0	4	5
Recovery	1	1	2	4
Professional				
Permanent paralysis	0	1	0	1
Recovery	0	0	1	1
Total	9	18	16	43

In 1979 there were 4 football fatalities (high school, 3; college, 1), an all-time low (Table 1). This contrasts with an all-time high of 36 deaths in 1968. Incidence of direct fatalities was 0.23 and 1.33 per 100,000 participants for high school and college football, respectively. Three of the 4 deaths were caused by head injuries; 1 resulted from a fractured neck. Of 43 catastrophic, nonfatal head and neck injuries reported in 1977–1979, 23 resulted in permanent paralysis (Table 2). Tackling was by far the most common activity causing catastrophic injury.

Various factors are cited as contributing to the dramatic decrease in football fatalities. These include the prohibition of "butt blocking" and "spear tackling," establishment of a football helmet standard, and improved physical examinations and physical conditioning programs.

▶ [This is an ongoing pattern of reporting that should be compared with the data of the prior year included in the 1980 YEAR BOOK, pages 174–176. There were 4 deaths in 1979, compared with 9 deaths in the prior year. These figures must be taken in perspective and with the proverbial grain of salt. Comparison really is meaningless when the data base is as small as it is and when a single fatality can influence the statistical rates so meaningfully. Suffice it to say that fatalities still occur; tackling continues to be the most common activity causing catastrophic injury. The skeptical spectator is not impressed that spear tackling is a thing of the past. One would also like to believe that each generation of football players is increasingly better trained and that the coaching staffs are more perceptive of the risks of hyperthermia. There may be favorable trends for all of these factors, but the data have yet to prove it. Football will remain a dangerous sport. The ideal preventive measures will never be reached, but the goal is sound.

The growth of club rugby bears comment. The casual observer also must sense that this is being played frequently as sandlot football was, with American intensity and habit patterns and the obvious absence of some of the protective equipment. I should like to see club rugby keep statistics of their injury rates, but such statistics are not yet available. I would guess the injury rate is rather high.—L.J.K.] ◀

4–13 **Relationship Between Exposure Time and Injury in Football** was investigated by Robert F. Dagiau, Charles J. Dillman, and E. Keith Milner. Data were collected at all practice sessions and games of the University of Illinois varsity football team during the 1976 and 1977 seasons. The 54 members of the traveling squad were the subjects used in collection of game and injury data. Games were divided

(4–13) Am. J. Sports Med. 8:257–260, July–Aug. 1980.

into three intervals and practice into five 25-minute intervals for data analysis. A likelihood ratio test was used to test the data for statistical significance.

Exposure time was defined as the time a player actually spent participating in a specific activity or specific play until an injury occurred. When both seasons were combined, the knee was the most frequently injured part, but the ankle was also often injured. Sprains were the most prevalent injury (44% of all injuries). Outside and inside tackle runs and pass plays caused most injuries. The interval of low exposure (25 plays or less) accounted for most injuries, and an inverse relationship was found between exposure time and injury in games for both seasons. Most offensive injuries occurred in the low interval, whereas defensive injuries were evenly distributed over the low and intermediate (26 to 49 plays) intervals for the two seasons. The interval of high exposure (more than 50 plays) accounted for the fewest injuries. Preseason drills accounted for a disproportionate share of the practice injuries. Therefore, restructuring of the practice session should be considered. The third and fourth intervals in practice accounted for highest injury totals, suggesting that contact scrimmages and 3+ person contact drills should take place in the second interval of practice, to allow sufficient warm-up and permit players better to withstand mentally and physically the severity of the contact inherent in the drills.

▶ [The authors correctly identify the use of a statistical analysis based on the Poisson distribution, then something goes wrong. To illustrate, Poisson would predict that the 1976 game data would be distributed as 12, 8, and 3 injuries in the three successive time intervals. The authors observed 12, 7, and 4. They conclude that the observations are significantly different from what was expected! They repeat this same error in analyzing their 1977 game data and the 1976 practice data. The 1977 practice data are, in fact, statistically significant, but not to the degree stated by the authors.

The correct interpretations of this research are that the exposure time-versus-injury relationship follows the classic Poisson distribution in both game years and the one practice year. The 1977 practice year shows a significant deviation occuring in the fourth of the five intervals. What the authors present is simply the way such events are expected to occur.—J.S.T.] ◀

4-14 **Touch Football: Friendly Game?** John R. McCarroll and Roy Riddle (Naval Regional Med. Center, Charleston, S.C.) prospectively studied the incidence of injuries sustained by 270 players of two-hand touch football during a 5-week period. Games consisted of two 20-minute halves, and 3 officials were present. No protective equipment was worn and only soccer-style cleats were allowed.

The 30 injuries that occurred resulted in an injury rate of 11.1%. Surgery was required in 7 of the 19 injuries classified as serious. The knee was the most frequently (26.7%) and most seriously (31.6%) injured area. The shoulder, hand, and ankle were the next most seriously injured areas (21.1% each). Overall, the injuries caused a loss of 1,332 days from full duty, an average of 44.4 days per injury. Approximately 47% of the injuries caused a time loss of less than 14 days, whereas 53% caused a loss of more than 14 days. Everyone injured was wearing soccer-style cleats, and most injuries resulted from collisions.

Further studies are needed to prevent injuries in touch football and to return the game to the friendly competition it was meant to be.

▶ [The authors point out that theirs is the highest injury rate of any touch football report to date, with 73% of the injuries due to "collision with another player." To put these observations into proper perspective, it should be noted that in this study all of the participants had played high school or college football and all had the incentive of going on to further Navy-wide competition.

The definition of a serious injury "as one that is not normally expected to occur as a result of the game" is certainly unique. Noteworthy is the fact that an anterior cruciate ligament injury was not observed.—J.S.T.] ◀

4–15   **Injuries in Karate.** Today, there are hundreds of variations of karate being practiced, each with its own training methods and attitudes toward competition. Harvey L. Kurland (Natl. Athletic Health Inst., Inglewood, Calif.) discusses various forms of karate and identifies four phases of training in which different types of injuries can occur.

Solo practice, the first stage of training, includes warm-up, flexibility exercises, and shadow boxing. Improper training methods and insufficient warm-up time are related to most of the injuries sustained during this phase. Injury to the knees, shoulders, and elbows are common and strains are prevalent, although rarely reported. Few injuries are associated with kicking and striking objects—the second phase of training—and beneficial adaptive changes of the hands often occur. In prearranged and free sparring, strains are the predominant injuries and result from improper technique in which the digits are hyperextended, hyperflexed, or jammed. Misjudgment can result in rib fractures and contusions of the torso. Most of the chronic problems in karate are related to inadequate rehabilitation. The most significant injuries in karate are concussions and trauma to the liver, spleen, heart, and kidneys. In a study of 49 karate students over 931 practice hours, 18 injuries occurred. Women had a higher injury rate than men.

About 72% of the injuries in this karate class could have been prevented by the use of hand, foot, and chest protectors.

▶ [An interesting essay on the history of Chinese martial arts is included in the original article. The author reports 18 injuries occurring among 49 students, for an injury rate of 19 per 1,000 practice hours. There were 18 injuries per 1,000 practice hours for men and 21 injuries per 1,000 practice hours for women. From these data, the author concludes a higher injury rate among the women. This does not represent a statistically significant difference, and such a comparison cannot be made between the two injury rates. Also, the author's contention that about 72% of the reported injuries could have been prevented by hand, foot, and chest protectors is not supported by the data presented.—J.S.T.] ◀

4–16   **Mountain Rescue and Preparation** are discussed by Edward C. Geehr (Univ. of California, Los Angeles). Fewer than 10% of mountain accidents are caused by natural phenomena or equipment failure; most result from inexperience and lack of proper preparation.

(4–15)   Physician Sportsmed. 8:80–85, October 1980.
(4–16)   Top. Emerg. Med. 2:119–125, October 1980.

Fatigue and poor judgment, often aggravated by the effects of cold or altitude, are the final common pathway to tragedy. A slip or fall results in 60%–70% of cases, whereas hypothermic exposure complicates 10% of cases. Protection against cold, wetness, and wind is fundamental, as is protection against ultraviolet injury to the eyes and skin. The cardinal rule of rescue work is not to become a victim oneself. Helicopters should be considered unreliable. In considering supplies for mountain rescue work, anticipation of the "worst possible" circumstance is tempered by practical considerations of size and weight.

Victims of severe crush injuries should, after volume expansion, receive mannitol and bicarbonate. Cimetidine may be used to prevent stress ulceration. In cases of head trauma, the integrity of the spinal axis must be considered. Adequate hydration of the immobilized patient is essential. Disorientation in the victims must be watched for. The issue of glucocorticoid support is unresolved. Evidence of cerebral edema calls for immediate descent. High-altitude pulmonary edema is managed by oxygen and descent. A lightweight portable oxygen system is useful in mountain rescue work. Time is a critical factor in avalanche rescue. Solar injury may present as ultraviolet keratitis or photic retinopathy. Disoriented or disabled victims with underlying vitamin A deficiency due to malnutrition are particularly vulnerable to photic retinopathy.

▶ [This is an excellent review. The reader is referred to the original article.—J.S.T.] ◀

4–17 **Injuries in High School Physical Education Classes.** Gregory J. Austin, Kenneth D. Rogers, and Grace Reese (Pittsburgh) examined the occurrence of injuries in a population of about 1,870 predominantly white, middle-class high school students in 1976–1978. The students were required to participate in physical education classes 2 hours a week; the usual activity time in a class was about 40 minutes. Students were allowed to select from among several types of physical education activities.

A total of 134 injuries were reported officially during the study period, for a rate of 3.6 per 100 participants per year. Rates were about equal for boys and girls, although ninth grade girls had almost 4 times the injury rate of ninth grade boys and 12th grade boys had approximately twice the injury rate of 12th grade girls. Over half the injuries were sprains and about a third were contusions or abrasions. The proportions of various types of injury were similar for the two sexes and for all grades. Just over one fourth of the injuries occurred in interactions with other participants. About half the 71 sprains affected the ankle. The greatest cause of contusions and abrasions in girls was being struck by a field hockey stick. There were 4 fractures. Basketball was the activity most often associated with ankle and foot injuries. In a group of 484 subjects sampled for injuries that were not reported, 26 had sustained injuries in physical education class, for a rate of 5.4 per 100 pupil-years.

(4–17) Am. J. Dis. Child. 134:456–458, May 1980.

Physical education class-related injuries were relatively infrequent in this survey, and their severity was mild. Most often injuries were due to falling or tripping; the next most common cause was contact with a ball. Both these circumstances reflect musculoskeletal skills, conditioning, and experience. Protective equipment might reduce injuries in field hockey. Adolescents in physical education programs are always at risk of injury, but such injuries were not a major health problem in this setting.

▶ [The apparent advantage of this report over the National Center for Education Statistics survey is the breakdown of injuries by type and location, while maintaining a comparable injury rate. The order of magnitude of this rate is less that what has been reported for competitive high school sports activities.—J.S.T.] ◀

4–18 **Injuries Presenting From Rugby Union Football.** Peter T. Myers (Mater Misericordiae Hosp., Brisbane, Australia) surveyed adult rugby union injuries in 271 players who presented with injury to the medical officer on duty in 221 club and representative matches played at Ballymore in Brisbane in the 1979 season. The rate of injury was 0.032 injuries/player hour (1.23 injuries/game, or 0.041 injuries/player appearance). Facial lacerations accounted for one third of all injuries. Of the 271 players, 140 (52%) suffered 146 injuries to the head and neck; 24 of these sustained head injuries (defined as any period of unconsciousness, state of confusion, etc.); 10 sustained clinically fractured noses; 2 patients had a cauliflower ear; 3 suffered fractured mandibles. Lower limbs accounted for 57 injuries (21%), including 28 knee injuries and 18 ankle injuries. There were 51 injuries to the upper limb (19%), 14 of which were to the acromioclavicular joint. Four patients had shoulder dislocations. There were 22 injuries to the hands and fingers, including several fractures. Most of the 23 trunk injuries (8%) were to the chest wall. There was no significant injury to an abdominal viscus. Two thirds of the injuries were of a minor nature. There were no deaths and no permanently incapacitating injuries. One patient required emergency reduction of a dislocated hip; 8 patients had semielective surgery, and 1 had elective surgery. The 31 serious injuries (11%) comprised mainly fractures and dislocations; 9 of these were to head and neck, comprising 6 nasal and 3 mandibular fractures.

There was a significant trend of increasing incidence of injury from the lower to the higher grades of play. There was no correlation between injury and age of the player. Representative players at maximal fitness suffered the highest rate of injury. Serious injuries as well as minor injuries could perhaps be prevented by wearing full or three-quarter-length sleeves instead of short sleeves, soft padded headgear, and molded mouth guards. There must be improved player, coach, and referee awareness of injury-prone phases of play, for example, rucks and mauls.

▶ [This article is noteworthy because of the authors' recognition that, for the purpose of scientific comparison of injuries, suitable standards for the rate and severity are necessary.—J.S.T.] ◀

(4–18) Med. J. Aust. 2:17–20, July 12, 1980.

4–19 **Trends in Skiing Injuries: Analysis of a 6-Year Study (1972 to 1978)** was made by Robert J. Johnson, Carl F. Ettlinger, Robert J. Campbell, and Malcolm H. Pope (Univ. of Vermont), with emphasis on effects of age, sex, and equipment. There were 11,041 skier interviews; 998 control skiers and 1,711 injuries were evaluated during 407,600 skier-days. The overall injury rate was 4.2/1,000 skier-days, dropping from 5.3 to 3.3 from the first to the last year. Injuries of the upper part of the body (pelvis, trunk, neck, head, and upper extremities) totaled 713 (42%) and lower extremity injuries totaled 998 (58%). Of the lower extremity injuries, 796 (80%) were classified as lower extremity equipment-related (LEER). From the first to the last year the overall injury rate decreased 41% (upper part of the body, 25%; LEER, 43%; lower extremity nonequipment related, 71%). Among LEER injuries, fractured tibias decreased 72%, sprained ankles 71%, and sprained knees 28%. Boot-top contusions showed no change.

The Vermont release calibrator was used to determine the release characteristics of the equipment of a control population and of those skiers who sustained a LEER injury. Below-knee injuries caused by twisting moments decreased more than those caused by bending moments, possibly because the release characteristics of equipment in twist have been improved, whereas the function of the forward lean release mechanism has not changed. Most bindings are sensitive only to a forward lean torque applied from the skier's leg through the boot, but lateral and backward bending moments are ignored. Improvements in boot design may be required to change some injury rates. A decline was observed in the median release torques of the bindings of both the control population and the LEER group, but the greatest reductions occurred in the LEER group. The percentage of skiers who exceeded their recommended release torques also diminished in both groups. Better binding function was directly related to the decreases in LEER injuries and in the overall injury rate. The absence of twist at the heel, shear, and roll release modes may result in knee ligament injury in certain loading configurations that occur in ski accidents. Binding design criteria have been based solely on protection of the tibia; improvement in the knee ligament injury rate will require a more complex model on which to base the design of future bindings. More emphasis must be placed on better understanding of the mechanisms of knee sprains and the development of equipment and procedures to prevent them.

▶ [The Vermont release calibrator was used the first 3 years to determine binding release characteristics, and an American Society for Testing and Materials ski binding evaluation system was used in the latter 3 years. No correlation of the equivalency of these devices is offered, and so the conclusions on binding trends are open to criticism. The injury trends do give direction to persons involved in prevention and mitigation of skiing injuries.—J.S.T.] ◀

4–20 **Skiing Lacerations: Preventability by the Use of Ski Brakes.** Thomas G. Colmey and F. Jack Eck reviewed reports of all ski inju-

(4–19) Am. J. Sports Med. 8:106–113, Mar.–Apr., 1980.
(4–20) J.A.M.A. 244:1699, Oct. 10, 1980.

ries recorded at Vail, Colorado, in the 1973–1974 season and found 178 instances in which the skier was lacerated by his or her own ski. This represents about 1 in every 10 ski injuries, a ratio which remained constant from 1972 to 1978. More than two thirds of the injuries were above the waist, and 57% involved the head or face. No injuries to skiers were attributed to skis equipped with ski brakes in this 6-year period.

The newer type of runaway strap is attached to the ski in only one place rather than at two, and this permits the ski to bounce further upward, often striking the skier about the head. The runaway strap is designed to keep a detached ski from sliding unchecked down a hill or falling on someone below a lift, but it is dangerous when a binding releases and the ski does not fully disengage from the skier. The ski brake is an acceptable alternative to the runaway strap, and it allows the ski to be disengaged completely from the skier at the time of binding release. There appears to be a wide lack of knowledge that ski brakes are available and that they are safer than runaway straps.

▶ [Although this is certainly not a controlled study, it is interesting to note that no injuries to skiers could be attributed to skis equipped with ski brakes during the 6-year period from 1972 to 1978.—J.S.T.] ◀

4–21   **Sledding Injuries.** Jerris R. Hedges and Michael I. Greenberg reviewed 61 sledding accidents that occurred during a 3-week period in 1978, involving 39 male patients, with a mean age of 14.4 years, and 22 female patients, with a mean age of 18 years. Injuries tended to occur primarily in the young, but 7 injuries occurred in the 21 to 30 year age range and 5 in the 31 to 42 year age range. Whereas 21% of patients seen for contusion, laceration, or abrasion were over age 21, only 13% seen for fracture, dislocation, or abdominal injury were over that age. Minor abrasions or lacerations were seen in 27 patients (44%), contusions in 15 (25%), fractures in 10 (16%), and a dislocation in 1. There were 2 ankle sprains (4%), 4 knee injuries (7%), 5 head injuries (8%), and 4 abdominal injuries (7%). One patient with multiple traumas was dead on arrival.

The driver of a sled can obtain considerable velocity and hence kinetic energy on a modest slope. Injuries occur when the sled overturns, when sled and rider strike an object, when the rider attempts to stop the sled too quickly, or when the rider falls off. Minor contusions and abrasions may be produced by the metal runners. When a stationary object is struck, most of the kinetic energy is absorbed by the rider's body; impact forces may then fracture bones or rupture viscera. The position of the rider can also predispose different anatomical regions to injury.

To guide evaluation of the accident victim, the following information should be obtained: height of the hill to estimate velocity of impact, position of the rider on the sled, type of contact (direct impact, protruding object), and preexistent medical problems. The number of extremity injuries suggests that moment forces generated in stopping

(4–21) Ann. Emerg. Med. 9:131–133, March 1980.

of the sled are more often the cause of injury. The 1 death and 8 admissions in this small series underscore the respect with which sledding injuries should be treated. Four of the 8 patients admitted sustained abdominal injuries including blunt trauma, ruptured spleen, and renal contusion. Other injuries requiring admission included dislocated hip, fractured femur, fractured ribs and fractured L3 (compression).

Patients with serious thoracic, abdominal, or extremity injury may present in shock or with airway compromise. In the stable patient, a screening examination is useful to ascertain rotational and translational movement at impact.

▶ [This article represents the first published report of a large series of what appears to be relatively unappreciated injuries resulting from this particular form of recreational activity.—J.S.T.] ◀

4–22 **Evaluation of Injuries in Youth Soccer.** Soccer is the fastest growing team sport in the United States, yet little information is available on the incidence of soccer injuries. J. Andy Sullivan, Richard H. Gross, William A. Grana, and Carlos A. Garcia-Moral (Oklahoma City) conducted a prospective study of soccer injuries in youth soccer programs (for boys and girls less than age 19 years), involving 80 teams with 1,272 players, 341 of whom were girls.

A total of 34 injuries were reported for an overall injury rate of 2.6 per 100 participants. Based on the number of injuries per 1,000 hours of participation, the injury rates were 0.51 for boys and 1.1 for girls. The injury rate for those less than age 10 was 0.8 per 100 participants, whereas that for older players was 7.7 per 100. Most of the injuries were not serious. They included 13 contusions, 12 sprains, 3 strains, 2 fractures, and 1 dislocation.

It is concluded that soccer is a relatively safe activity for children and adolescents.

▶ [The general impression would be that the injury rate for youth soccer should be lower than for other sports, particularly those involving a greater degree of contact. There have been no data available in the United States on this sport, and this article provides the findings corroborating the anticipation.—L.J.K.] ◀

4–23 **Diving Emergencies** are reviewed by Ronald D. Stewart (Univ. of Pittsburgh). The scuba apparatus has increased the number of divers; over 200,000 divers are licensed each year in the United States. Diving-related illness is not seen only in the sunnier climates. Alcohol is a major predisposing factor in diving accidents. Other risk factors are hypothermia and toxic animals or plants. The use of thermal wetsuits has decreased the incidence of progressive underwater hypothermia. Compressed-air diving may cause "rapture of the deep," with euphoria, poor judgment, and inability to concentrate.

Type I decompression sickness, or the bends, consists of extremity pain, usually in the larger joints. Type II decompression sickness may include back pain, joint pain, ataxia, muscle weakness, and loss of sensation in the extremities. Shallow-water blackout may occur in breath-hold divers who hyperventilate before the dive.

(4–22) Am. J. Sports Med. 8:325–327, Sept.–Oct. 1980.
(4–23) Top. Emerg. Med. 2:77–88, October 1980.

The bends are managed by recompression; the prognosis is good. Type II decompression sickness is treated with immediate oxygenation by nonrebreathing mask, saline infusion, and intravenously administered dexamethasone. Recompression is carried out in a hyperbaric chamber facility. This treatment offers the possibility of complete recovery. The efficacy of steroids has not been definitely demonstrated, but many clinicians favor their use in type II decompression sickness. Repetitive treatment may be useful for conditions that respond to hyperbaric therapy. Air embolism is managed by left-lateral positioning, inhalation of a high oxygen concentration, and recompression.

▶ [This is an excellent review. The reader is referred to the original article.—J.S.T.] ◀

4-24 **Drowning and Near Drowning** are discussed by Ronald D. Stewart (Univ. of Pittsburgh). An estimated 8,000 persons in the United States drown each year, and many thousands may have a near-drowning episode and recover, some with neurologic or other sequelae. Nearly 90% of drownings occur only 10 yards from safety. Drowning victims aspirate water in an estimated 80%–90% of cases, whereas laryngospasm keeps the lungs dry in the others. Victims with dry lungs may respond better to resuscitation procedures. Shallow-water blackout predisposes to drowning in swimmers who hyperventilate before starting a long underwater swim. Immersion syndrome consists of sudden death after contact with very cold water. The "postimmersion syndrome," or "secondary drowning syndrome," is an adult respiratory distress syndrome following submersion, preceded by a relatively asymptomatic interval lasting hours to days.

Risk factors for submersion accidents include inadequate swimming ability, age, cervical spine injury, seizures, decompression sickness, and air embolism in scuba divers. Alcohol also may be a risk factor. Drowning can result directly from hypothermia. Risks can be reduced through drownproofing, swimming instruction, and education in dealing with exposure and in wilderness rescue. There is growing evidence that alcohol use can increase the risk of trouble during water recreation.

The real problems in human submersion accidents are acidosis and hypoxia. The real target organ is the lung. Hypoxia can be expected in all cases. Patients may respond to initial resuscitative measures and require high oxygen concentrations and constant attention to vital signs and to the possibility of vomiting. Drainage of the lungs may improve the chance of survival, especially in seawater submersion incidents. Positive-pressure ventilation should be started as soon as possible. Conservation of body heat is important. Prolonged resuscitative attempts at the scene without apparent progress are not wise. In most instances, the time of submergence is not a reliable guide to the outcome; the state of consciousness in the emergency room is a better indicator. Modern measures for treating pulmonary failure and

(4–24) Top. Emerg. Med. 2:63, October 1980.

preventing or ameliorating neuronal damage may improve the outlook for victims of submersion accidents.

▶ [Although this is a fine review, it should be noted, however, that the author has
failed to deal adequately with the status of the mammalian diving reflex.

Martin Nemiroff, at the University of Michigan Medical Center, has made us aware
that persons who drown in cold water, that is, 70 F or colder, and who remain submerged for up to an hour can be successfully resuscitated. The key to resuscitation is
that it be aggressive and be continued for at least 2 hours.

Nemiroff had studied 11 near drownings in which he explains survival as due to a
combination of coldness, which lowers the body's requirement for oxygen, and a bod-
ily response knows as "mammalian diving reflex."

The mammalian diving reflex was first noted in seals, whales, and other air-breath-
ing aquatic mammals. They are normally able to remain submerged up to 30 minutes
without suffering any damage. The reflex itself is stimulated by cold water. Breathing
stops and blood flow is redistributed from the skin, muscles, gut, and other tissues
that are not necessarily affected by low oxygen levels and is sent to the heart, lungs,
and brain.

In human beings, the reflex is most active in children aged 1 to 2 years and becomes
less active in the later teens. It is probably not very active in middle age or after.

Nemiroff has emphasized the importance of initiating resuscitation immediately,
once the victim is out of the water. The mammalian diving reflex starts automatically
when a person's face goes underwater and also stops immediately when the face
comes out of the water.

Aggressive resuscitation includes simultaneous closed chest massage and mouth-
to-mouth breathing. This must be done continuously until the patient is seen by a
physician in a hospital and either recovers or is pronounced dead.

The basic guideline is: In young victims submerged in cold water of 70 F or less for
up to an hour, initiate and sustain aggressive cardiopulmonary resuscitation techniques for at least 2 hours.—J.S.T.] ◄

4–25 **Injuries in Interscholastic Wrestling.** Joseph J. Estwanik III,
John A. Bergfeld, H. Royer Collins, and Richard Hall have reviewed
records of 666 wrestling injuries sustained from 1972 through 1976
in patients treated at the Cleveland Clinic. Knee, shoulder, and ear
injuries (62.2% of the total) were further investigated by telephone
interview with the wrestler to determine present status, mechanism
of injury, and duration of disability. Knee injuries (38.4% of the total)
numbered 256 and involved 282 structures. The most common injuries were medial meniscus tear, medial collateral ligament sprain,
lateral meniscus tear, and prepatellar bursitis. Medial meniscus tears
resulted from a sudden twist or valgus stress on a weight-bearing leg;
79% were weight-bearing injuries, and 68% occurred during take-
downs. Lateral meniscus injuries were non-weight-bearing, and hy-
perflexion and hyperflexion/twisting were incriminated. Injuries of
the shoulder girdle (16.2% of the total) included subluxation and dislocation (25%), acromioclavicular sprain (24%), sternoclavicular
sprain (14.8%), muscular strain (14.8%), and capsular sprain (13.9%).
No common hold was incriminated in dislocations. Almost all acromioclavicular injuries occurred during a takedown and were related
to a fall on the shoulder. whereas sternoclavicular injuries occurred
on the mat. Few serious back injuries occurred (6.2%), and head and
neck injuries were also low in this series (5.7%). The true incidence

(4–25) Physician Sportsmed. 8:111–121, March 1980.

of the latter is usually higher. They included cauliflower ears, cervicospasm (sprain), pinched nerve syndrome, and nasal contusion. Patients with pinched nerve syndrome are advised to substitute isometric resistance neck exercises for neck bridging exercises. Seventy percent of hematomas occurred while ear guards were not being worn. Fourteen of the 35 elbow injuries were sprains, and of these, 86% were caused by hyperextension. These injuries are protected with extension-stop adhesive taping. Hand injuries (33, or 5%) were primarily sprains and fractures. The thumb was the most frequently involved digit, and the metacarpophalangeal joint was injured most frequently. Chest injuries (5%) included costochondral sprains (24), intercostal sprains (5) and manubrium sterni sprain (1). There are two mechanisms for the first sprain: direct compression force and torsional strain. Ankle injuries (3.9%) were mostly sprains, occurring when the foot was gripped by the opponent.

It was concluded that more injuries occur during practice, but when participation time is considered, the wrestler is at higher risk during a competitive match. The takedown phase is a short but high-risk period.

▶ [Noteworthy is the authors' failure to convert their data into injury rates.—J.S.T.] ◀

4–26 **Sudden Death in Young Athletes.** Barry J. Maron, William C. Roberts, Hugh A. McAllister, Douglas R. Rosing, and Stephen E. Epstein (Natl. Inst. of Health) investigated the sudden death of 29 highly conditioned competitive athletes ages 13 to 30 years. Sudden death occurred during or just after severe exertion in 22, and death was instantaneous in 28. Structural cardiovascular alterations were identified at autopsy in 28 athletes, but no significant abnormality was found in any organ besides the heart. Only 1 patient had a normal heart on both gross and histologic examination. Of the 28 athletes with structural alterations, 22 had unequivocal cardiovascular disease causing sudden death; the diseases were congenital in 19 and acquired in 3.

Hypertrophic cardiomyopathy was present in 14 athletes who also had at least one of the associated features of asymmetric septal hypertrophy, marked disorganization of cardiac muscle cells in the ventricular septum, and clinical or echocardiographic evidence of hypertrophic cardiomyopathy in at least 1 closely related family member.

Four athletes had anomalous origin of the left coronary artery from the right (anterior) sinus of Valsalva, including 1 patient with hypertrophic cardiopathy. The left main coronary artery appeared to be narrowed and obstructed by virtue of its oblique course.

Acquired abnormalities of the coronary arteries were present in 3 patients and included severe atherosclerosis in the three major extramural coronary arteries in 2 and 50% luminal narrowing of the left anterior descending coronary artery by atherosclerotic plaque in the third.

Two athletes died of aortic rupture with massive mediastinal hem-

(4–26) Circulation 62:218–229, August 1980.

orrhage. The ascending aorta was markedly dilated and had a linear tear in its wall.

Six of the 29 subjects had cardiovascular alterations considered to be probable but not definitive evidence of cardiovascular disease. Five had a hypertrophied, nondilated left ventricle with none of the characteristic features associated with the disease previously cited. Mild to moderate right ventricular dilatation was present in 3 of these with idiopathic concentric left ventricular hypertrophy. Another patient had a heart of normal weight with diminished coronary arterial distribution to the posterior wall of the left ventricle.

Of the 29 athletes, 21 had been entirely asymptomatic, the other 8 had had transient symptoms including syncope, presyncope, chest pain, mild fatigue, or palpitations. In 5 asymptomatic and in 2 transiently symptomatic athletes, cardiovascular disease was suspected by a physician. Six of these had hypertrophic cardiomyopathy at autopsy, but in only 1 of the 6 was the correct diagnosis made clinically. The seventh patient had obvious signs of Marfan's syndrome, and diagnosis was established during life. The other 5 subjects with hypertrophic cardiomyopathy in whom cardiovascular disease was suspected had distinctly abnormal ECGs. Echocardiograms could have established the diagnosis during life. The 5 patients with ventricular hypertrophy without other evidence of a primary, genetically transmitted cardiomyopathy are a diagnostic dilemma. In 3 of them the wall thickening exceeded the physiologic hypertrophy associated with athletics.

Definitive identification of hypertrophic cardiomyopathy without obstruction could be made noninvasively in athletes only by echocardiography, but routine comprehensive screening is impractical.

▶ [This excellent article is required reading for physicians involved in the medical care of the athlete. To be noted is the authors' conclusion, "The data in this study do not provide definitive information regarding the feasibility of screening programs for detecting cardiovascular disease in competitive athletes. However, the basic knowledge and awareness of the diseases that may cause sudden death in athletes help to create the groundwork necessary for the initiation of studies that will provide such answers."—J.S.T.] ◀

▶ [There have been many reports of ventricular septal thickening in athletes, and more work is necessary in order to decide how commonly it is linked to adverse pathologic sequelae, as here. It is only recently that the concept of athlete's heart (a radiographic diagnosis) has been set in correct perspective, and there may need to be a similar cortical examination of echocardiographic diagnoses of septal hypertrophy.—R.J.S.] ◀

HEAD, NECK, AND SPINE INJURIES

4–27 **Computed Tomography of the Musculoskeletal System.** Harry K. Genant, John S. Wilson, Edwin G. Bovill, Francis O. Brunelle, William R. Murray, and Juan J. Rodrigo (Univ. of California, San Francisco) reviewed experience with more than 250 computed tomography (CT) studies done for musculoskeletal disorders since 1977 with the use of the GE 7800 or the EMI 5005 body scanner. Seventy-eight

(4–27)   J. Bone Joint Surg. [Am.] 62-A:1088–1101, October 1980.

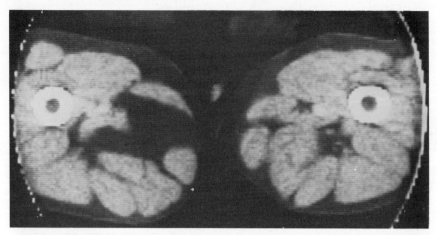

Fig 4–2.—The CT scan defines a sharply marginated soft tissue mass with the density of fat, diagnostic of lipoma. The CT number for the mass was comparable to that of subcutaneous fat (approximately – 100 Hounsfield units). (Courtesy of Genant, H. K., et al.: J. Bone Joint Surg. [Am.] 62-A:1088–1101, October 1980.)

patients had neoplasms of orthopedic interest; 51 had primary tumors. Computed tomography scanning was useful in localizing primary bone tumors and defining their relationship with nerves and blood vessels. Scans often are important in the diagnosis of soft tissue tumors (Fig 4–2). Suspected metastatic lesions can be confirmed and their intramedullary and extraosseous extent assessed. Local recurrences of neoplasms can also be identified by CT scanning. The study was also useful in distinguishing nonneoplastic masses and anatomical variations. Computed tomography scanning is useful in evaluating patients with spinal stenosis, dysraphic lesions of the spine, and problems involving total hip arthroplasty. Quantitative bone mineral analysis is possible in vitro with CT.

Computed tomography scanning facilitated the diagnosis in 29% of patients with neoplastic disease and aided treatment in 68%. Treatment of nonneoplastic disorders was aided by CT scanning in 69% of the patients so affected. The usefulness of the study will increase when faster scanning times and near-instantaneous image reconstruction are available. There will be more situations in which multiplanar reconstructions of lesions will be of value. Options are now available on prototype scanners that provide for extremely high spatial and density resolutions, permitting better visualization of fine details of bone and joints anywhere in the skeleton and direct visualization of structures such as the spinal cord, nerve roots, and intervertebral disks. The CT scout film, or computed roentgenography, provides precise anatomical localization for subsequent conventional transverse CT scanning.

► [This is an excellent discussion of the present applications and future potential for CT examination in the evaluation of musculoskeletal abnormalities. The review of current literature is extensive.—J.S.T.] ◄

4–28   **Cineradiographic Study of Football Helmets and the Cervical Spine.** Herbert Virgin (Mercy Hosp., Miami, Fla.) investigated the possible role of the posterior rim of football helmets in the occurrence of neck injuries in 16 men (4 professional football players, 5 high school athletes, and 7 hospital personnel). A series of lateral view cineradiograms of the path and position of the posterior rim of the helmet relative to the cervical spine was taken while each person's head was moved from the fully flexed to the full extended position under different loading conditions. The study group included short persons with chunky necks as well as tall persons with elongated necks. Five helmets from 5 different manufacturers were used.

There was no cineradiographic evidence that the posterior rim of the helmet ever impacted on the C1 through C6 spinous process. In fact, the helmet rim moved away from the cervical spine as the neck became hyperextended. If impingement did occur, it would have been on the thoracic spine. The findings were similar for all of the persons studied.

The results clearly demonstrate that it is impossible for the posterior rim of a modern football helmet to strike the C1 through C6 spinous process; therefore, the rim is not involved in injuries to the hyperextended cervical spine.

▶ [The conclusion of this radiographic study has been substantiated by a biomechanical analysis by Carter and Frankel (*Am. J. Sports Med.* 8:302, 1980) of the proposed "guillotine" effect of the posterior rim of the helmet. The importance of these studies is to refute the misconception that the football helmet is a causative factor in fractures or dislocations of the cervical spine.—J.S.T.] ◀

4–29   **Biomechanics of Lumbar Invertebral Disk: A Review.** Low back pain is one of the most common of human disabilities, and evidence suggests that degenerative and mechanical changes within the invertebral disk are a cause of this problem. Because physical therapy is often recommended for patients with low back pain, the physical therapist should understand the mechanics of the normal and abnormal invertebral disk. Gail M. Jensen (Stanford Univ.) reviewed the literature on the biomechanics of the lumbar invertebral disk. The areas in which the therapist should be knowledgeable include the following: disk structure and disk properties; biomechanical principles and their relevance to the disk; biomechanics and pressures within the disk as they relate to posture, work, and exercise; and prophylactic measures in the treatment of patients with low back pain. Numerous graphics are included to illustrate the anatomical components of the invertebral disk, the strain-stress curve, compression loading in normal and degenerated disks, tensile and compressive stresses in the disk during bending, tension and shear stresses resulting from torsion loading, pressure on the third lumbar disk in loaded and unloaded postures and during various exercises, the effect of backrest inclination and lumbar support on disk pressure, and forces generated in pushing and pulling.

▶ [This is a well-written, concise, and nicely illustrated basic review of the biomechan-

(4–28)   Am. J. Sports Med. 8:310–317, Sept.–Oct. 1980.
(4–29)   Phys. Ther. 60:765–773, June 1980.

ics of the lumbar invertebral disk. The original article is recommended for those desiring such elementary information.—J.S.T.] ◄

4–30 **Spondylolysis in Athletes.** Hitoshi Hoshina (Doshisha Univ., Kyoto, Japan) examined x-ray films of the lumbar spines of 677 male high school and university athletes to determine the incidence of spondylolysis.

Spondylolytic neural arches were detected in 140 (20.7%) athletes. University athletes had a slightly greater incidence of the defect than high school athletes (22.4% vs 20.0%). Spina bifida of the fifth lumbar vertebra was found in 8.9% of those with spondylolysis, compared to 2.1% in the normal group. Spondylolysis was more common in athletes who were heavier and had stronger back musculature. This was also the case for those with spina bifida of the fifth lumbar vertebra. Lower back pain was reported by 24.1% of those with spondylolysis and by 14.4% of those with intact neural arches. Spondylolysis was most common in sports requiring forcible hyperextension or rotation of the lumbar spine.

The incidence of spondylolysis in this study was approximately three times the estimated occurrence in the adult Japanese population. The chances of spondylolysis occurring in athletes can be diminished by correcting poor technique that results in excessive hyperextension or rotation of the spine. Early recognition of the fracture and support of the lumbar spine with a brace until healing is radiologically confirmed are important.

▶ [An interesting report is presented here on the relatively high incidence of spondylolysis in a group of Japanese athletes. To attribute the relatively high occurrence of back pain (14%) in those with no evidence of spondylolysis as being due to soft tissue origin is not valid. Radionuclide bone scans were indicated, but were not performed in this group. The suggestion that correcting the "poor technique" will prevent the lesion is not substantiated by the data presented.—J.S.T.] ◄

4–31 **Epidural Cortisone Injections in the Young Athletic Adult.** Lumbar epidural injection of cortisone can be a useful adjunct in the conservative management of athletes with a symptomatic lumbar disk and irritated neural elements. Douglas W. Jackson, Arthur Rettig, and Leon L. Wiltse (Meml. Hosp. Med. Center, Long Beach, Calif.) reviewed the findings in 32 competitive athletes with a clinical diagnosis of symptomatic lumbar disk and associated sciatica who received epidural steroid injections by the translumbar or sacral-hiatus route. Injections consisted of 120 mg of methylprednisolone in 6–10 ml of saline solution. The 26 men and 6 women had an average age of 24.5 years. All had low back pain and radiating leg pain distal to the knees; 82% had positive nerve root tension signs on physical examination. Ten patients had definite disk space narrowing at L4–L5 or L5–S1. Average duration of symptoms was 3.6 months. Average follow-up was $10^{1}/_{2}$ months.

Fourteen patients had relief from disabling radicular pain within 2–4 days after injection, and 6 had definite improvement but were

(4–30) Physician Sportsmed. 8:75–79, September 1980.
(4–31) Am. J. Sports Med. 8:239–243, July–Aug. 1980.

still restricted by pain. Twelve patients had no response within 2–4 days of steroid injection. Of 17 patients with a good or fair initial response who were followed up for more than 3 months, 13 had a good or fair final result. Two others were operated on. Of 9 patients with a poor initial response, on follow-up, 3 had a good result and 3 others were operated on. A good response was most frequent in patients with symptoms for less than 2 months at the time of epidural injection. Five patients (16%) were operated on within a year of onset of symptoms.

These results are encouraging, although the success rate in this study was lower than has been reported in larger groups of the general population. The selective use of metrizamide myelography, epidural lumbar venography, and computerized axial tomography in athletic patients who do not respond to conservative measures and epidural cortisone injections has been of considerable value in making decisions on management.

▶ [It would appear that an average follow-up of 10½ months is inadequate. Also to be noted is that the success rate in this group was less dramatic than for larger reported series in the general population.—J.S.T.] ◀

4–32 **Use of Modified Boston Brace for Back Injuries in Athletes** is described by Lyle J. Micheli, John E. Hall, and M. E. Miller (Children's Hosp. Med. Center, Boston). A spinal brace that maintains adequate immobilization or positioning of the spine and allows continued participation in normal adolescent activities is advantageous. The Boston brace system is a modification of the Milwaukee brace system. Low curves are treated without a metal superstructure and high curves retain it. There are 20 sizes of prefabricated thermoplastic body brace modules. Fitting of lumbar and thoracolumbar curves with an underarm brace results in increased functional activities and improved cosmesis (Fig 4–3). A module that opens posteriorly and is made for forward flexion on the anterior surface of 30 degrees and on the posterior surface of 15 degrees reduces lumbar lordosis.

Fifty-two young athletes were treated with the Boston brace in the past 3 years; 31 have completed brace treatment and have been followed for an average of 15 months. Eight of 12 patients with spondylolytic back pain had excellent results from brace treatment, and 4 had good results. (Good results implied full sports participation with some residual pain). Three of 6 adolescents with discogenic low back pain had good results, 2 had fair results, and 1 had a poor outcome. Three patients with apophyseal changes and low back pain had good or excellent results. Treatment of mechanical back pain resulted in 8 excellent and 2 good results. The combined average of good or excellent results for the group was 81%.

Good or excellent results have been obtained with the Boston brace in most young athletes. Most have continued full participation in athletics while wearing the brace. The stability afforded by thermoplastic orthotics and the reduced lumbar lordosis have helped in the treat-

(4–32) Am. J. Sports Med. 8:351–356, Sept.–Oct. 1980.

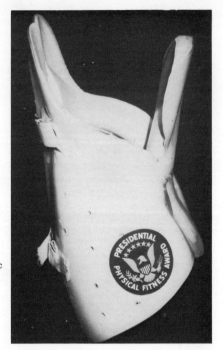

Fig 4–3.—Boston brace showing antilordotic contour. Physical fitness award was won while patient was wearing this brace. (Courtesy of Micheli, L. J., et al.: Am. J. Sports Med. 8:351–356, Sept.–Oct. 1980.)

ment of back injuries in these patients. The brace functions as both a therapeutic and a protective apparatus. Use of a semirigid lumbosacral orthosis lessens axial loading of the spine by increasing intra-abdominal pressure and limits pelvic torsion of the trunk.

▶ [The statement that a semirigid lumbosacral orthosis lessens axial loading of the spine by increasing intra-abdominal pressure requires an explanation. Is the brace acceptable to persons who participate in activities requiring a high degree of mobility, such as gymnastics? The authors fail to state when the brace is worn. Is it worn night and day? Is it worn during the daytime only and removed for activity? Is it worn only during activity? A comparison of the 52 youngsters treated with the Boston brace with a similar group not treated is necessary to determine the efficacy of the device.— J.S.T.] ◀

UPPER EXTREMITY INJURIES

4–33 **CT Evaluation of Intra-articular Fractures.** David H. Carlson (Newton-Wellesley Hosp., Newton Lower Falls, Mass.) has reviewed 2 cases in which computed tomographic (CT) scanning was useful in evaluation of intra-articular fractures.

CASE 1.—Man, 37, suffered an open comminuted fracture of the distal tibia and fibula in a fall (Fig 4–4, A and B). Better confirmation of the position of the intra-articular component was achieved on CT scanning, in which the position of the fragments appeared acceptable (Fig 4–4,C). Internal fixation could not be used because of the open nature of the fracture.

(4–33) South. Med. J. 73:820–821, June 1980.

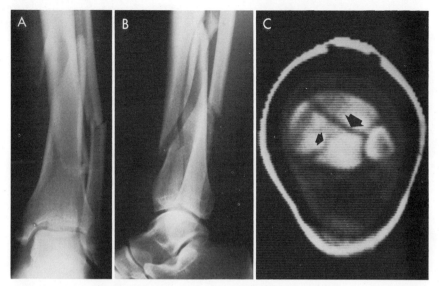

Fig 4–4.—**A** and **B,** roentgenograms of the left ankle show a comminuted fracture of the distal tibia and fibula, with extension into the joint space. **C,** a CT scan 1 cm above the ankle mortise shows transverse *(large arrow)* and sagittal *(small arrow)* tibial fractures with satisfactory alignment. (Courtesy of Carlson, D. H.: South. Med. J. 73:820–821, June 1980.)

CASE 2.—Woman, 68, sustained a comminuted fracture of the proximal tibia when she fell from a ladder. The extensive degree of comminution was better demonstrated on CT scanning, and the fracture was treated conservatively, since there were no major fragments to support an internal fixation device.

Thus in both cases, CT scanning helped in evaluation of the separation and size of the fracture fragments. Also, the unique cross-sectional anatomy seen on the CT scan gave a better sense of the orientation of the fragments. The presence of plaster does not limit detail, as it does on a roentgenogram. The mean and window may be manipulated to heighten certain areas of interest.

▶ [Computed tomography is an expensive method to determine information obtainable on oblique views of upper and lower extremities. A plaster cast does not interfere with determining the position of fracture fragments if the radiographs are exposed adequately and the cast material is radiolucent.—J.S.T.] ◀

4–34 **Digital Perfusion of Handball Players: Effects of Repeated Ball Impact on Structures of the Hand.** Decreased digital perfusion to the index finger of the catching hand of professional or collegiate baseball catchers has been described. Bradley C. Buckhout and Mark A. Warner used thermography and roentgenography to study the effects of repeated ball impacts on the hands of handball players to determine alterations in perfusion or other tissue changes. Twenty-two league and tournament handball players were examined and compared with 22 controls who had not played handball.

(4–34) Am. J. Sports Med. 8:206–207, May–June 1980.

Multiple areas of decreased perfusion were found in 17 of the players. Most of these cool areas were located over the metacarpal heads and in the fingers. A definite correlation between symptoms (coldness, numbness, or paleness) and thermographic findings was found in 8 of 12 players with symptoms. There was no correlation between bony abnormalities and symptomatic areas. Temperatures of the players' hands were considerably lower than those of controls. Players with more than 2 years' experience or 200 hours of accumulated playing time had a greater chance for the development of symptoms and thermographic changes.

These findings may provide a baseline for evaluating the efficacy of modifications in the design of handball gloves and balls.

▶ [The authors state that no skeletal or articular changes were noted. However, no mention is made of the presence of palmer calluses, fibrous subcutaneous thickening, or edema secondary to trauma. If present, what effects would these have on the thermographic display? Also, the authors have not discussed the quantitative relationship between actual profusion and thermographic findings.—J.S.T.] ◀

4–35 **Index Metacarpal Fractures in Karate.** Douglas W. Kelly (Torrance, Calif.), Michael J. Pitt (Tucson, Ariz.), and David M. Mayer (Grand Junction, Colo.) evaluated 18 male subjects suspected of having karate-related hand fractures. Eleven had metacarpal fractures, 5 of which involved the index metacarpal. There were 2 nonarticular fractures of the proximal portion of the thumb metacarpal, 1 avulsion fracture of the distal radial aspect of the thumb metacarpal, 2 fractures of the little finger metacarpal (more proximal than the common punch fracture), and 1 fracture of the ring finger metacarpal. Most injuries occurred in the dominant hand and resulted from missed blows. Nine of the 11 metacarpal fractures showed elements of axial compression. Ten patients returned to competition within 3 months of injury. Two patients with index metacarpal fractures had depressed knuckles.

Statistics show that the index metacarpal fractures occur uncommonly. In karate, the correctly executed thrust and hand strike places axial compression forces on the index and long finger metacarpal heads; these forces are transmitted to the distal carpal row, which is dynamically splinted by taut wrist extensors and flexors. This mechanism may have caused intra-articular fractures. Inaccurate thrusts transmit angular and torsional forces to the metacarpals, causing, when combined with axial loading, oblique diaphyseal fractures. Slight irregularities of metacarpal subchondral articular bones and subtle narrowing of joint spaces in metacarpophalangeal joints were also found in some individuals. Thrusts executed with equal axial compression of the index and long finger metacarpal heads, without torsional or angular stresses, could eliminate all fracture patterns observed, except those occurring from blocked kicks or board breaking.

▶ [No mention is made of the methods of treatment used. Also, the fact "all the patients except for one were able to return to competition within three months of injury" is not a suitable criterion by which to judge the results of management.—J.S.T.] ◀

(4–35) Physician Sportsmed. 8:103–106, March 1980.

4–36 **Fracture and Dislocation About the Carpal Lunate.** James R. Ryan (Wayne State Univ.) reports a case of delayed diagnosis of dislocation of the carpal lunate.

Man, 23, a gymnast, had injured the right wrist 3 months previously. Radiographs had been interpreted as normal by the emergency physician and radiologist, but the patient was unable to participate in athletics because of continued pain. The right wrist was diffusely swollen, and there was tenderness to palpation over the volar aspect. Radiographs revealed a volar dislocation of the carpal lunate. The original emergency room radiographs also confirmed the dislocation. Because the patient was young and a gymnast, open reduction rather than excision of the carpal lunate was undertaken. The bone was fixed with two Kirschner wires and held in place for 6 weeks. The wires were then removed and range-of-motion exercises begun. There was no avascular necrosis, and the patient regained almost normal motion.

The lunate may dislocate in relation to the radius and other carpal bones. The dislocation is usually in a volar direction. The lunate may retain its normal relation with the radius even when the other carpal bones dislocate. This is called a perilunate dislocation. The carpal bones then dislocate dorsally. With lunate dislocations, if the lunate rotates 90 degrees, it is seen as a triangular shape rather than its normal quadrilateral shape. In a lateral view the lunate appears displaced volarward and usually rotated. Without an associated navicular fracture, the dislocation is best interpreted in the lateral radiograph, which shows that the capitate is displaced dorsally and the head of the capitate does not articulate with the lunate. An abnormal gap between the carpal navicular and lunate is seen on an anteroposterior radiograph, where the space should bear the same relationship as the space between the other carpal articulations. The injury usually requires surgical reduction.

▶ ["Patients with injuries about the wrist should not be diagnosed as having sprains and released from the emergency department until the physician is confident in interpreting the radiographs of these injuries."—J.S.T.] ◀

4–37 **Evaluating Carpal Instabilities With Fluoroscopy.** Jacob M. Protas and William T. Jackson (Univ. of Texas) evaluated 4 patients (5 wrists) in whom wrist movement caused pain and a clicking sound, suggesting carpal instability. In all, radiographic and arthrographic studies showed either normal or nonspecific findings. Fluoroscopy was undertaken to observe the wrist in motion.

CASE 1.—Man, 21, injured the right wrist when a door slammed against the dorsal aspect of the hand and wrist. Radial and ulnar deviation produced a painful audible "pop." Radiographs were normal, but an arthrogram revealed abnormal communication between the radiocarpal and the lunate-triquetral space. Fluoroscopic examination revealed asymmetric widening of the scapholunate space. Continued smooth exertion toward ulnar deviation produced a rapid lurch of the proximal pole of the scaphoid into normal position, causing pain. A ligament reconstruction was done with the use of a split segment of extensor carpi radialis brevis. Immobilization was discontinued after 6 weeks. The patient returned to work after 3 more weeks. Fluoroscopy showed normal scaphoid movement 5 months later.

(4–36) Ann. Emerg. Med. 9:158–160, March 1980.
(4–37) AJR 135:137–140, July 1980.

CASE 2.—Boy, 16, had a 3-year history of clicking wrists on ulnar deviation. The right wrist remained asymptomatic, but pain had developed in the left wrist. Fluoroscopic findings in the right wrist were similar to those in case 1. Findings in the left wrist revealed a more dramatic lurching motion because the entire proximal carpal row jerked as a unit. Reconstruction of the dorsal radiocarpal and the scapholunate intercarpal ligaments was undertaken, using one half of the extensor carpi radialis brevis. Normal synchronous movement was restored, with some limitation in range of motion.

CASE 3.—Man, 39, injured the right wrist while working with a sledgehammer. He had injured the same wrist 1 year previously. Plain radiographs showed a healed fracture of the scaphoid with an exostosis on the proximal border of the midbody. The osteophyte on the scaphoid was excised 2½ months after the second injury. Excision of residual osteophytes 2 months later still produced no relief. Fluoroscopy showed severe radial deviation limitation due to impingement of the residual scaphoid osteophyte against the styloid process of the radius. A radial styloidectomy and limited carpal fusion were done.

CASE 4.—Man, 19, fell on the right hand. Fracture of the right medial malleolus was demonstrated, and after 3 weeks of immobilization, static radiographic examinations were normal. Clicking persisted, and fluoroscopic examination revealed the dyssynchronous movement observed in case 1, but only with the hand in a clenched fist. At operation, radioscapholunate articulations were stabilized by passing tendon graft from the extensor carpi radialis brevis through adjacent drill holes in these bones.

These cases demonstrate that ligamentous damage can occur and yet not be demonstrated by plain film study or by arthrography. Fluoroscopic examination can document such injuries.

▶ [The art of fluoroscopy is presently underutilized. With the advent of videotape recording, fluoroscopy is a readily available procedure for evaluation and documentation of joint motion unobtainable by other means.—J.S.T.] ◀

4–38 **Elbow and Tennis.**—*Part 1. An analysis of players with and without pain.*—Although "tennis elbow." or lateral humeral epicondylitis, was first described more than 100 years ago, only two statistical studies of this entity among average tennis players have been published. James D. Priest, Vic Braden, and Susan Goodwin Gerberich (Inst. for Athletic Medicine, Minneapolis) statistically analyzed the differences between tennis players with and without elbow pain.

In all, 2,633 completed questionnaires were returned by 1,343 male and 1,290 female tennis players, 31% of whom reported having had elbow pain at some time during their playing history. The frequency of elbow injury was almost 4 times as great as the next most frequently injured area (ankle, 8%). The variables most significantly associated with elbow pain were increased age and a greater frequency of play ($P < .005$). Other factors significantly associated with elbow pain were greater body weight, advanced level of ability, increased years of play, and the occurrence of other tennis injuries. Height, hand dominance, and two-handed strokes were not significantly related to elbow pain; in fact, there is some evidence that the two-handed backhand stroke may be effective in treating or preventing

(4–38) Physician Sportsmed. 8:81–91, April 1980.

tennis elbow. Shoulder and knee injuries were more common in men, whereas forearm and wrist injuries were more common among women.

The results contradict the supposition that beginners, weekend players, and players with low ability are more susceptible to the development of tennis elbow. Rather, it appears that the harmful effects of tennis are cumulative and that many factors may interact before elbow pain develops.

4–39 **The Elbow and Tennis.**—*Part 2. A study of players with pain.*— Priest, Braden, and Gerberich investigated 2,633 tennis players for the presence of elbow pain by questionnaire and physical examination over a 2-year period. In part 1 of the study, age, weight, level of ability, years of play, and frequency of play were all found to be significantly greater in players with elbow pain. Of the 2,633 players (1,343 men and 1,290 women), 31% had experienced elbow pain at some time in their careers; of these 811, 41% were currently experiencing pain. Players had begun playing tennis at a mean age of 30.1 years; elbow pain was noted 9.1 years after beginning. The percentage of players with elbow pain history increased almost linearly from ages 21 through 25 to ages 51 through 55 and increased with increasing years of play, especially after 10 years. Frequency of play was a factor; the incidence of pain was 5 times greater for individuals playing once a day than for those playing once a month. The lateral humeral epicondyle was the most frequent site of discomfort (75%), but 17% had pain over the lateral or extensor muscle mass. The backhand was the most painful stroke among players with lateral epicondylitis, while serve and forehand were cited as most painful among players with medial epicondylitis. Pain was episodic in 39% of participants, but 61% had a single occurrence of pain. Only 14% of participants had ever had generalized muscle, bone, or joint disease. Patients identified 37 different forms of treatment; the most common were rest, exercises, and alteration of tennis stroke, while the most frequent were tennis elbow support or brace (131) and cortisone or steroid (130), rest (95), and heat (50). Alteration of tennis stroke was the most successful form of treatment, and exercise the second most successful. Steroids were successful in 75%. Cold and ultrasound were least helpful.

Results of the study suggest that the harmful effects of tennis may be cumulative and many variables may interact before elbow pain occurs. In most players, tennis playing was a significant factor in the production of elbow symptoms. It is also worth noting that among girls between ages 11 and 15, 23% reported pain. Also, medial symptoms were more than twice as common in men than women, possibly due to their more strenuous service motion.

▶ [This study correlates a symptom, elbow pain, with a number of variables involved in playing tennis. To be noted is the fact that the article deals solely with a symptom, and no attempt is made to account for this subjective finding on the basis of a pathologic diagnosis.—J.S.T.] ◀

(4–39) Physician Sportsmed. 8:70–85, May 1980.

4–40 **Osseous Manifestations of Elbow Stress Associated With Sports Activities.** The elbow is the focus of musculoskeletal stress in throwing and racket sports and is particularly prone to injury. Richard M. Gore, Lee F. Rogers, Jack Bowerman, Jacob Suker, and Clinton L. Compere (Northwestern Univ., Chicago) reviewed the elbow radiographs of 29 symptomatic professional, amateur, and juvenile athletes, aged 8–82 years; 9 were aged 15 and younger. The adults included 16 professional baseball players. Comparison views of the nondominant elbow were available in 24 cases.

Osseous abnormalities were seen in all but 1 of the baseball players and in 5 of the 9 juvenile athletes. Most adults showed generalized bony hypertrophy in the region. Loose bodies were commonly found in the elbow joints of pitchers. One amateur thrower had a spiral fracture of the humerus with a butterfly component. Most adults had an ulnar traction spur arising from the medial aspect of the coronoid tubercle. Avulsion of the medial epicondylar apophysis was seen in 3 juveniles. One professional pitcher had an osteochondral fracture of the capitellum. Two adolescents had similar injuries. Loose bodies were found in the olecranon fossa in 2 professional pitchers.

Osseous changes at the elbow may result from diffuse generalized stress from overuse of the extremity or may be secondary to a specific, localized stress unique to a phase of the pitching act. Diffuse stress is believed partly responsible for loose bodies in the elbows of professional pitchers. Most localized injuries in both professional and juvenile pitchers and in tennis players are due to medial tension stress. The most common focal osseous manifestation of stress in professional pitchers and tennis players is a traction spur arising from the medial aspect of the coronoid tubercle. The most common significant injury of the juvenile pitcher is avulsion of the medial epicondylar apophysis. Most permanently disabling elbow injuries in adolescents are lateral compression injuries. Stress fracture or acute avulsive injury may result from extension stress in adults. Avulsion fracture of the olecranon apophysis due to pull of the triceps has been reported in adolescents.

4–41 **Myositis Ossificans of the Upper Arm** is a benign condition due to severe muscle contusion and heterotopic bone formation. It is seen most often in men and boys aged 15–30 years, particularly after football injuries. Symptoms include pain in the affected muscle, a palpable mass, and a flexion contracture. Charles D. Huss and James J. Puhl report the findings in 10 cases of myositis ossificans in the upper arm in 9 patients, all a result of football injuries. Median age was 17 years. Seven patients presented with flexion contracture of the elbow. Eight patients had a palpable mass, and pain was prominent in 7.

Seven patients were significantly improved or asymptomatic within 3 months of the start of conservative treatment. Three patients underwent surgery for a persistent painful mass. Two of them had clinical and radiographic evidence of recurrence postoperatively despite

(4–40) AJR 134:971, May 1980.
(4–41) Am. J. Sports Med. 8:419–424, Nov.–Dec. 1980.

delaying excision until there was radiographic evidence of maturation. One patient had complete disappearance of pain, mass, and contracture after surgical treatment. All 5 patients managed nonsurgically and with restricted activity had resolution of the flexion contracture. One of the 5 was completely free of signs and symptoms, 3 were asymptomatic but had palpable masses at the end of the observation period, and 1 was improved but still complained of some pain.

The exact mechanism of injury in these cases is not clear, but the predilection of injuries for the lateral or anterolateral aspect of the middle or distal part of the arm indicates that the player's own shoulder pads may transmit the blow of a tackle or block to this area. The ban on "spearing" and increased use of the arm in lieu of the helmet may increase the occurrence of these injuries. It is not clear whether continuation of contact sports with padding of the affected area in the convalescent period worsens or lengthens the process.

▶ [The authors have failed to differentiate between myositis ossificans, as manifested histologically by heterotrophic bone formation, and tackler's exostosis, as reported by Diamond and McMaster (*J. Sports Med.* 3:238, Sept.–Oct. 1975). The latter lesion is often bilateral and is characterized by lack of involvement of the anterior mass of the brachialis muscle or elbow. Perhaps the failure to differentiate between a mature exostosis and myositis ossificans is related to the 66% recurrence rate in those treated surgically.

The authors also have failed to comment on the histologic pattern of the three lesions removed surgically. The value or lack thereof of a radionuclide bone scan has also not been considered. Correlation of alkaline phosphotase studies with resolution of the lesion or timing for excision would be interesting and should be a part of a prospective study dealing with this problem.—J.S.T.] ◀

4–42 **Treatment of Acromioclavicular Separations: Retrospective Study.** John P. Park, James A. Arnold, Tom P. Coker, Walter Duke Harris, and David A. Becker (Univ. of Arkansas) made a follow-up study of 134 patients with types I, II, and III acromioclavicular separation. The mechanism of injury was a direct blow in 92% of patients, whose average age was 30.1 years. Average follow-up was 6.3 years. A standard rating system for the shoulder and humerus was used; the total for perfect recovery was 100. Type I separations (24 patients) were immobilized for a mean of 19.5 days. Disability lasted an average of 6 weeks. The mean rating was 94. Type II separations (25) were immobilized for a mean of 27 days. The average disability period was 6 weeks. The mean rating was 90. Eighty-five patients with type III separations were followed. Seven treated conservatively were immobilized an average of 22 days, had a mean disability period of 13 weeks, and had a mean rating of 82. For the 20 patients who underwent surgical repair excluding Dacron graft substitution, mean immobilization was 6 weeks, mean disability period was 12 weeks, and mean rating was 80. Fifty-eight patients underwent repair with double velour Dacron prosthetic substitution for the coracoclavicular ligaments, combined with distal clavicular resection in all but 2. Average immobilization lasted 1 week and average disability lasted 3

(4–42) Am. J. Sports Med. 8:251–256, July–Aug. 1980.

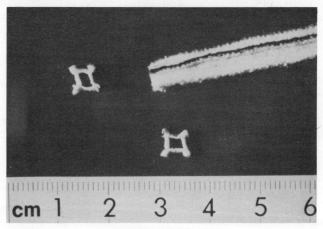

Fig 4–5.—Figure H-beams made of 0.6×3.2-cm piece of double velour Dacron. Such H-beams are used to form grafts in knee for repair of ligaments and prosthesis in shoulder for treatment of acromioclavicular separations. (Courtesy of Park, J. P., et al.: Am. J. Sports Med. 8:251–256, July–Aug. 1980.)

Fig 4–6.—Appearance at end of operation. (Courtesy of Park, J. P., et al.: Am. J. Sports Med. 8:251–256, July–Aug, 1980.)

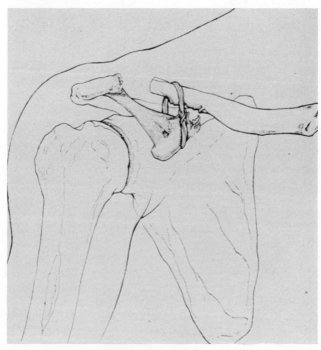

weeks. The average rating was 96; 24 patients had a rating of 100. Among those with a rating of less than 100, slight to moderate pain was present, which persisted in a few, but which was only occasional and associated with a particular activity. One infection occurred, which required graft removal 5 months after operation. Calcification in the area of the coracoclavicular ligaments did not affect the final rating, and the deformity did not recur.

The surgical technique of Henry was modified by use of a straight incision from the coracoid process to the acromion. The clavicular origin of the deltoid was exposed, and the distal 1 cm of the clavicle, with its meniscus, and the acromioclavicular joint were excised. Traction on the clavicle permitted exposure of the coracoid process. Periosteum beneath the coracoid was elevated and the graft was passed around the clavicle and beneath the coracoid process. The graft was placed posterior to the tendon or origin on the coracobrachialis muscle and was tied in a square knot deep within the substance of the wound (Fig 4–5), while the clavicle was held in reduced position. The double velour Dacron graft with an H-beam configuration (Fig 4–6) was thought to approach the modulus of elasticity of the human ligament. This procedure is relatively easy, reduces the time of immobilization, and allows earlier resumption of normal activities, and gives good results.

▶ [Although the authors, in reporting this series of 134 patients with acromioclavicular separations of types I, II, and III, state a mean follow-up of 6.3 years for the group, they have failed to specify the length of follow-up for the 58 patients who underwent repair with the double velour Dacron prosthetic substitution for the coracoclavicular ligaments. For the critical reader evaluating the worthiness of this prosthetic substance, this oversight is a major problem. Also, the authors' conclusion, "The procedure we have developed with the use of the double velour Dacron graft seems to be the most effective for the patient of any treatment we have in our armamentarium at this time," is not substantiated by the data presented.—J.S.T.] ◀

4–43 **Repair of Recurrent Anterior Dislocation of the Shoulder Using Transfer of the Subscapularis Tendon.** Over 150 operations for recurrent anterior shoulder dislocation have been described. J. Karadimas, G. Rentis, and G. Varouchas (Naval Hosp., Athens) report the treatment of 154 cases by transfer of the subscapularis tendon, as described by Magnuson and Stack. This operation, which resembles the Putti-Platt procedure, may be ideal for treating recurrent anterior shoulder dislocation because it is simple, prevents further dislocation in a high proportion of cases, and causes no significant loss of shoulder motion. One of 152 patients operated on in 1952–1978 had both shoulders operated on, and another required a second operation for recurrent dislocation after a new injury. All patients were male, with an average age of 23 years. A violent injury had caused initial dislocation in 70.4% of cases.

The tendon is transferred not only laterally but also distally, about 1 cm past the greater tuberosity. A bone wedge is not transplanted with the tendon insertion, rather, the insertion itself is transferred.

(4–43) J. Bone Joint Surg. [Am.] 62-A:1147–1149, October 1980.

The shoulder operated on is placed in a Velpeau dressing for about 3 weeks, when physiotherapy is begun.

Limited abduction and external rotation were noted in most cases for 6 months after surgery, but the range of motion gradually improved in all cases. No serious complications occurred. Results were excellent in 87.7% of shoulders, with no pain and less than 10 degrees of limitation of external rotation. Another 10.3% of shoulders had satisfactory results, whereas 3 had unsatisfactory results with recurrent dislocation. The only patient previously operated on elsewhere had had recurrent dislocation.

Follow-up of these patients has been long enough to have revealed most recurrences, were these to occur. The rate of postoperative recurrence has been only 2%. Transfer of the subscapularis tendon distally as well as laterally may be an improvement on the original technique of Magnuson and Stack.

▶ [An average follow-up of 7.6 years is certainly adequate to evaluate this surgical procedure. The 2% recurrence rate compares very well with other reported series for the Magnuson-Stack method, as well as other procedures. Subjects of this report were members of the Greek War Navy and not necessarily involved in competitive athletics or contact activities.—J.S.T.] ◄

4–44   **The Shoulder in Competitive Swimming.** The most common orthopedic problem in competitive swimming is shoulder pain. Allen B. Richardson, Frank W. Jobe, and H. Royer Collins (Natl. Athletic Health Inst., Inglewood, Calif.) surveyed and examined 137 highly competitive swimmers to investigate this problem. The group comprised 83 female and 54 male swimmers aged 14–23 years. Of 58 swimmers who reported a history of shoulder pain, 53 (91%) responded to a detailed questionnaire.

Symptoms were more common during the early and middle season. The incidence of shoulder problems increased with the ability of the swimmer, was somewhat more common in males, and was associated with sprint rather than distance swimming. Analysis of the shoulder mechanics involved in swimming showed that freestyle, butterfly, and backstroke require similar motions, and that a swimmer using any of these strokes is susceptible to shoulder pain (table and Fig 4–7 to 4–9). Most of the swimmers reported that pain occurred during both the pullthrough and recovery phases of the stroke. The pain was more likely to occur on the dominant, the right, or the breathing side. More than 80% of the swimmers stated that hand-paddle training exacerbated symptoms. The most common forms of treatment were ice packing, decreasing yardage, heat, complete rest, massage, ultrasound, oral medication, and steroid injections. Several swimmers felt that weight work and stretching decreased the shoulder pain.

It is believed that shoulder pain in swimmers is the result of chronic irritation of the humeral head and rotator cuff on the coracoacromial arch during abduction of the shoulder. If treatment is directed to the biceps tendon alone, symptoms will persist. It is hypoth-

(4–44) Am. J. Sports Med. 8:159–163, May–June 1980.

SHOULDER MECHANICS IN SWIMMING

Stroke and phases	Description
Freestyle	
Pull-through phase	
Hand entry	Shoulder external rotation and abduction. Body roll begins
Midpull-through	Shoulder at 90° abduction and neutral internal-external rotation. Body roll is at maximum of 40–60° from horizontal
End of pull-through	Shoulder internally rotated and fully adducted. Body has returned to horizontal
Recovery phase	
Elbow lift	Shoulder begins abduction and external rotation. Body roll begins in opposite direction from pull-through
Midrecovery	Shoulder abducted to 90° and externally rotated beyond neutral. Body roll reaches maximum of 40–60°. Breathing occurs by turning head to side
Hand entry	Shoulder externally rotated and maximally abducted. Body has returned to neutral roll
Backstroke	
Pull-through phase	
Hand entry	Shoulder external rotation and abduction. Body roll begins
Midpull-through	Shoulder at 90° abduction and neutral internal-external rotation. Body roll maximum
End of pull-through	Shoulder internally rotated and abducted. Body roll horizontal
Recovery phase	
Hand lift	Shoulder begins abduction and external rotation. Body roll allows arm to clear water
Midrecovery	Shoulder at 90° abduction. Body roll maximum
Hand entry	Shoulder at maximum abduction. Body roll neutral
Butterfly	
Pull-through phase	Same as freestyle with the absence of body roll in all stages. To avoid shoulder flexion or extension, the hands are spread apart at the mid pull-through stage
Recovery phase	Again, similar to freestyle with the absence of body roll. Body lift allows both arms to clear the water. Shoulder flexion-extension does not occur.

esized that body roll in freestyle and backstroke and body lift in butterfly will be significant determinants of pain.

▶ [Of 137 competitive swimmers questioned, 58 had symptoms of "swimmer's shoulder." Of the 53 in this group who responded to the authors' questionnaire, 29 had pain severe enough to seek a physician's help. The efficacy of treatment, including stretching, rest, ice therapy, oral anti-inflammatory agents, and injectible steroids, was not evaluated; therefore, no conclusion can be drawn with regard to these modalities. Also, attributing shoulder pain in swimmers to result from chronic irritation of the humeral head and rotator cuff on the coracoacromial arch during abduction of the shoulder is suppositional.—J.S.T.] ◀

4–45 **Impingement Syndrome in Athletes** is discussed by R. J. Hawkins and J. C. Kennedy (London, Ont.). In athletes involved in sporting

(4–45) Am. J. Sports Med. 8:151–158, May–June 1980.

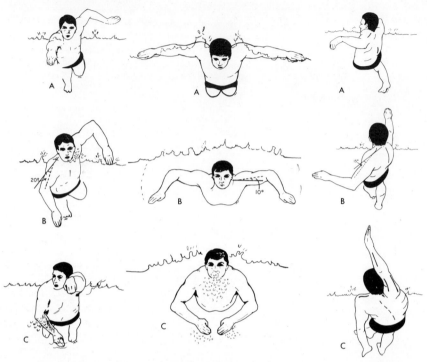

Fig 4–7 (left).—Illustration of shoulder mechanics in freestyle competitive swimming. For the right arm, three stages are identified: hand entry (**A**), mid-pull-through (**B**), and end of pull-through (**C**). For the left arm, three stages can be identified: elbow lift (**A**), midrecovery (**B**), and hand entry (**C**).

Fig 4–8 (center).—Illustration of shoulder mechanics in butterfly competitive swimming. Three stages are shown: midrecovery (**A**), mid-pull-through (**B**), and end of pull-through (**C**).

Fig 4–9 (right).—Illustration of shoulder mechanics in backstroke competitive swimming. For the right arm, three stages are identified: hand lift (**A**), midrecovery (**B**), and hand entry (**C**). For the left arm, three stages can be identified: hand entry (**A**), midpull-through (**B**), and end of pull-through (**C**).

(Courtesy of Richardson, A. B., et al.: Am. J. Sports Med. 8:159–163, May–June 1980.)

activities requiring repetitive overhead use of the arm (tennis players, swimmers, baseball pitchers, and quarterbacks), a painful shoulder may develop because of impingement in the vulnerable avascular region of the supraspinatus and biceps tendons. With time, degeneration and tears of the rotator cuff may result. Pathologically, the syndrome has been classified into stage I (edema and hemorrhage), stage II (fibrosis and tendonitis), and stage III (tendon degeneration, bony changes, and tendon ruptures). The syndrome may be a problem for the young, competitive athlete as well as for the casual weekend athlete.

Positive clinical signs in stage I include: point tenderness over the greater tuberosity and usually the anterior acromion; painful arc of abduction, maximum at 90 degrees; and a positive "impingement sign," which reproduces the pain and resulting facial expression when the arm is forcibly forward flexed (jamming the greater tuberosity against the anteroinferior surface of the acromion). A less reliable method of demonstrating this impingement is described in Figure 4–10.This maneuver drives the greater tuberosity farther under the coracoacromial ligament, reproducing the impingement pain. The biceps tendon may be involved in addition to the supraspinatus tendon. At stage II, there is more commonly a stiffer shoulder, sometimes with acromioclavicular tenderness, and the lesion is not reversed by avoidance of activity. Pain-related weakness and stiffness increase in stage III, and roentgenograms often show sclerosis and osteophyte formation in complete-thickness rotator cuff tears. Differential diagnosis includes acute traumatic bursitis, the apprehension shoulder, primary acromioclavicular pathology, cervical disk, calcific tendinitis, and frozen shoulder. Diagnosis of the apprehension or unstable shoulder in the absence of dislocation is shown in Figure 4–11.

Warm-up exercises, isokinetic equipment for developing strength and endurance in the shoulder, and modification of training practices may prevent or be useful in treatment of impingement syndrome. Treatment in stage I includes icing of the shoulder after workouts, ultrasound, anti-inflammatory agents, or transcutaneous nerve stimulation. In some cases, total rest may be necessary for a period of time. Steroids should be avoided. Surgical treatment involves dividing the coracoacromial ligament; however, relief may not be long lasting. Prolonged use of anti-inflammatory agents with range of motion

Fig 4–10.—In this method of demonstrating the impingement sign, the arm is flexed forward at about 90 degrees and the shoulder is then forcibly internally rotated, impaling the supraspinatus tendon against the anterior surface of the coracoacromial ligament, reproducing the patient's pain. This test might be helpful when resection of this ligament is being considered. (Courtesy of Hawkins, R. J., and Kennedy, J. C.: Am. J. Sports Med. 8:151–158, May–June 1980.)

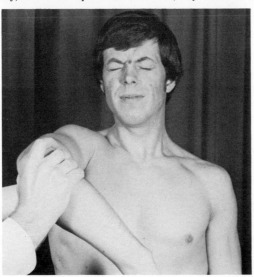

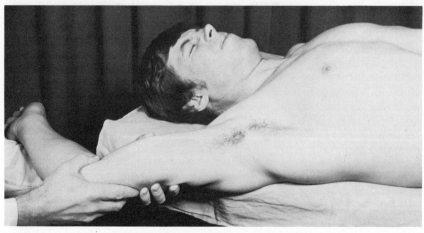

Fig 4–11.—A positive apprehension sign. This test is a method of determining anterior instability of the shoulder and is performed with the athlete lying supine. The humeral head is externally rotated and abducted and stressed anteriorly, in an attempt to sublux it out of the joint. The patient will have immediate feelings of misgiving and anxiety, sometimes associated with pain. (Courtesy of Hawkins, R. J., and Kennedy, J. C.: Am. J. Sports Med. 8:151–158, May–June 1980.)

exercises are recommended in treatment of stage II. In stage III, a complete-thickness rotator cuff tear with pain lasting for more than 3 months might suggest that decompressive anterior acromioplasty be performed, with preservation of the deltoid and repair of the rotator cuff. Anterior acromioplasties performed in young athletic subjects with absence of rotator cuff tears over a 2-year period have shown good results for stage II. Resecting the coracoacromial ligament through a deltoid split is a lesser procedure and might be attempted first in stage II. With biceps involvement in the presence of a history of shoulder problems, anterior acromioplasty, exploration of the rotator cuff, and surgical attack on the biceps tendon itself may be necessary.

▶ [The reader is referred to the original article, which is informative, well written, and well illustrated.—J.S.T.] ◀

4–46 **Pack Palsy in Backpackers.** Upper limb numbness, weakness, and atrophy have been associated with use of a heavy backpack in military personnel. The condition is termed pack palsy or rucksack paralysis. The cause is presumed to be compression of the upper trunk of the brachial plexus or the peripheral nerve supply to the shoulder girdle. Guy Corkill, James S. Lieberman, and Robert G. Taylor (Univ. of California, Davis Med. Center, Sacramento) have treated 3 male civilians with weakness or atrophy of the shoulder muscles, or both, associated with backpacking. The cause in all 3 cases appears to have been peripheral nerve injury, although most other reported cases have been attributed to brachial plexus compression. One patient had accessory nerve involvement as well as involvement of muscles innervated by the suprascapular and long thoracic nerves; the latter nerves were involved in the other cases. One patient had hepatitis B infection, and 1 may have had an abnormal sleep posture.

The prognosis for complete recovery within 3 months approaches 90%. Treatment consists primarily of removing the source of trauma. A sling may be helpful when trapezius or deltoid weakness allows shoulder separation. Heavy therapeutic exercise may be harmful. Pack palsy should be considered in civilians as well as military personnel who present with weakness and wasting of the arm and shoulder girdle without an obvious cause. Electrodiagnostic testing may help localize the process to the upper trunk of the brachial plexus or the nerves to the shoulder musculature. Recovery usually is good, although prolonged dysfunction may occur if the condition is not recognized.

▶ [An excellent discussion is presented here of a relatively unappreciated problem. The reader is referred to the original article.—J.S.T.] ◀

4–47 **Pain in Avulsion Lesions of Brachial Plexus.** Traction lesions of the brachial plexus are occurring more frequently, especially among motorcyclists. Avulsion of nerve roots from the spinal cord is often involved and is associated with a severe burning pain in the anesthetic area. This type of pain and the difficulty in managing it have been discussed in the literature, but there has been no long-term study of the nature of this pain and the efficacy of various therapies. C. B. Wynn Parry (Royal Natl. Orthopaedic Hosp., London) reports on the long-term follow-up of 275 patients with traction lesions of the brachial plexus who were followed for at least 3 years and, in some cases, for 30 years. From this group, 108 were selected who had evidence of avulsion of one or more roots of the brachial plexus. A significant degree of pain was experienced by 98 of these patients. Virtually all sustained their injuries in motorcycle accidents.

Descriptions of the pain and the various activities affecting it were similar among the patients. External stimuli do not affect this type of pain, and treatment with analgesics is of little value. Cannabis produced remarkable relief in 5 patients, but because of its side effects, none continued to use it. Transcutaneous electric stimulation was the most effective method of treatment; self-absorption in a job or hobby was the most effective maneuver to reduce pain. Transcutaneous electric stimulation was not effective in 12 patients whose lesions were total, which suggests that there must be some afferent input for this treatment to be effective. In 12 patients, the pain continues to be as severe as it was at the time of injury or is growing steadily worse; these patients are being considered for cerebral electric stimulation.

Early return to work and participation in community activities offer the best prospects for relief, as distraction from the pain appears to be the most potent analgesic.

▶ [The authors have differentiated among three main types of traction lesions of the

(4–47) Pain 9:41–53, August 1980.

brachial plexus. First is a traction lesion in continuity, in which the nerve fibers are stretched and degenerate while the epineural sheath remains intact and there is a possibility of spontaneous regeneration. The second type, rupture of the spinal nerves between the two points of anchorage of the plexus, the intervertebral foramina and the clavipectoral fascia, is amenable to surgical repair, at least in the upper part of the trunk. In the third type, avulsion of roots from the cord, there is no hope of recovery. This article provides a classic description of the features of an avulsion of one or more roots secondary to trauma.—J.S.T.] ◀

4–48   **Closed Injuries of the Pectoralis Major Muscle** are discussed by Ronald Tietjen (Danbury, Conn.). Review of the literature revealed about 100 cases. Injuries occur most commonly between ages 20 and 35 years, are mostly on the right side, and thus far have been reported only in male patients. X-ray films can reveal loss of the pectoralis major shadow and loss of the normal soft tissue anterior axillary fold when ruptures are complete. Symptoms include sudden, snapping, tearing pain in the area of the muscle, followed by persistent discomfort. Clinical signs vary and depend on the location and extent of injury. Pain and tenderness over the injured part increase with forced adduction of the arm. Weakness is common in complete tears, and swelling is seen in severe injuries. Ecchymosis is common in injuries involving the muscle belly. Indirect trauma most often causes the injury. Forced adduction against resistance and involuntary contraction or a severe pull on the arm may cause the injury.

A classification based on the extent and anatomical location of the tear is proposed. Contusion or sprain (type I) is the most common injury. A partial injury (type II) may compel patients to seek medical attention because of severe, persistent symptoms. Complete injuries (type III) are rare. A complete tear at the muscle origin (IIIA) is indicated by cosmetic deformity, swelling, and bunching of muscle away from the origin. Tears of the muscle belly (IIIB) are indicated by swelling and tenderness associated with hematoma. In tears of the musculotendinous junction (IIIC), bunching of the muscle is seen medial to the tear. Tears of the muscle tendon (IIID) are indicated by marked weakness of adduction and ecchymosis extending down the arm.

Treatment suggested for type I injury is activity as tolerated. Rest and immobilization are recommended in type II and type IIIA injuries. Type IIIB requires rest and immobilization with consideration of evacuation of the hematoma if it is significant and possible attempted repair of the muscle belly. If cosmetic or functional deformity is severe, type IIIC may require attempted establishment of continuity of the musculotendinous junction, besides the treatment recommended for type IIIB. Type IIID injuries are the best candidates for surgical repair followed by immobilization until healing takes place.

▶ [It is difficult to understand how the authors have developed their elaborate classification with specific recommendations for treatment, which includes surgical repair, on the basis of the three cases that they have presented, all treated conservatively and having full functional recovery.—J.S.T.] ◀

(4–48)   J. Trauma 20:262–264, March 1980.

LOWER EXTREMITY INJURIES

4–49 **Achilles Tendon Disorders in Runners: A Review.** G. W. Smart, J. E. Taunton, and D. B. Clement (Simon Fraser Univ., Burnaby, B. C.) point out that the increase in fitness activities has led to an increase in injuries to runners that may hamper training. Both recreational joggers and competitive athletes are affected. The dynamic imbalance that develops between active muscles during training is an important biomechanical factor in Achilles tendon disease. Most Achilles tendon disorders attributable to poorly designed footwear arise in the shoe heel because of inadequate heel wedging. Changes in foot plant or in the type of training surface can lead to microtrauma in the Achilles tendon. Training errors also may lead to tendon damage, as can the resumption of training after a long period of relative inactivity. Achilles tendon ruptures often are preceded by local steroid injections. Various rheumatic conditions have been implicated in Achilles tendon disease. Injuries may result from pushing off at the start of a sprint or jump or from the violent dorsiflexion of the plantar-flexed foot.

Peritendinitis with or without tendonisis requires immediate withdrawal from all activities that increase symptoms. Crutch immobilization may be necessary. Oral anti-inflammatory agents, ice massage, heel wedges, and foot orthoses also may be helpful. Release of the paratenon has been recommended for chronic peritendinitis. Repair of a partial rupture can be reinforced with the plantaris tendon or flaps from the tendon aponeurosis. Surgical repair of a total rupture appears to provide superior tendon reconstitution and restoration of function. Relative inactivity is recommended for 7–10 days after symptoms subside and should be followed by a gradual return to the preinjury level of activity. The training shoe should be modified or replaced to provide maximum protection to the Achilles tendon. Exercises to restore tendon function must follow removal of a cast. Swimming exercise is helpful. The athlete can resume running after 2–3 weeks of successful therapy. A staged program of progressive intensity is recommended.

▶ [With a virtual epidemic of injuries occurring in runners, this article presents a timely review of those problems involving the Achilles tendon. It is recommended reading for those caring for the running athlete.—J.S.T.] ◀

4–50 **Thompson Test for Ruptured Achilles Tendon.** H. Bates Noble and F. Harlan Selesnick (Northwestern Univ.) review an easy method to diagnose this injury promptly. The Thompson test is performed with the patient prone or kneeling on an examining table with feet extended beyond the table's edge. The examiner should squeeze both calves just below the widest calf circumference (Fig 4–12). The test is positive when the foot on the injured side cannot perform plantar flexion.

Studies have reported that 22% to 46% of Achilles tendon ruptures

(4–49) Med. Sci. Sports Exercise 12:231–243, October 1980.
(4–50) Physician Sportsmed. 8:63–64, August 1980.

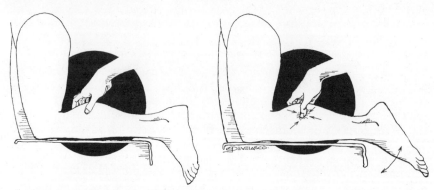

Fig 4–12.—Performing the Thompson test. (Courtesy of Noble, H. B., and Selesnick, F. H.: Physician Sportsmed. 8:63–64, August 1980.)

are initially misdiagnosed by physicians. Two case reports are presented to typify the problem. Both patients heard a loud noise on injury and found that the injured foot could not support weight. Both experienced calf pain and slight swelling. Both cases were misdiagnosed, and the patients experienced continued weakness, even after several weeks, when the Thompson test permitted accurate diagnosis of rupture.

The high rate of misdiagnoses may partly stem from the variable physical findings with this injury. Classic findings are a palpable gap in the back of the ankle, calf swelling, ecchymosis, and inability to plantar flex the foot actively. Patients may delay seeking medical assistance because their only symptom is ankle weakness that does not improve with time. The delay may make classic findings even more variable. Moreover, the examiner may also fail to recognize that the

Fig 4–13.—The posterior tibial, peroneal, and toe flexor tendons can plantar flex the foot, even when the Achilles tendon is ruptured. (Courtesy of Noble, H. B., and Selesnick, F. H.: Physician Sportsmed. 8:63–64, August 1980.)

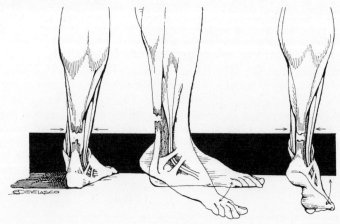

posterior tibial, peroneal, and toe flexor tendons can plantar flex the foot even when the Achilles tendon is ruptured (Fig 4–13), as in the case of the second patient.

▶ [The facts that the posterior tibial, peroneal, and toe flexor tendons can plantar flex the foot when the Achilles tendon is ruptured completely and that the Thompson test has uniform reliability are worthy of reiteration.—J.S.T.] ◀

4–51 **Surgical Repair of Ruptured Achilles Tendon: Analysis of 40 Patients Treated by Same Surgeon** between 1947 and 1971 is presented by Thomas B. Quigley and Arnold D. Scheller (Tufts Univ.). Average follow-up was 19 years. Ninety percent of the patients were men, with an average age 37.5 years, who were engaged in recreational sports. Most denied a physical conditioning program.

For acute ruptures, a 15-cm incision was made on the medial aspect of the tendon with either the plantaris muscle being woven clockwise through the Achilles tendon or a pullout wire, supplemented with silk mattress sutures, being used to repair the ruptured tendon. The wound was closed and the patient's leg was immobilized. The wire was removed at 6 weeks. The rehabilitation plan consisted of ambulation with a heel lift and elastic stocking (the height of the lift was gradually reduced) and toe exercises. Patients began walking downstairs backward at 3 months and continued exercises until full range of motion was attained.

Results were excellent, as graded by the patients. Objectively, there were some minor deficits, but they did not impede overall function. Clinical results were rated excellent in 42% of cases, good in 36%, fair in 15%, and poor in 6%. Ratings were based on comparison of calf atrophy, range of motion, and toe raise on the affected side and unaffected side.

The Thompson test is a reliable indicator of Achilles tendon rupture. The test was 100% positive in this group of patients. The next most reliable sign was swelling and a palpable gap at the site of rupture. The main objective of treatment is restoration of normal length and tension to the tendon complex. When rupture is complete, with no evidence of independent activity of the tendon complex, the tendon is reconstructed surgically. In this series there were no incomplete ruptures.

Six of the 40 patients had seven complications in the immediate 6 months after operation. The two major complications were ruptures; both were associated with severe blunt trauma. Both were successfully treated surgically. The complication rate is not a contraindication to the treatment described. Normal tension and length of the tendon complex is best restored when the problem is identified correctly and when a rational rather than a dogmatic treatment is introduced.

▶ [The average follow-up of 19 years in this study is impressive. Forty-two percent excellent and 36% good results speak in favor of operative intervention in instances of complete Achilles tendon rupture. However, a comparison with a group of similar injuries treated conservatively would be more meaningful. The authors' conclusion,

(4–51) Am. J. Sports Med. 8:244–250, July–Aug. 1980.

". . . [T]he normal tension and length of the Achilles tendon complex can best be restored when the problem is identified correctly, and when a rational rather than dogmatic mode of therapy is introduced," cannot be disputed.—J.S.T.] ◄

4–52 **Achilles Tendon Injury: 3. Structure of Rabbit Soleus Muscles After Immobilization at Different Positions.** Many patients exhibit myopathic changes in the soleus muscle after surgical treatment for total Achilles tendon rupture, and these sometimes coincide with a marked decrease in static and dynamic plantar flexion strength. It is not clear to what extent conventional tendon suture and immobilization contribute to these abnormalities. Michael Sjöström, Lennart Wählby and Axel Fugl-Meyer (Univ. of Umeå) examined the effects of varying periods of immobilization and passive tension over the muscle during immobilization on the structure of soleus muscle fibers. Rabbit ankles were unilaterally immobilized for 1 or 3 weeks, with the knees semiflexed and the feet in either the plantar or dorsal flexed position. The animals were killed after removal of the plaster or after a further 6 months.

Fibers that were slack when immobilized showed marked degenerative changes, and type 1 fibers often were necrotic. The relative number of type 2 fibers was increased after cast removal. Stretched fibers exhibited essentially normal structure. The contralateral soleus muscle fibers, which bore excessive weight during the time in plaster, showed small, sometimes necrotic type 2 fibers and splitting of type 1 fibers.

Whatever the basic cause of these structural changes, the surgeon should know that too much emphasis on the state of the tendon carries certain risks. Strenuous attempts to unload the tendon safely during the time of immobilization after repair of a ruptured Achilles tendon may result in long-standing damage to the muscular structures and decreased strength. In addition, conservative treatment of Achilles tendon ruptures may result in even greater myopathy involving the triceps surae as a result of prolonged immobilization.

► [This excellent study has marked implications that raise several questions. Are the changes observed in the muscle immobilized in the slack position reversible? Do similar changes occur in other muscle groups during immobilization, i.e., the quadriceps after operation on the knee? The original article is recommended reading for the orthopedic surgeon.—J.S.T.] ◄

4–53 **Operative Treatment of Chronic Calcaneal Paratenonitis.** Helmer Kvist and Martti Kvist (Univ. of Turku) present a new surgical technique performed between 1961 and 1978 in 182 patients (201 operations), 62 of whom were top-ranking athletes. All patients suffered from chronic calcaneal paratenonitis. The commonest history was tenderness or burning pain above the heel. The interval between first symptoms and operation ranged from 2 months to 10 years for all patients (mean 7.5 months). Conservative management had included local steroid injections and heparin. Patients refrained from exercise wholly or partly for 1–2 weeks before surgery.

(4–52) Acta Chir. Scand. 145:509–521, 1979.
(4–53) J. Bone Joint Surg. [Br.] 62-B:353–357, August 1980.

TECHNIQUE.—The crural fascia on both sides of the tendon was incised and left open, and adhesions around the tendon were trimmed away. The strongly hypertrophied portions of the paratenon were removed. If the epitenon had been damaged during the freeing procedure, it was sutured with the finest catgut. The smallest bleeding points were cauterized or ligated. The crural fascia and subcutaneous layer were not sutured. All adhesions were trimmed away on the lateral side of the tendon first; the tendon was then retracted and the procedure repeated on the medial side. The most important feature of postoperative care is that the leg was not splinted; the patient began dorsiflexion and plantar flexion of the ankle after recovery from the anesthetic. Sutures were removed after 10 days.

All cases revealed thickened paratenon with fibrous adhesions between the tendon and surroundings. The adhesions were strongest where definite nodules were observed. Results were excellent in 169 patients, good in 25, and poor in 7. Good results were indicated in those whose minor pain did not prevent them from undertaking physical activities. Excellent results were indicated by total recovery. In 26 cases of recurrence some months after operation, 20 patients had a further operation with good results. Three patients could not continue athletics, 4 had bilateral second operations, and 6 had recurrence of symptoms, which was successfully treated with conservative management. In most instances the affected tendon remained thicker than the healthy one for some months, but resolution to almost normal thickness usually occurred.

A small rupture may be difficult to distinguish from chronic paratenonitis. Fourteen cases in this study probably represent the sequelae of small tendon ruptures; all these patients had excellent results. Good results could be due simply to removal of the adhesions or to circulatory factors, especially venous circulation.

4–54 **Stenosing Tenosynovitis of the Pseudosheath of the Tendo Achilles.** An increasing number of reports of heel cord complaints in runners have appeared in recent years. Nathaniel Gould and Roy Korson (Univ. of Vermont) report data on 9 patients aged 25–67 years with stenosing tenosynovitis of the pseudosheath of the Achilles tendon. This condition consists of a chronic inflammatory process of the peritenon, usually bilateral and near the insertion of the tendon. Six patients have had bilateral involvement at one time or another. Two had a past history of spontaneous rupture in the other leg, and 2 had had a recent partial rupture. Four patients had received steroid injections.

These patients present with gradually increasing discomfort in one or both Achilles tendons, worsening with activity. Conservative measures have given only transient benefit. Eventually nodular thickenings appear in the tendon, and the patient walks with a shortened stride. The earliest change appears to be fragmentation of collagen fibers within the substance of the tendon. Proliferation of capillaries and perithelial cells and mild inflammation also are noted. The end stage is fibrosis with irregular new collagen deposition. The thick-

(4–54)   Foot Ankle 1:179–187, November 1980.

ened peritenon is stripped off and removed. Prominent hatchet-shaped bone spurring at the upper end of the os calcis is removed if present, as is a regional retrocalcaneal bursa. Ambulation is begun the second day after surgery. Bandaging and crutches are continued for 3 weeks after surgery.

All but 1 of the 9 patients followed for at least 1 year recovered without pain and with unrestricted activity in a few months. The rate of recovery appears to depend largely on the ambition of the patient.

▶ [Operative treatment may well be conservative treatment for this problem. The original articles are recommended reading for those dealing with problems of the tendo Achilles.—J.S.T.] ◀

4–55 **Isolated Lateral Compartment Syndrome.** Murray J. Goodman (Harvard Med. School) presents a case report of a lateral compartment syndrome after an inversion injury to the ankle. A proximal peroneal muscle injury resulted in isolated increased lateral compartment pressure and peroneal nerve compression.

Woman, 25, who sustained an inversion injury to the right foot and ankle, initially had pain just distal to the fibular head and complained of swelling of the right calf, difficulty in walking, and persistent "charley horse." She had been treated at other hospitals for muscle strain for 1 week. Physical examination revealed symmetrical dorsalis pedis and posterior tibial pulses, swelling of the right calf, intact sensation to pinprick, and no active peroneal function. Active plantar flexion of more than 20 degrees and active dorsiflexion beyond neutral were prevented by pain. Laboratory studies revealed myoglobin in the urine and elevated levels of serum lactic acid dehydrogenase, glutamic-oxaloacetic transaminase, and direct bilirubin. Roentgenograms were negative. Peroneal nerve conduction velocity was 37 m/second in the right leg and 58 m/second in the left. Conduction across the popliteal fossa was equal and normal bilaterally. Compartment pressure was elevated to 70 mm Hg in the lateral compartment of the right leg and was less than 15 mm in all other compartments.

A fasciotomy of the lateral compartment and debridement of the necrotic peroneus longus and peroneus brevis were performed with the patient under general anesthesia. The superficial peroneal nerve was edematous. Around 50% of the muscle in the lateral compartment was necrotic and was removed. The wound was loosely packed open, the leg was supported in a posterior splint, and dressings were changed frequently. The wound was allowed to close secondarily, and after 2 weeks a plastic below-the-knee orthosis was used and gait training was begun. By 2 months postoperatively the peroneus brevis muscle was rated good and gait was normal.

While neurapraxia from inversion injury at the ankle is rare, it is important to determine whether the neurapraxia is caused by a stretch injury or by increased intracompartmental pressure. Whereas nerve conduction velocity studies document nerve injury, measurement of intracompartmental pressure should be done to determine if a compartment syndrome is present. Only in the presence of increased compartment pressure is neurapraxia an indication for decompression. Myoglobinuria suggests myonecrosis and is an indica-

(4–55)   J. Bone Joint Surg. [Am.] 62-A:834–845, July 1980.

tion for debridement. Careful wound management prevents secondary wound infection in the presence of necrotic muscle.

▶ [This article makes the point: "Neurapraxia in the presence of increased compartment pressure is an indication for decompression. In the presence of normal pressure, neurapraxia is *not* an indication for decompression."—J.S.T.] ◀

4–56 **Recurrent Anterior Compartmental Syndromes.** Muscle volume may expand 20% during exercise from both increased capillary filtration and blood content. If muscle blood flow is compromised by a sufficient rise in tissue pressure, a compartment syndrome results. Both acute and recurrent forms of compartment syndrome are seen. Recurrent syndromes of the leg usually occur in athletes and military recruits. The anterior and lateral compartments are most often involved. Robert G. Veith, Frederick A. Matsen III, and Stanley G. Newell (Univ. of Washington, Seattle) reviewed the findings in 7 patients seen in 1977–1979 with 11 recurrent anterior compartment syndromes of the leg. Twelve control subjects also were evaluated. Compartmental pressures were evaluated by the continuous infusion technique.

Patients typically had a painful tight sensation in the anterolateral leg with weak dorsiflexion on excessive exercise of the anterior compartment. Paresthesia sometimes was noted on the dorsum of the foot. No traumatic events were noted. The findings often were normal in the nonexercising patient. Fascial hernias were noted in 6 legs of 5 patients. Symptoms could be reproduced by the patient's dorsiflexing the foot repeatedly against resistance. Pulses were normal before and after exercise. The resting anterior compartment pressure averaged 18 mm Hg in patients and 11 mm Hg in control subjects. Postexercise pressures were higher in the patients and did not return to baseline within 6 minutes after exercise.

Apart from a modification of the exercise program, surgery is the only effective treatment of recurrent compartment syndromes of the leg. Surgery is elective. One compartment usually can be clearly implicated. The anterior compartment fascia is incised distally through a small incision, avoiding the superficial peroneal nerve, and then proximally; the proximal fascial incision is completed through a second incision. Eight compartments have been decompressed in 5 patients, all of whom improved significantly after surgery and returned to their activities. Infusion study showed a normal response to exercise in 1 case after subcutaneous fasciotomies.

Fascial hernias are present in a majority of patients with recurrent compartment syndromes. This is not a common cause of recurrent leg pain on exercise. The condition can be distinguished clinically from tendinitis, fatigue fracture of the tibia, and shin splints.

▶ [Athletic trainers must recognize the symptoms of and be able to differentiate between an anterior compartment syndrome and shin splints. All cases of suspected anterior compartment syndrome must be referred immediately to a physician for evaluation. A delay in treatment of anterior compartment syndrome can result in permanent nerve and muscle damage. A characteristic that may help differentiate between an anterior compartment syndrome and "shin splints" is that with the former, pain usually persists or may even increase after activity ceases; also, there is usually pain, tenderness, swelling, an increase in temperature and a tightness of the structures of the anterior compartment. If passive plantar flexion of the ankle or toes causes a referred pain to the anterior compartment, this is considered a good indicator of the problem. Joseph Torg commented in the 1980 YEAR BOOK, "Anterior compartment intermittent claudication is chronic and occurs after specific periods of exercise. Pain and symptoms are relieved with rest. Although the syndrome is not an acute emergency, fasciotomy may be indicated to rectify a potentially disabling condition."—F.G.] ◄

4–57 **Atypical Stress Fracture of Tibia in Professional Athlete.** The incidence of stress fractures of the tibia is approximately 20% in athletes. Malcolm A. Brahms, Robert M. Fumich, and Victor D. Ippolito (Cleveland) describe a suspected stress fracture of the tibia in a professional football player which 3 years later fractured to completion.

In May 1972, the patient was found to have a palpable deformity over the midportion of the right tibia. He had no history of associated trauma or pain, and completed the 1972 season without complaint referable to the right leg. X-ray films revealed a well-healed, stable, stress fracture of the anterior lateral cortex of the midshaft of the right tibia. The patient played the 1973 and 1974 seasons without related problems. However, in November 1975, while returning a kickoff, the player suddenly fell and sustained a comminuted fracture of the right tibia through the previously noted lesion. Motion pictures confirmed that the patient had not been tackled. In January 1978, x-ray films indicated consolidation of the fracture without complete healing.

These findings support the theory that when the muscular system fatigues, it loses its shock absorption efficiency, allowing biomechanical forces to be transmitted to the bone. The attending physician should be aware that the lack of pain and local tenderness is not 100% reliable in predicting prognosis and that a stress fracture on the tension side of a bone may suddenly fracture to completion.

► [The statement by the authors, ". . . [T]he muscular system provides shock absorption, fatigues, loses its shock absorption efficiency, and thus allows the biomechanical force to be transmitted to bone," is not supported by the data presented. However, the position that a stress fracture of the shaft of the tibia, occasionally misdiagnosed as "shin splints," can go on to complete fracture is well taken and is supported by the clinical experience by others.—J.S.T.] ◄

4–58 **Problems Associated With Tibial Fractures With Intact Fibulas.** Carol C. Teitz, Dennis R. Carter, and Victor H. Frankel followed 68 patients who were treated for a tibial shaft fracture without concomitant fibular fracture. The follow-up period was 2 to 7 years. The 45 patients younger than age 20 (group A) had fewer complications than the 23 patients older than age 20 (group B); thus, the two groups were analyzed separately. Initial fracture management, the development of tibial angulation, the presence of delayed union or nonunion, the need for secondary treatment, and the final result were studied.

(4–57) Am. J. Sports Med. 8:131–132, Mar.–Apr. 1980.
(4–58) J. Bone Joint Surg. [Am.] 62-A:770–776, July 1980.

Most fractures were in the distal one third to one half of the tibia, and the predominant fracture pattern was spiral-oblique in both groups. Forty-four (98%) of group A fractures and 15 (65%) of group B fractures were closed. Weight-bearing casts were used from the onset of treatment in 74% of fractures in both groups. The mean time for healing was 9 weeks in group A and 13.2 weeks in group B.

In group B, 6 (26%) had delayed union or nonunion and 6 (26%) had varus malunion of the fractured tibia. Pain and roentgenographic changes developed in the ipsilateral ankle within 2 years of injury in 2 of the 6 patients with malunion. In group A, 1 patient had delayed union and 12 (27%) had varus malunion. Pain in the ipsilateral ankle was observed in 2 of these 12 patients. A bent fibula was observed in 13 patients in group A.

Clinical observations were corroborated by biomechanical studies on an experimental model in which a fresh human lower limb was loaded before and after fracture of the tibia. It was found that when the fibula remains intact, a tibiofibular length discrepancy develops and causes altered strain patterns in the tibia and fibula. These may lead to delayed union, nonunion, or malunion of the tibia with the sequelae of joint disturbances. The deformation before fracture reflects the ability of soft tissues to yield with compression; the increase in deformation observed after fracture reflects shortening occurring at the fracture site in the form of angulation and separation of the fragments. In patients younger than age 20, the greater compliance of the fibula compensates for the tibiofibular length discrepancy and allows approximation of the fracture surfaces of the tibia. Some authors suggest that the intact fibula holds the tibial fracture surfaces apart. This report suggests that the tibial fracture with an intact fibula is an insidiously dangerous fracture pattern, especially in patients older than age 20 in whom bone and soft tissues are less compliant.

▶ [This well-documented study calls attention to the problem inherent in managing this particular fracture. The authors did not mention whether any of the patients had been treated with short-leg weight-bearing casts. The implication of such treatment in preventing delayed union or nonunion or causing varus deformity could be interesting. Also, how might these complications be prevented? What is the role of fibular osteotomy and at what point in time should it be performed? Is there a role for electric stimulation of osteogenesis and, if so, when should this therapy be implemented?— J.S.T.] ◀

4–59 **Avulsion Fracture of the Proximal Tibial Metaphysis: Report of a Case.** L. Danielsson and G. Theander (Malmö, Sweden) discuss radiologic diagnosis of avulsion of a tibial metaphyseal fragment and the mechanism of this exceptional injury.

Girl, 13, missed a jump while vaulting the buck horse, hitting the anterior surface of the left knee against the top of the horse. She had increasing pain and difficulty in walking 10 days after injury. Pain was located to the dorsal aspect of the medial tibial condyle, provoking a 20-degree extension deficit of the joint. Radiography of the left knee was reported to show osteolytic and sclerotic abnormalities of the tibial metaphysis and a periosteal reaction.

(4–59) Acta Radiol. [Diagn.] (Stockh.) 21:293–296, 1980.

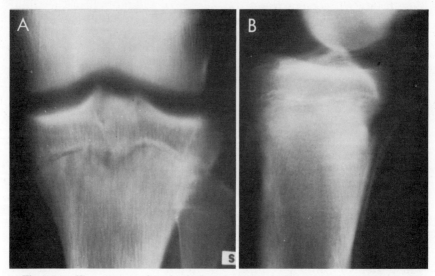

Fig 4–14.—Views (tomography) of metaphyseal avulsion fracture in left knee of girl, aged 13. **A,** anteroposterior view; **B,** lateral view. The posteromedial fragment of the metaphysis is slightly displaced. (Courtesy of Danielsson, L., and Theander, G.: Acta Radiol. [Diagn.] (Stockh.) 21:293–296, 1980.)

Findings suggested tumor or osteomyelitis, but repeat radiography 15 days after the accident showed that the trabecular disarrangement was caused by fracture with incipient callus. The fracture, confirmed by tomography, extended from the epiphyseal plate 4 cm distally, separating a posteromedial fragment of the metaphysis. The knee was immobilized in plaster, which was removed 10 days later. Joint motion became normal, but left thigh circumference had decreased and periarticular demineralization had occurred. After 1 more month, healing was complete and erythrocyte sedimentation rate (ESR) was normal.

The posteromedial fragment of the metaphysis was wedge shaped, tapered distally, and consisted of trabecular as well as cortical bone. Slight tilting of the fragment had resulted in a diastasis, which also tapered distally (Fig 4–14, A). Figure 4–14, B, shows the posteromedial fragment of the metaphysis slightly displaced. The dorsal position of the fragment and the diastasis clearly indicate avulsion fracture.

Metaphyseal avulsion has not been reported previously. Vaulting the horse requires a combination of abduction and outward rotation of the hips and extension of the knees. The hips are not normally in flexion, but if the legs hit the horse, the body is tilted forward with resultant flexion of the hips and avulsion fracture at the ischial tuberosity or at the tibial insertion of the hamstring tendons. The tibial fracture here suggests an extraordinary kind of strain on the medial hamstring. The accident was claimed to have been caused by skewing and slipping of the springboard. The maneuver used to overcome these difficulties implies exaggerated abduction of the left leg. When hitting the horse, the leg was thus in an unusual position known to favor avulsion.

The initial erroneous evaluation of the injury may have been due partly to an abnormal ESR (which was 38 mm in 1 hour), but was also due to the extreme rarity of metaphyseal avulsion.

▶ [To this observer, it appears that the lesion in question might well be a nondisplaced Salter-Harris II fracture involving the proximal tibial epiphyseal line and metaphysis.— J.S.T.] ◀

4–60 **High Stress Fractures of the Fibula.** Pan P. Symeonides (Genl. Air Force Hosp., Athens) describes a high stress fracture of the fibula that occurred in 48 of 120 recruits doing a difficult jumping exercise. Fractures of the uppermost third of the fibula occurred as a result of an exercise begun 2 weeks after the start of training in which recruits jumped across the gymnasium in a squatting position several times daily. Two recruits were referred with pain, swelling, and tenderness at the lateral aspect of the uppermost third of both fibulas. Radiography confirmed stress fractures in these patients and in 40% of the recruits (Fig 4–15); 14 cases were bilateral. In most patients the stress fracture was oblique or transverse, with the line of fracture running downward and outward. In some patients the fracture line was not visible as such, but there was callus formation comparable to that seen in shin soreness of the tibia.

It is believed that the jumping exercises produced the stress fractures. In runners the powerful contraction of the flexor muscles of the ankle and foot approximate the fibula to the tibia, possibly causing stress fractures. In the recruits the knee was fully flexed and ankle

Fig 4–15.—Bilateral comminuted stress fractures of the fibula. There is slight displacement and good callus formation. (Courtesy of Symeonides, P. P.: J. Bone Joint Surg. [Br.] 62-B:192–193, May 1980.)

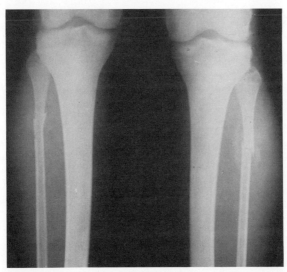

dorsiflexed, bringing the insertion of the calcaneal tendon to some 5 cm posterior to the lateral malleolus, so that the direction of the muscular force on the fibula was obliquely and posteriorly toward the tibia. Whereas in athletes the lowermost end of the bone is most often affected, in recruits it is usually the middle third. This report confirms the theory that different muscular activities cause different stress fractures. Most of the fractures occurred in recruits who had given up exercise. If the recruits had been brought up to proper athletic standard before the start of the particular exercise, the fractures might not have occurred. Bone does not gain strength as rapidly as does muscle, which possibly explains why most recruits who had kept in training did not get a stress fracture.

▶ [The author's contention, "The importance of this report is that it confirms the theory that different muscular activities cause different stress fractures," is not substantiated by the data presented.—J.S.T.] ◀

4–61 **Anterior Dislocation of the Head of the Fibula** is reported by B. Conforty, E. Tal, and Y. Margulies (Univ. of Tel-Aviv). Dislocation of the proximal tibiofibular joint is rare and may be overlooked when it does occur. It has been described in parachutists. Anterior dislocation is by far the most common type.

Man, 28, was tackled hard while playing soccer. As he was ready to kick, he twisted the body, the right knee flexed and "gave in," and he fell onto the right leg, with sudden pain. A fusiform bulge was noted in the outer aspect of the right knee. The x-ray films showed anterior displacement of the proximal end of the right fibula. When moderate pressure was applied to the fibular head with the knee flexed and the foot inverted, a snap was heard, and the bone resumed its normal place, with disappearance of all abnormal signs and complaints. Mobility of the knee was entirely normal. A plaster tutor cast was applied for 3 weeks. When it was removed, the knee was completely normal.

This dislocation usually occurs in a fall with the knee flexed and adducted. Harrison and Hindenach (1959) stated that every anterior dislocation is initially a lateral one, occurring when external force causes a fall with the leg in flexion and adduction and the hamstrings and biceps contract suddenly and violently, freeing the fibular head from its anchoring elements and bringing it into lateral subluxation and then anteriorly. Falls from a height can also produce this injury. Posterior dislocation is much rarer. Knee motion is unrestricted, but the patient does not move because of the pain. Motor neurologic complications are rare, but sensory changes have been described.

The dislocation is reduced easily by flexing the knee, inverting the foot, and applying direct anteroposterior pressure on the fibular head. The authors suggest immobilization in a plaster tutor cast for 3 weeks to allow complete healing of the ligaments and soft tissues. Certain patients may develop recurrent dislocation if treatment is not carried out.

▶ [Subtle x-ray changes require comparison with comparable lateral projections of the opposite uninvolved knee.—J.S.T.] ◀

(4–61) J. Trauma 20:902–903, October 1980.

4–62   **Tourniquet-Induced Nerve Ischemia Complicating Knee Ligament Surgery.** C. H. Rorabeck and J. C. Kennedy (Univ. Hosp., London, Ont.) describe paralysis to the sciatic nerve in 5 patients after the application of a pneumatic tourniquet for knee ligament surgery. The tourniquet pressure in all patients measured 500 mm Hg. A standard Kidde pneumatic tourniquet was used. Tourniquet time varied from 45 minutes to $1^{1}/_{2}$ hours. Clinical deficit observed postoperatively ranged from complete absence of function of both lateral and posterior divisions of the sciatic nerve in 1 patient to a partial foot drop in 4 patients. Four patients recovered full clinical and electric function in the territory of the injured portion of the nerve within 6 months of surgery. One patient had weakness of dorsiflexion persisting beyond a 6-month period.

Experimental investigation in hind limbs of adult dogs showed that impairment of sciatic nerve conduction velocity occurs with every tourniquet application of either 250 mm Hg or 500 mm Hg pressure. The portion of the nerve directly under the tourniquet is the portion most susceptible to extrinsically applied tourniquet pressure. However, the portion of the nerve most susceptible to injury is the portion lying directly underneath the proximal edge of the cuff. The standard tourniquet is designed to fit a perfect cylinder, but the shape of most lower extremities is more like a cone. Thus, uneven pressure distribution is likely to occur, with high forces delivered at the proximal edge of the cuff and much lower forces delivered at the distal edge (Fig 4–16). The more uneven the pressure distribution, the greater the potential for shear stress in the underlying tissue. A peripheral nerve might be more susceptible to longitudinal or shearing stresses than to compression. The excessive shear caused by the uneven force distribution may account for asymmetric nerve damage underneath and distal to the tourniquet. The fact that some patients have irreversible paralysis while others do not might be accounted for by the "cone theory" or by a calibration error within the tourniquet itself.

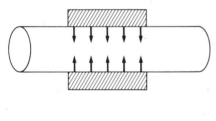
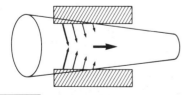

Fig 4–16.—A diagram of the "cone theory" of the shape of the lower extremity to show how uneven pressure distribution against the limb can cause shear stresses on the underlying tissues and the sciatic nerve. (Courtesy of Rorabeck, C. H., and Kennedy, J. C.: Am. J. Sports Med. 8:98–102, Mar.–Apr. 1980.)

(4–62)   Am. J. Sports Med. 8:98–102, Mar.–Apr. 1980.

The experimental investigation gave results suggesting that a tourniquet should not be left continuously inflated at 500 mm Hg for more than 75 minutes. If that period is reached during surgery, the tourniquet should be released and not reinflated during the rest of the procedure. It follows from the cone theory that the period of inflation should be considerably less in a fat conical thigh.

▶ [This report of data on five patients with sciatic nerve paralysis after knee ligament surgery alleged to be due to the application of the pneumatic tourniquet is noteworthy. The data would be of greater interest had they been presented in terms of rate per number of tourniquet applications. The suggestion that a peripheral nerve (sciatic nerve) is more susceptible to longitudinal shearing stress than it is to compression is interesting, original, and deserves further investigation. On the basis of personal experience, it is difficult to understand why tourniquet pressure need be increased beyond 300 mm Hg for knee surgery.—J.S.T.] ◀

4–63 **Systemic and Local Effects of the Application of a Tourniquet.** L. Klenerman, Meenakshi Biswas, G. H. Hulands, and A. M. Rhodes (Northwick Park Hosp., Harrow, England) have investigated the effect of the application of a tourniquet to a limb and the release of the accumulated metabolites with reference to the acid-base level in the blood from the limb and in the right atrium. Studies were carried out experimentally in rhesus monkeys and clinically in patients undergoing reconstructive operations on the knee.

PROCEDURE.—In monkeys the right atrium was catheterized through the internal jugular vein, and a cannula was passed retrograde into the femoral vein of the limb to which the tourniquet was to be applied. An infant-sized Kidde tourniquet cuff was applied to the experimental limb and inflated to a pressure of 300 mm Hg for a predetermined time. At regular intervals, samples were taken from the cannula in the right atrium to establish control values for acid-base status and for potassium. After release of the tourniquet, samples were taken simultaneously from the internal jugular route and femoral vein. Samples were measured for PCO_2, pH, and excess of base and standard bicarbonate. In the clinical studies a cannula was passed via the right internal jugular vein into the atrium. An Esmarch bandage was used to exsanguinate the site of operation, and a 10-cm Kidde tourniquet cuff was inflated to occlude the arterial flow at a pressure of twice the preinduction systolic pressure. Samples were taken from the atrium and from the femoral vein of the surgically treated limb both just before and when the tourniquet was released.

In a limb that has been rendered ischemic, metabolites accumulate as a result of hypoxia in the tissues. Although potassium levels in the blood leaving the limb were raised, no significant rise was detected in the right atrium in animals or in patients, possibly due to a dilutional effect. Similarly, the fall in pH in the venous blood leaving the acidotic limb was not reflected in the acid-base status of blood samples from the right atrium, a result of the dilution effect and buffering capacity of the blood. In animals, the acid-base balance in the limb returned to normal within 20 minutes of the release of a tourniquet in place for 1 hour, and within 40 minutes after 4 hours of ischemia. When buffering capacity is reduced by anemia, hypovolemia, meta-

(4–63)   J. Bone Joint Surg. [Br.] 62-B:385, 388, August 1980.

bolic acidosis, or vascular disease, the period during which a tourniquet is used should be reduced to the minimum, and full cardiovascular monitoring must be available. Results suggest that a period of 3 hours with the use of a tourniquet is safe and that systemic changes are readily reversible, provided blood pressure and acid-base status of the subject are stable.

▶ [In view of the observations of Rorabeck and Kennedy (*Am. J. Sports Med.* 8:98–105, 1980) regarding impairment of sciatic nerve conduction velocity with every tourniquet application in their experimental investigation on the hind limbs of adult dogs, the conclusion of this article that 3 hours is the upper time limit for the safe use of a tourniquet must be viewed with skepticism. The local acid-base changes in the limb rendered ischemic by a tourniquet is hardly the only factor for determining safety criteria.—J.S.T.] ◀

4–64 **Iliotibial Band Friction Syndrome in Runners.** Clive A. Noble (Rosebank Clinic, Johannesburg, South Africa) discusses the musculoskeletal abnormalities and clinical signs that permit accurate diagnosis, as well as general principles of treatment and observations on a series of 100 patients, in this syndrome. Iliotibial band friction syndrome is an overuse injury, found especially in long-distance runners, which is caused by friction of the iliotibial band over the lateral epicondylar prominence. It is characterized by pain on the outer aspect of the knee in close relation to the lateral femoral epicondyle. The pain is usually poorly localized, is aggravated by running long distances or by excessive striding, and is more severe in running downhill. It may be prevented by walking with a stiff knee.

The series included 100 consecutive knees, including 6 patients with the syndrome in both knees (age range, 19–48 years; average, 31 years). Of these, 73 were available for follow-up evaluation. The condition resolved in only 30 patients on the initial regimen of a single injection of local steroid and reduction in the training program. Twenty-one patients had two injections, and 8 patients required a third injection. The other 14 patients were placed on a regimen of total rest from running for 4–6 weeks. Nine patients returned to training and had no recurrence of pain. Five patients consented to surgery and returned to long-distance running 2–7 weeks later. One of these patients had iliotibial band release and removal of the lateral epicondyle, while the other 4 had release of the posterior portion of the iliotibial band.

Incorrect training and structural abnormalities are possible etiologic factors in this syndrome. Incorrect training includes excessive distance, speed, or hill training, as well as sudden alterations in routine. Possible structural abnormalities include excessive prominence of the lateral epicondyle and excessive tightness of the iliotibial band, which abnormally increases pressure. The tightness may be structural or functional. Excessive genu varum may increase the tightness of the iliotibial band. Excessive internal rotation of the tibia on the femur also causes increased tension on the iliotibial band. Repeated flexion and extension of the knee in long-distance running may pro-

(4–64) Am. J. Sports Med. 8:232–234, July–Aug. 1980.

duce inflammation due to iliotibial band friction. In this series, 16 patients showed heel valgus of more than 5 degrees, indicating excessive pronation on weight-bearing, and genu varum measurements showed that 8 patients had a gap of more than 3 cm, with a maximum of 10 cm. The most frequent sign in this group was tenderness over the lateral epicondyle and, occasionally, swelling at the site.

4-65 **Stress Fracture in Soldiers—A Multifocal Bone Disorder: A Comparative Radiologic and Scintigraphic Study.** Kalle O. A. Meurman and Sirkka Elfving (First Central Military Hosp., Helsinki) investigated the correlation between radionuclide images and radiographs in 42 military recruits with suspected stress fractures, referred because of pain during or after exercise. Pain became worse with continued stress and ceased at rest. Tenderness was found at the painful site, and swelling was observed in such regions as the metatarsals and calcaneus. A painful longitudinal protuberance could sometimes be felt at the medial border of the tibial diaphysis. The interval between onset of symptoms and the first radiograph averaged 28 days. Conventional radiographs of suspected fractures were obtained first, then radionuclide images of legs and pelvis. Sites showing increased activity were then reexamined radiographically if initial radiographic and scintigraphic results did not correspond. If repeat radiography was negative, follow-up studies were done 10 and 20 days later.

There was positive correlation between the radiographic and radionuclide image in 6 cases, with most sites of increased radionuclide uptake corresponding to lesions found radiographically. When sites of increased uptake were radiographed a second time, 15 additional abnormal views were obtained, but half of the scintigraphic foci still gave negative results on the radiogram. Bilateral stress fractures of the pubic arch were found radiographically in 2 patients in whom the gamma camera image showed increased activity on only one side. In all other cases, both studies were positive. Bilateral positive scintigraphic findings were obtained in 28 patients, bilateral positive radiographic findings in only 8. Seventeen patients had more than 2 foci, including 2 patients with 6 and one with 7. Fifteen patients had 1 or more foci in the small tarsal bones, but the radiogram was positive in only 2 (Fig 4–17). The gamma camera images demonstrate several sites of increased uptake in both tarsal regions (Fig 4–17,A) and in the right metatarsal area (Fig 4–17,B). The corresponding radiogram showed only a slight stress fracture in the left calcaneus and was negative on the right. The finding that half of the foci with increased radionuclide activity remained radiographically negative, while only a third were asymptomatic, may be due to the fact that most symptoms in these patients were slight, transitory, and subjective; some were not noticed until later, on meticulous reexamination. From the numerous foci of marked intensity in the tarsal region, it would seem that stress damage of the tarsus is not rare; however, these small

(4–65) Radiology 134:483–487, February 1980.

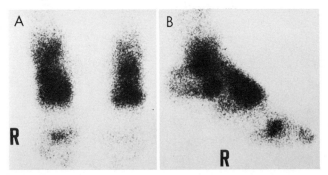

Fig 4–17.—Sites of increased uptake in both tarsal regions **(A)** and the right metatarsal area **(B)**. (Courtesy of Meurman, K. O. A., and Elfving, S.: Radiology 134:483–487, February 1980.)

bones partially overlap, and the lesion may therefore be difficult to find on a plain radiogram.

Results suggest that the possibility of multifocal stress fractures should be kept in mind when planning appropriate therapy, training, and stationing of young recruits.

▶ [A radionuclide bone scan is more sensitive to bone abnormalities than a radiographic study. Roentgenograms may never demonstrate the specific finding; however, tomography and/or coned views should be requested before radiographic documentation can be totally excluded.—J.S.T.] ◀

4–66 **Early Confirmation of Stress Fractures in Joggers.** Joseph F. Norfray, Lawrence Schlachter, William T. Kernahan, Jr., Donald J. Arenson, Stephen D. Smith, Ivar E. Roth, and Barbara S. Schlefman (Chicago) confirmed stress fractures in 4 of 5 joggers by clinical findings, a radionuclide bone scan (RBS), and delayed conventional roentgenograms.

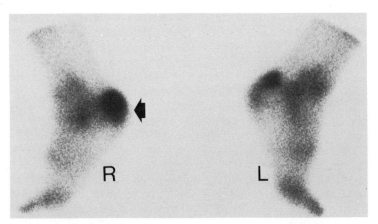

Fig 4–18.—Radionuclide bone scan of both feet showing increased uptake in right *(R)* calcaneus *(arrow)*; *L*, left. (Courtesy of Norfray, J. F., et al.: J.A.M.A. 243:1647–1649, Apr. 25, 1980; copyright 1980, American Medical Association.)

(4–66) J.A.M.A. 243:1647–1649, Apr. 25, 1980.

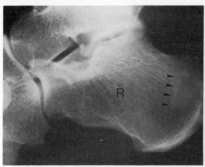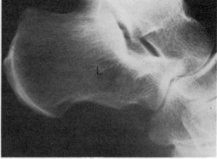

Fig 4–19.—Lateral views of right *(R)* and left *(L)* calcaneal bones demonstrating slight medullary sclerosis on right *(arrowheads)*. (Courtesy of Norfray, J. F., et al.: J.A.M.A. 243:1647–1649, Apr. 25, 1980; copyright 1980, American Medical Association.)

One runner with referred pain to the knee had an abnormal RBS with increased uptake in the middle third of the femur. The initial routine roentgenograms of the femur did not identify the stress fracture; however, the coned-down views in the area of the scintigraphic findings showed subtle endosteal and periosteal callus consistent with stress fracture. Two patients had tibial stress fractures of the middle third of the tibia, with 1 patient having bilateral involvement. The RBS was abnormal as early as 6 weeks before appearance of conventional roentgenographic changes. One patient had an abnormal RBS of the calcaneus (Fig 4–18). The subtle medullary sclerosis was appreciated only because the bone scan was abnormal (Fig 4–19). One patient had hip pain, but stress fracture was ruled out since the RBS and conventional roentgenograms were normal.

Stress fractures occur during remodeling of normal bone when resorption of bone exceeds repair. Unusual physical activity causes remodeling. The symptom of stress fractures is pain which recurs with activity and is relieved by rest. Clinical examination will usually demonstrate point tenderness of the bone at the site of the fracture and localized swelling. When a stress fracture is suspected clinically and conventional roentgenograms are normal, an RBS is indicated. The RBS detects stress fractures earlier than conventional roentgenograms and is also used to indicate the area for coned-down roentgenograms. Conventional roentgenograms are still required since they are more specific and can identify causes of falsely abnormal bone scans, i.e., tumors and infections, and since findings of a stress fracture would obviate the need for a bone scan. Early detection of stress fractures is essential since they may proceed to complete fractures if undiagnosed. Rest from any activity causing pain is the best treatment. Rest allows the reparative phase of remodeling to catch up to the resorptive phase. Internal fixation may be required in stress fractures of the neck of the femur and midshaft of the tibia in the elderly.

▶ [Bone pain without roentgen findings is a valid indication for obtaining a radionuclide bone scan in nonjoggers as well as joggers. A radionuclide bone scan is a safe, noninvasive procedure that is extremely sensitive to bone lesions.—J.S.T.] ◀

4–67 **Stress Fracture of the Pubic Arch in Military Recruits.** K. O.
A. Meurman (Helsinki) surveyed 49 pubic arch stress fractures in 39
military recruits. These fractures represented 8% of all stress fractures seen at one military hospital between 1971 and 1979. They
were more common than fractures of the femoral neck. Twenty percent were bilateral, and 8 patients had stress fractures in other bones.
Median age of the patients was 22 years. Of the 49 patients, 37 were
nonathletes and 2 were noncompetitive sportsmen. Basic training
was the same for all. In all patients the pelvis had a normal physical
structure.

There were 30 fractures on the right side and 19 on the left; 9 were
bilateral (Fig 4–20). In 26 patients, symptoms began after marches
or terrain exercises at a time of year when the terrain was hard.
Skiing was not thought to be an important factor. The main symptom
was progressive pain in connection with exercise. The pain was felt
in the sacral, inguinal, perineal, or gluteal regions or in the region of
ischial tuberosity. Limping and local tenderness on palpation over the
groin, the proximal part of the thigh in adductor regions, and over
the pubic arch or ischial tuberosity were present. Abduction was limited and painful. The first roentgenographic sign was a slight transverse fissure, a small cloudlike callus, or both. Fracture occurred invariably at the inferior ischiopubic junction. Callus formation was
first seen in the cranial border in the obturator foramen. In some
patients, x-ray films showed bizarre, bubble-like formations. Bilateral
fractures usually did not occur simultaneously.

Stress fractures in the pubic arch are not common. Diagnosis seems
to have been made relatively late. Confusion with various muscular
causes is common, and in this group the primary diagnosis varied
from muscular pain, myalgia, and arthralgia to suspected stress frac-

Fig 4–20.—Bilateral pubic arch stress fractures. Pain was on left side. Rectal examination
disclosed pain on the left side and a palpabale mass on the right side. Only a little callus is seen on
left side *(arrow)*. (Courtesy of Meurman, K. O. A.: Br. J. Radiol. 53:521–524, June 1980.)

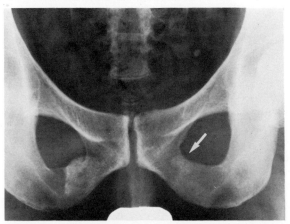

(4–67) Br. J. Radiol. 53:521–524, June 1980.

ture. Hard ground, snow, slipperiness, and heavy winter equipment might have been important contributors to the injury. The nonspecific symptoms and lack of knowledge of the fracture may explain why pubic arch stress fractures are often not diagnosed correctly.

▶ [This fracture is identical in location and radiographic appearance to that seen in marathon runners. The delay in diagnosis of this fracture in either the runner or the recruit can be avoided by obtaining a radionuclide bone scan whenever there is a clinical suspicion of a fracture.—J.S.T.] ◀

4–68 **Groin Pain in Soccer Players,** according to Vojin N. Smodlaka (SUNY, Downstate Med. Center), is possibly due to the extremely forceful movements of the leg that affect the adductor muscles and pelvic ring. A groin injury may be caused by sudden, powerful over-stretching of the leg in abduction and external rotation, especially if there is an opposing force (the ball, the ground, or an opponent's foot). These forces may overstretch the fibers of the muscles or tendons, the bony tissue of the pelvic ring, and the pubic symphysis. Although groin pain in soccer players was rare and was caused by acute injury, soccer has become more popular and dynamic and the players more aggressive, so the forces are greater and collisions more dangerous. Thus, groin injuries are now common.

X-ray films may demonstrate traumatic myositis or tendinitis of the adductor muscles, arthritis of the symphysis, osteitis and necrosis of the pubis, ossification along the pubis or in the attached muscles, exostosis in the symphysis, or a combination of these. Groin pain may develop suddenly or gradually, and it may be sharp or dull, localized or diffuse. It may radiate in different directions, but the principal pathway is the sensory division of the obturator nerve. Rest relieves and may eliminate pain; movement, especially abduction with external rotation of the hip, aggravates it. Diagnosis is made by considering the biomechanics of the movement and the location, radiation, and duration of the pain. Passive and active assisted movements of the hip with the leg extended are performed with movement in all directions. Rispoli has recommended anteroposterior, lateral, and oblique roentgenograms of the pubis and symphysis.

Professional soccer players should be treated with rest, physical therapy, medication, and rehabilitation. Immediate treatment consists of rest combined with local pressure with a small ice bag for 30 minutes to 1 hour and aspirin for pain. Analgesics and anti-inflammatory agents are used with 5 to 10 ml of 0.5% to 1% lidocaine. Cortisone may aggravate the existing local necrosis in chronic cases or initiate a new one and is therefore not recommended. After 36 hours, heat is applied with warm compresses, hydrocollator pads, whirlpool, diathermy, and underwater ultrasonic treatment for 10 to 15 days. Rehabilitation begins with range-of-motion exercises, performed lying down without weight-bearing until pain subsides. To prevent groin injuries, careful conditioning of the pelvis and lower extremities is accomplished by exercises against resistance through the maximal

(4–68)   Physician Sportsmed. 8:57–61, August 1980.

range of motion and with repetition to develop maximal flexibility and strength.

▶ [This is an interesting account of a problem that in many instances is extremely difficult to manage in a physically active person.—J.S.T.] ◀

KNEE INJURIES

4–69 **Arthroscopy Today.** S. Ward Casscells (Thomas Jefferson Univ.) assesses the importance of arthroscopy in diagnosis, research, and surgery in contemporary orthopedics. Clinical diagnostic accuracy ranges from 70% to 75%, whereas arthroscopic diagnostic accuracy exceeds 95% in the hands of experienced physicians. However, few orthopedic procedures require experience with so many cases to achieve the necessary expertise. Synovial lesions can be visualized, biopsied and evaluated. The mechanics and the tracking of the patella on the femur can be studied. The anterior cruciate ligament can be seen and tested. The entire lateral meniscus, the posterior horn of the medial meniscus, and at times the posterior cruciate ligament can be evaluated. Arthroscopy is useful in follow-up studies on damaged articular cartilage of the knee.

With anesthesia, arthroscopy is usually acceptable to the patient. However, there is a tendency to overuse arthroscopy. Although pain relief may follow lavage of an arthritic joint, the benefits are questionable. Arthroscopy has great potential as a research tool but has been little used for this purpose. Arthroscopic surgery has attracted great attention. Simpler procedures include shaving of the patella, release of a tight lateral capsule, division of a thickened shelf or plica, and removal of a loose body. Arthroscopy is often used to evaluate the lesions of osteochondritis dissecans, but it is of doubtful value in these cases. Partial or even complete arthroscopic meniscectomy requires great skill. Its advantages are the lower morbidity rate, the shorter hospitalization, and the absence of any appreciable scar. Its disadvantages are the increased likelihood of damage to the articular cartilage and longer anesthesia. A danger inherent in arthroscopic surgery is that with the overemphasis on removing the menisci, the possibility of suturing peripheral tears may be overlooked, a procedure that can be done more often, especially in the teenage patients. Fewer needless meniscectomies are now being performed, and the evidence suggests that limited meniscectomy, where possible, is best for integrity of the knee.

▶ [This excellent essay places the arthroscope in the proper perspective. Casscells has cogently noted, "Unfortunately, there are few orthopaedic surgeons in this country who presently have sufficient experience with diagnostic arthroscopy to realistically attempt to perform meniscectomies through the scope. It is likely that this may remain a restricted field, not only because of the large volume of clinical experience needed in order to become a proficient arthroscopist, but also because some orthopaedic surgeons don't seem to possess the necessary hand-eye skills to learn even diagnostic arthroscopy." He also notes, with regard to arthroscopic meniscectomy, "From a pragmatic point of view, six months postsurgery the essential difference to the average

(4–69) Contemp. Orthop. 2:389–395, August 1980.

patient between an arthroscopic meniscectomy and one performed by conventional arthrotomy is the length of the scar."—J.S.T.] ◀

4–70 **Arthroscopy of the Knee Under General Anesthesia: An Aid to the Determination of Ligamentous Instability.** F. Martin Ivey, Martin E. Blazina, James M. Fox, and Wilson Del Pizzo (Sherman Oaks, Calif.) have made a retrospective comparison between preoperative evaluation and operative examination under general anesthesia in 790 patients who underwent arthroscopic examination of the knee under general anesthesia during a 34-month period (March 1976 through December 1978). Of all patients, 114 (14%) had an increased grade or additional component of instability noted under general anesthesia. Of 601 patients with no preoperative instability, 46 (8%) first demonstrated ligamentous instability under general anesthesia. Of 189 patients known to have preoperative instability, 68 (36%) had an increase in grade or additional components of instability when examined under general anesthesia. Of 259 patients who had undergone previous surgery, 70 (27%) also showed a change in assessment. Of 11 patients with acute injuries, 18% had additional information gained during ligamentous examination under anesthesia. The types of instability that increased in grade were variously distributed, but the most frequently appearing instability was the anterolateral rotary type associated with a positive jerk or pivot shift test.

Patient anxiety or fear of impending subluxation during a maneuver, acute pain, or normal muscle tone may disguise the true degree of instability or mask an individual component unless the knee is examined under anesthesia. However, diagnostic arthroscopy under local anesthesia on an outpatient basis is suitable in certain circumstances. Patients at high risk, including those with acute injuries, preoperative instability, or previous surgery, may require the more comprehensive examination.

▶ [To be reiterated is the authors' position that arthroscopy of the knee has not replaced a thorough history and physical examination, standard roentgenograms, or arthrography; rather, arthroscopy is complementary to them. Amen!—J.S.T.] ◀

4–71 **Arthroscopy and Arthrography of the Knee: Critical Review.** John Ireland, E. L. Trickey, and D. J. Stoker (London) reviewed 135 knee arthroscopies performed between 1973 and 1977 to determine the accuracy of detection of meniscal lesions. Fifty-six patients also had double-contrast arthrograms and 94 underwent arthrotomy. Arthroscopy was indicated only when a meniscal lesion was suspected but the clinical diagnosis was inconclusive or when a meniscal lesion had to be excluded as a cause of instability. Final diagnosis was based on findings at arthrotomy and on examination of excised menisci. Forty-one patients did not undergo arthrotomy. No meniscal tears were demonstrated by arthroscopy in their knees.

In 15 knees, abnormalities were found that were unrelated to the menisci; there were 2 arthroscopic errors in this group. Among the other 120 knees there were 7 false negative results: in these knees tears of the posterior horn were demonstrated at meniscectomy. Arthroscopy and double-contrast arthrography achieved similar accuracies (84% and 86%) in the diagnostically more difficult knees of the series. The combined accuracy of both examinations was 98%. Arthroscopic errors were primarily failures to demonstrate tears of the posterior horn of the medial meniscus in a few patients. The diagnosis is revealed in these cases only at meniscectomy, when the anterior two thirds of the meniscus has been detached or when the knife point enters the tear and the meniscus displaces laterally. The common primary medial meniscal tear is almost always posterior, and the normal line of view with the arthroscope is obstructed in the relevant arc by the femoral condyle. The undersurface of the medial meniscus is not generally seen with the arthroscope. In arthrography a slightly lesser accuracy in detection of detachment of the posterior horn of the lateral meniscus, compared with posterior tears of the medial meniscus, is reported in the literature. This is due to the greater mobility of the lateral meniscus and to the less secure peripheral attachment of the posterior part of the meniscus because of the intervening sheath of the popliteal tendon. Since the main areas of error in the two procedures are different, the methods are complementary in the diagnosis of difficult meniscal problems, giving a combined error rate of 1.7% in this series. When a medial lesion is suspected, a double-contrast arthrogram is appropriate before arthroscopy is considered, but "problem knees" require both procedures.

▶ [Arthrography and arthroscopy are complementary procedures. However, the accuracy of either procedure depends on the expertise of the persons performing and interpreting the respective findings. The accuracy rates reported in this series are based on 135 knees, although only 94 had arthrotomies. The results, therefore, include arthroscopic and arthrographic studies of normal menisci that were accepted as correct without surgical confirmation.—J.S.T.] ◀

4–72 **Comparison Between Transpatellar Tendon and Lateral Approach to the Knee During Arthroscopy.** The standard arthroscopic approach to the knee is 1.5 cm above the lateral tibial plateau proximal to the lateral edge of the patellar tendon. Recently, a central approach through the patellar tendon approximately 1 cm below the apex of the patella has been proposed. It is claimed that this approach does not require multiple insertions and affords an excellent view of the posterior compartment. Ejnar Eriksson and Ahmet Sebik (Karolinska Sjukhuset, Stockholm) compared the central transpatellar tendon arthroscopic approach and the standard lateral approach in 200 unselected cadaver knees. A dummy arthroscope 5 mm in length was used.

With the transpatellar approach, the dummy arthroscope penetrated the infrapatellar fat pad in 198 knees. It failed to reach the medial posterior compartment of 7 knees using the transpatellar approach and in 22 using the lateral approach. Insertion of the arthroscopic dummy into the posterior fossa was usually easier when the

(4–72) Am. J. Sports Med. 8:103–105, Mar.–Apr. 1980.

knee was held at 35 degrees to 40 degrees of flexion rather than at 90 degrees of flexion. The dummy arthroscope could be passed into the lateral posterior fossa in 88 of 100 knees with the transpatellar approach and in 77 of 100 knees with the lateral approach. Patella baja was present in 16 knees. Because the transpatellar approach is contraindicated in these conditions, it is not universally employable.

The transpatellar tendon approach seemed to facilitate insertion of the dummy arthroscope medial to the cruciates into the medial posterior compartment of the knee. However, from an anatomic point of view, the transpatellar tendon approach did not demonstrate a significant advantage over the standard lateral approach.

▶ [The fact that the authors have attempted to relate an in vitro situation, using cadaver knees and "dummy" arthroscopes (Steinmann's pins), with clinical arthroscopy without considering the aspect of arthroscopic lens obliquity (0, 30, and 70 degrees) raises questions regarding the validity of their conclusions.—J.S.T.] ◀

4–73 **Operative Arthroscopy for the Treatment of Problems of the Medial Compartment of the Knee.** Wilson Del Pizzo, James M. Fox, Martin E. Blazina, Marc J. Friedman, and William C. Loos (Sherman Oaks, Calif.) reviewed the early results in 1,158 patients who had arthroscopy in 1976–1979, 628 of whom had operative arthroscopy. The study group included chiefly middle-aged patients. Of these, 51 had 54 operations for meniscus and articular lesions associated with middle age, involving only the medial compartment. The age range was 25–75 years. A total of 119 procedures were done (an average of 2.2/operation), including 47 partial medial meniscectomies, 41 shavings of the medial femoral condyle, 24 shavings of the medial tibial plateau, and 7 removals of loose bodies. The meniscectomies excluded bucket-handle tears. About half the patients were operated on within a year of the onset of symptoms. Arthrography was done preoperatively on 32 knees and results were positive in 27 instances. Surgery was done with the use of tourniquet ischemia and aided by a video camera with video tape recorder.

Good results were obtained in 67% of patients, with marked improvement in symptoms, a return to recreational sports, and no need for medication. Another 20% of patients improved subjectively but did not have a good objective outcome. Poor results were obtained in 13% of cases. Two patients with fair or poor results had a good outcome after secondary surgery. Most patients with fair or poor results had marked arthritis involving the medial femoral condyle and medial tibial plateau.

The results of operative arthroscopy in these middle-aged patients were comparable to those achieved by formal arthrotomy in similar patients. Operative arthroscopy is generally well tolerated by such patients. Poorer results are obtained in patients with more marked arthritis. If a patient does not respond or if symptoms recur, operative arthroscopy can be repeated with a chance of improving the outcome.

▶ [The observation that the results of operative arthroscopy in dealing with medial compartment lesions of the middle-aged knee are dependent on the amount of preex-

(4–73) Orthopedics 3:984–986, October 1980.

isting degenerative arthritis is valid. The conclusion of the authors that results in the middle-aged patients "are comparable with those results achieved by formal arthrotomy in this particular age group" may well be true, but has not been established by the data presented.—J.S.T.] ◄

4–74 **Arthroscopy in Acute Traumatic Hemarthrosis of the Knee: Incidence of Anterior Cruciate Tears and Other Injuries.** Frank R. Noyes, Rick W. Bassett, Edward S. Grood, and David L. Butler (Univ. of Cincinnati) carried out a prospective study of knee injuries with acute traumatic hemarthrosis but no, or negligible, instability on initial clinical evaluation. The knees were reexamined under general anesthesia and by arthroscopy. The injuries generally represented typical grade I ligament sprains with hemarthrosis. Eighty-five knees of 83 patients (11 female and 72 male) were examined in a 125-week period in 1976–1978. Patients ranged in age from 14 to 43 years; mean patient age was 21. The most common antecedent activities were football, basketball, and baseball. About one third of injuries involved contact with an opponent.

The anterior cruciate ligament was completely intact in only 28% of knees. It was partially disrupted in 28%, and completely disrupted in 44%. Only 12% of patients had a normal range of motion without guarding on initial clinical examination, and all but 3 knees were acutely tender to palpation. Both the anterior drawer test and the flexion-rotation drawer test, a modification of the pivot-shift test for anterior subluxation of the lateral tibial plateau, proved most reliable when performed under anesthesia in knees with complete anterior cruciate disruption. The anterior drawer test was less accurate than the flexion-rotation drawer test, which made it possible to diagnose correctly 89% of the disruptions verified at arthroscopy. This test was more than twice as sensitive as the anterior drawer test in knees with partial ligament disruption. Associated injuries were present in 82% of patients with anterior cruciate disruption and in 79% of those with an intact anterior cruciate ligament. Twenty-five knees with complete anterior cruciate disruption had surgical repair.

Traumatic hemarthrosis frequently is associated with a tear of the anterior cruciate ligament or other ligament injury and joint derangement. Arthroscopy is very useful in making a proper diagnosis in these cases. An anterior cruciate tear in itself does not justify reconstruction, especially in less active or older subjects. A "trial of function" approach is useful. Arthroscopy is contraindicated in knees with identifiable major collateral ligament and capsular tears.

► [This excellent prospective study documents the high incidence of anterior cruciate ligament disruption (72%) in acutely traumatized knees. O'Donoghue (*J. Bone Surg.* [*Am.*] 37-A:1–13, 1955), reporting on the end results of his series of major injuries to the ligaments of the knee, observed that of 69 patients with disruption of the medial joint structure, 50, or 72%, had tears in the anterior cruciate ligament. Kennedy et al. (ibid. 56-A:223–235, 1974) studied 50 patients with anterior cruciate ligament tears. He concluded that isolated tears of this ligament do occur and that there is a high incidence of associated medial meniscus injury (19 of 40, or 50%). Torg et al. (*Am. J. Sports Med.* 4:84–93, 1976), in a retrospective study of 250 knees that came to operation,

(4–74) J. Bone Joint Surg. [Am.] 62-A:687–695, July 1980.

254 / SPORTS MEDICINE

demonstrated that there was a high incidence of anterior cruciate ligament disruption, (172 of 250, or 69%). It has been little appreciated that in the knee of the athlete, the anterior cruciate ligament is one of the most frequently injured structures. Also, injuries to this structure can occur as an isolated entity.—J.S.T.] ◄

4–75 **Arthroscopy of the Patellofemoral Joint.** Fleming Lund and Bo E. Nilsson (Univ. of Lund) examined the diagnostic efficacy of arthroscopy in 126 patients presenting with patellofemoral joint symptoms. The Storz arthroscope was used. Arthroscopy was done under general anesthesia with a tourniquet on the thigh. Chondromalacia was graded from I (discoloration only) through IV (erosion down to subchondral bone). Arthrotomy was performed within 3 months after arthroscopy in 58 cases, usually for treatment of chondromalacia patellae.

Chondromalacia of grades I–III was present in 37% of cases and grade IV changes, indistinguishable from patellofemoral arthrosis, in 29% of cases. The latter patients were significantly older than the others. Findings outside the patellofemoral joint which might produce pain were observed in 35% of patients. Degenerative changes were seen in the tibiofemoral joint in 24 patients; these patients also were older. A torn medial meniscus was seen in 7 patients, a torn lateral meniscus in 4, and a ruptured anterior cruciate ligament in 1. Two patients had an osteochondral fracture, and 1 had rheumatoid arthritis. Two had loose bodies. The degree of patellofemoral joint involvement seen at arthroscopy was confirmed at surgery in all but 4 of 58 joints. In most instances the other findings also were confirmed at operation. All the meniscal injuries were verified.

Arthroscopy showed changes at sites other than the patellofemoral joint in about one third of cases in this series. Chondromalacia patellae and other patellofemoral processes may be mistaken for lesions of the medial semilunar cartilage, and the reverse also is true. Arthroscopy appears to be an adequate means of diagnosing and classifying degenerative changes of the patellofemoral joint. Arthrotomy and direct inspection of the patella appear to add little further information. Selection of patients for arthrotomy in the present study, however, usually was based on pathologic arthroscopic findings, and false negative results cannot be entirely excluded.

► [Almost all experienced arthroscopists would agree with the authors' conclusion, "Arthroscopy appears to be an adequate tool for the diagnosis and classification of degenerative changes of the patellofemoral joint. Arthrotomy and direct inspection of the patella appear to add little further information."—J.S.T.] ◄

4–76 **Diagnosis and Treatment of Plica Syndrome of the Knee.** William T. Hardaker, Jr., Terry L. Whipple, and Frank H. Bassett, III (Duke Univ.) reviewed clinical data on 69 patients (73 knees) who had symptomatic plica of the knee. Plicae, inconstant remnants of the development of the synovial tissue, are classified as suprapatellar, mediopatellar, or infrapatellar, according to the membrane from which they arose. The suprapatellar plica, a remnant of the embryonic septum dividing the inferiorly placed medial and lateral com-

(4–75) Acta Orthop. Scand. 51:297–302, April 1980.
(4–76) J. Bone Joint Surg. [Am.] 62-A:221–225, March 1980.

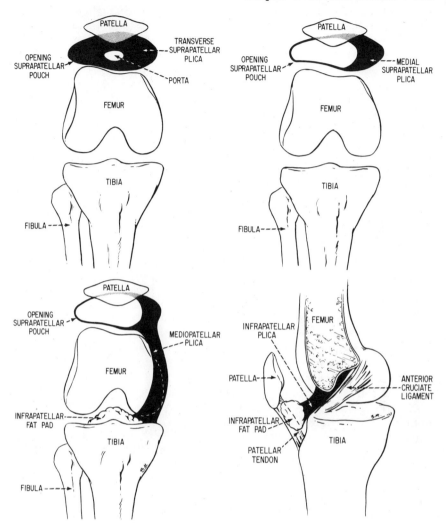

Fig 4–21(top left).—Transverse suprapatellar plica with porta, anterior view.
Fig 4–22 (top right).—Medial suprapatellar plica, anterior view.
Fig 4–23 (bottom left).—Mediopatellar plica, anterior view.
Fig 4–24 (bottom right).—Infrapatellar plica, lateral view.
(Courtesy of Hardaker, W. T., Jr., et al.: J. Bone Joint Surg. [Am.] 62-A:221–225, March 1980.)

partments from the suprapatellar pouch, commonly pinches off most of the pouch except for a centrally placed opening of variable diameter, the porta (Fig 4–21). The medial suprapatellar plica, the configuration of which varies with the position of the knee, appears as a crescent-shaped fold originating beneath the quadriceps tendon and extending to the medial wall of the joint (Fig 4–22). The mediopatellar plica, originating at or near the suprapatellar plica and coursing obliquely downward relative to the patella to attach distally to the synovial membrane covering the infrapatellar fat pad (Fig 4–23), lies along the medial wall of the joint. The infrapatellar plica originates in the intercondylar notch and sweeps through the anterior part of the joint space to attach distally to the infrapatellar fat pad; posteriorly it borders the anterior cruciate ligament (Fig 4–24).

Although most synovial folds are asymptomatic, a single episode of blunt trauma, repetitive trauma of athletics, or an associated internal derangement can precipitate an inflammatory cycle, causing the plica to become relatively inelastic and symptomatic as it snaps over the femoral condyle, leading to synovitis with further edema and eventual replacement with fibrous elements of the elastic tissue. Diagnosis rests on a history of blunt or twisting trauma to the knee, athletics, and symptoms including swelling, pain, snapping, instability, atrophy of the thigh when symptoms are of long duration, and clicking within the knee. Arthroscopy is useful in corroborating a clinical provisional diagnosis.

Of the 69 patients with plicae of the knee, 11 had been treated for meniscal tears and 26 for chondromalacia patellae. All but 6 patients were engaged in sports or heavy labor when symptoms began. Chief symptoms were pain, swelling, and snapping. Most patients had atrophy of the thigh and tenderness to palpation about the medial or lateral suprapatellar region or associated femoral condyles. Conservative treatment with rest, anti-inflammatory agents and local heat, followed by hamstring-stretching exercises, was successful in 12 patients, but 57 patients (61 knees) did not respond. Among these, diagnostic arthroscopy was done in 53, and in 8 knees, the plica was released during arthroscopy; the other 53 knees underwent arthrotomy and partial synovectomy. Postoperatively, a posterior splint was applied and straight-leg raising was prescribed, followed by passive range-of-motion exercises on the third day, with splint removal. At a mean follow-up of 19 months, the condition of 53 knees was rated excellent, that of 6 good, and that of 2 poor.

Conservative therapy is most successful in younger patients whose symptoms are of short duration and are associated with repetitive trauma. It is not successful in patients with symptoms lasting 6 months or more and who have a history of blunt or twisting rather than repetitive trauma.

▶ [To be emphasized is the fact the "incidence of these persistent embryonic structures (plica synovialis) in the general population is approximately 20%." It would be interesting to know what the incidence of symptomatic plica is in the general population and in the population of patients with various forms of internal derangement of the knee.—J.S.T.] ◀

4–77 **Practical Guide to the Initial Evaluation and Treatment of Knee Ligament Injuries.** Lonnie Paulos, Frank R. Noyes, and Mehrdad Malek (Univ. of Cincinnati) reviewed a total of 186 patients with "typical knee sprains" in 2 separate studies. A retrospective review of 103 patients with knee instability due to anterior cruciate ligament (ACL) insufficiency was undertaken, since many cases of "mild knee

sprain" actually represent ACL injuries. In 85%–90% of these patients, the knee gave way, was painful, and swelled by 6 hours; knee
motion decreased by 24 hours, and sports activities could not be continued. Most patients received supportive therapy. The second study
was designed to evaluate prospectively all acute knee injuries with
traumatic hemarthrosis but with no or negligible instability. Each
knee fulfilling the criteria for minor sprain underwent examination
under general anesthesia, followed by immediate arthroscopy.

The flexion-rotation drawer test (FRD) was performed to detect rotatory instabilities. The leg is held in neutral rotation at about 20
degrees of knee flexion. Simply by holding the leg, the subluxated
position of the lateral femorotibial joint is produced (Fig 4–25). With
a gentle flexion motion of about 10 degrees, combined with a downward motion of the tibia, the reduced position is reached as the tibia
is allowed to move posteriorly into its normal relationship with the
femur. The test brings out both the anteroposterior and rotatory
translations of the femur in reference to the tibia. Motion in both of
these planes is helpful in the detection of ACL laxity in acute cases.

The stability examination was repeated preoperatively and under
anesthesia. With the patient awake, the clinical examination generally underestimated the extent of the injury and the amount of instability present. Examination under anesthesia increased the accuracy of diagnosis of major ligament rupture to 89% with the use of
the FRD test; without anesthesia, the Lachman test was more accurate. Arthroscopy permitted detection of the etiology of the acute hemarthrosis in all but 7 cases. A disruption of the ACL was shown in

Fig 4–25.—Flexion rotation drawer test. **A,** subluxated position; **B,** reduced position. The
change in the contour of the infrapatellar region is shown. Note that in **A,** the patella has rotated
externally with the femur and then back to neutral in the reduced position, **B.** (Courtesy of Paulos,
L., et al.: J. Trauma 20:498–506, June 1980.)

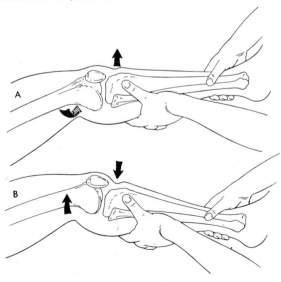

72% of these patients on arthroscopy. Correlation of the precise diagnosis with presenting history, symptoms, and clinical examination showed that the preoperative evaluation was too imprecise to be relied on completely. The limitations of the clinical examination must be recognized; great reliance should not be placed on a "negative" test. Pain, swelling, and inability to walk suggest a significant intra-articular problem. The location of swelling, the rate of accumulation of intra-articular fluid, the quantity of blood present, and the characteristics of blood aspirated should be documented. Aspiration should only be performed where diagnosis of hemarthrosis is questionable, where patient discomfort is severe, or where instillation of Xylocaine is used. Gross instability is easily detected, but lesser instability is difficult to demonstrate because of pain and muscular spasm. Radiographs give signs of fracture and ligamentous damage.

Immediate treatment of acute knee injury requires application of a soft compression dressing and coaptation splinting designed to decrease knee mobility. Weight-bearing is avoided, the involved leg is elevated, and ice packs are applied. Adequate analgesia aids rehabilitation. Because the initial examination is more reliable than any subsequent one, the initial examiner's impressions must be properly recorded.

▶ [The value of this article lies in the description of the flexion-rotation drawer test. Another one of the plethora of mechanical-gymnastic maneuvers for evaluating knee stability, it requires, at a minimum, disruption of the anterior cruciate ligament to be positive. Further identification and delineation of associated anatomical deficiencies appear to be in order.—J.S.T.] ◀

4-78 **Testing Anterior Cruciate Ligaments.** Kenneth L. Knight (Indiana State Univ., Terre Haute) compares four tests to evaluate anterior cruciate insufficiency. In the crossover test, the patient, standing upright with legs together, rotates the torso 90 degrees toward the side of the injured leg, while the physician stands facing the patient, stabilizing the foot of the injured leg by standing on the foot, while the patient rotates, the physician balances him by holding his arms or shoulders. Then the patient firmly contracts the quadriceps and, holding the contraction, bends the knees and dips toward the floor. The test result is positive if the patient feels definite discomfort, feels the knee giving out, or is unable to perform it.

In the anterior drawer test, the patient lies supine with the hip flexed 45 degrees, the knee flexed 80 degrees, and the foot flat on the table. The physician, sitting on the patient's foot to stabilize it, cups the hands around the proximal part of the tibia with the thumbs resting on the medial and lateral joint lines. With the hamstring relaxed, the tibia is pulled anteriorly. Significant anterior displacement of the tibia on the femur indicates a torn anterior cruciate ligament.

In the Lachman test, the patient lies supine with knee flexed 5 to 15 degrees and the tibia in slight external rotation. The physician, with the hand on the posterior aspect of the proximal part of the tibia and the thumb along the anteromedial joint line, attempts to trans-

(4–78) Physician Sportsmed. 8:135–138, May 1980.

late the tibia by stabilizing the anterior aspect of the distal end of the femur with one hand and lifting the tibia anteriorly with the other. A positive test is indicated by proprioceptive or visible anterior translation of the tibia in relation to the femur with a soft end point and by obliteration of the normal slope of the infrapatellar tendon when the anterior horizon of the knee is viewed from the lateral aspect.

In the pivot shift test, the patient lies supine with the knee and hip flexed 90 degrees and the foot in the air, and the physician grasps the ankle and internally rotates the tibia. With the other hand placed over the lateral joint line, fingers extending to about the midpatella, the physician exerts a valgus stress and extends the knee slowly. The lateral tibial condyle subluxates anteriorly on the lateral part of the femur if the ligament is compromised, and the test is positive if continued extension of the knee beyond 30 degrees of flexion results in sudden relocation of the tibia on the femur.

A complete examination probably should include the Lachman, the pivot shift, and the crossover tests.

▶ [The author has presented yet another test for evaluating the integrity of the anterior cruciate ligament. The crossover test deserves attention if for no other reason than curiosity. To be noted is both an incorrect description as well as illustration on how to perform the Lachman test. The author describes holding the "injured leg with the arm closest to it so that the patient's ankle is supported between your chest and humerus." This is incorrect and perhaps should be correctly described.

Lachman's test for anterior cruciate ligament instability is performed with the patient lying supine on the examining table with the involved extremity to the side of the examiner. With the involved extremity in slight external rotation and the knee held between full extension and 15 degrees of flexion, the femur is stabilized with one hand, and firm pressure is applied to the posterior aspect of the proximal tibia, lifting it forward in an attempt to translate it anteriorly. Position of the examiner's hands is important in performing the test properly. One hand should firmly stabilize the femur, while the other grips the proximal part of the tibia in such a manner that the thumb lies on the anteromedial joint margin. When an anteriorly directed lifting force is applied by the palm and four fingers, anterior translation of the tibia in relationship to the femur can be palpated by the thumb. Anterior translation of the tibia associated with a soft or a mushy end point indicates a positive test.—J.S.T.] ◀

4–79 **Acute Anterior Cruciate Ligament Injury and Augmented Repair: Experimental Studies.** The functional role of the anterior cruciate ligament as the principal stabilizer of the knee joint in the active athlete is now clear, and a means of primary ligament repair with augmentation is needed. H. Edward Cabaud, John A. Feagin, and William G. Rodkey transected the anterior cruciate ligament at the femoral origin of the stifle joint in 11 German shepherd-type dogs, repaired it primarily, and augmented the repair with the medial third of the patellar tendon by the Eriksson technique. The repairs were evaluated 4 or 8 months postoperatively. The ligament was repaired with 0 Dexon suture in a figure-eight pattern.

All the repaired, augmented anterior cruciate ligaments healed satisfactorily and provided clinical and functional stability to the knee joints. Ten joints operated on had 3 mm or less of anterior displacement on stress testing under anesthesia. Instron testing showed max-

(4–79) Am. J. Sports Med. 8:395, Nov.–Dec. 1980.

imal strength of 46.2 kg$_f$ at months and 64.3 kg$_f$ at 8 months, compared to a control value of 122.7 kg$_f$. By 8 months the ligaments operated on had healed by bony ingrowth. The collagen orientation of the ligament and patellar tendon was normal, and areas of interstitial failure were clearly seen. Abundant vascularity was common. The remaining part of the patellar tendon showed no abnormalities on gross inspection except for thickening of the undersurface where the fat pad had been dissected.

These observations are promising for the clinical management of the acutely torn anterior cruciate ligament. The transferred patellar tendon provided further blood supply, splinted the ligament to allow healing, and increased the strength of the repaired complex. The authors believe that clinical trials of augmentation of acutely injured and repaired anterior cruciate ligaments with the medial third of the patellar tendon are warranted.

▶ [A more valid evaluation of the technique used in this study should have included comparisons with determinations performed on transected and repaired but unaugmented anterior cruciate ligaments.—J.S.T.] ◀

4–80 **Intra-articular Substitution for Anterior Cruciate Insufficiency: A Clinical Comparison Between Patellar Tendon and Meniscus.** Loss of a functional anterior cruciate ligament may result in incapacitating symptoms of disabling degree, degenerative changes in the articular cartilage, abnormal extensor mechanics, and secondary meniscal tears. F. Martin Ivey (Univ. of Texas), Martin E. Blazina, James M. Fox, and Wilson Del Pizzo (Sherman Oaks, Calif.) treated 42 patients for moderate to severe anterior instability by replacing the anterior cruciate ligament with either the meniscus or the central third of the patellar tendon. In addition, extra-articular procedures aimed at specific components of combined one-plane and rotatory instability were done. The central patellar tendon was used in 17 cases, and the meniscus in 25. Three patients had augmentation of an acute anterior cruciate ligament repair. The 37 male and 5 female patients had an average age of 28 years. The average time from injury to reconstruction was 35 months. Twenty-five patients had had previous surgery.

The average follow-up period was 15 months. No patient felt that he or she was worse after the operation. Nine objective failures occurred. Successful results were most closely related to ability to correct anterior instability with all associated components of instability statically. An average loss of 6 degrees of flexion was noted in the patellar tendon group. All acute augmentations were considered successful. The failures were attributable to technical errors early in the series. Several of these patients had 90% or greater return of function when modifying their activities or using external support. Pain relief was unpredictable in individual cases. All patients reported improvement in climbing and walking ability.

All patients in this series improved subjectively after intra-articu-

(4–80) Am. J. Sports Med. 8:405–410, Nov.–Dec. 1980.

lar substitution for anterior cruciate insufficiency, and about 80% of patients had objectively successful results. Both the patellar tendon and meniscus appear to be successful intra-articular cruciate substitutes that can predictably correct moderate to severe anterior instability of the knee in a high proportion of cases.

4–81 **Macintosh Tenodesis for Anterolateral Instability of the Knee.** John Ireland and E. L. Trickey (Royal Natl. Orthopaedic Hosp., London) reviewed data on 50 patients who had undergone a MacIntosh type of repair for anterolateral instability of the knee due to a torn anterior cruciate ligament in the period 1973 to 1978. Mean duration of symptoms was 2 years. The medial meniscus had been removed in 25 patients and the lateral meniscus in 3, and 2 patients had undergone transfer of the pes anserinus, with no improvement in instability. Separate assessments were made of the severity of subjective instability and the degree of objective laxity. Objective assessment was based on the degree of jerk demonstrated under general anesthesia and in jerk tests in the conscious patient. Double-contrast arthrography was carried out to exclude meniscal tears as the primary cause of instability.

TECHNIQUE.—The MacIntosh repair involves use of an extra-articular distally based tenodesis. Fascia lata is used to limit anterior movement of the lateral tibial plateau by femorotibial tension in the tenodesis, which is obliquely placed to oppose the subluxation. The strip of fascia lata remains attached to the lateral tibial tubercle, but its proximal portion is freed and passed through a tunnel developed beneath the lateral collateral ligament. The strip is looped around the band of intermuscular septum that has been prepared and then pulled as tight as possible. After operation, the leg is elevated, having been placed in a padded cast from the groin to the ankle with the knee flexed to 60 degrees. Mobilization without weight-bearing is begun after a few days. No sport is permitted for 6 months.

There were 14 excellent results, 23 good, 4 fair, and 4 poor, as judged by the jerk test, participation in sports, and disappearance of instability. At review, after a mean follow-up of $2^{1}/_{4}$ years, 42 patients had a negative jerk test, and 37 patients (74%) were involved in some form of active sport, having regained functional and clinical stability.

Simultaneous undertaking of additional surgical procedures may invalidate the efficacy of a ligamentous reconstruction. Also, further injury may ruin an initially excellent result, as occurred in 12 patients in this series.

4–82 **Iliotibial Band Transfer for Anterolateral Rotatory Instability of the Knee: Summary of 54 Cases.** Robert A. Teitge, Peter A. Indelicato, Robert K. Kerlan, Martin E. Blazina, Frank W. Jobe, Vincent S. Carter, Clarence L. Shields, Stephen J. Lombardo, and Kimberley Kelly reexamined 48 patients 1 year after distal iliotibial band transfer (Ellison) for anterolateral rotatory instability, and another 6 patients completed a questionnaire. Only 5 patients had isolated lateral operations. Thirty-three also had anteromedial rotatory instabil-

(4–81)   J. Bone Joint Surg. [Br.] 62-B:340–345, August 1980.
(4–82)   Am. J. Sports Med. 8:223–227, July–Aug. 1980.

ity. Whereas 44% had had no previous operation, 36% had undergone one other procedure and 19% had undergone more than one. In combination with iliotibial band transfer, 74% had a lateral meniscectomy, 44% had a capsular reefing, 38% had a medial meniscectomy, and 44% had a pes anserinus transfer. Eight patients had prosthetic cruciate ligament replacement. Among these 8 patients, 5 prosthetic ligaments had fractured and were included; 3 were intact and were excluded. The knee was injured in football in 34% of the patients.

All patients had thorough knee and roentgenographic examinations; strength measurements by Cybex testing for knee extension and flexion; and strength measurement of external rotation of the tibia on the femur. Each completed a subjective questionnaire. Of the patients, 87% responded that they were improved. Ninety-one percent had positive jerk tests preoperatively; 46% had positive tests at follow-up. Whereas 53% reported no episodes of giving way, 28% reported monthly episodes, 9% weekly episodes, and 8% daily episodes. Only 15% had no difficulty cutting, 55% had some difficulty, and 26% had extreme difficulty. Only 23% reported no difficulty with jumping, 48% had some difficulty, and 30% were unable to jump or had extreme difficulty. Only 28% had returned to their desired level of activity, whereas 46% had reached 50% of their desired level. Only 13% expressed full confidence in the knee, 46% had 75% to 90% confidence, and 22% had less than 50% confidence. Of all patients, 29% had lost extension, and 57% had lost flexion; 91% had increased varus instability at follow-up, which did not seem to have clinical significance. Follow-up x-ray films showed osteophyte formation in 70% and joint space narrowing in 65%. Pain requiring aspirin was present in 46%. Eighty percent had atrophy averaging 1.72 cm. Thirty percent had tenderness at Gerdy's tubercle.

There were many variables in these patients, and poor results do not reflect failure of this one part of treatment. No patient was made worse by the procedure. There appeared to be definite reduction in anterolateral rotatory instability after iliotibial band transfer, which was maintained for more than 1 year after operation. The jerk test was considered to be diagnostic of anterolateral rotatory instability; 83% improved as measured by the jerk test, and in half of these the jerk test result became negative.

4-83 **Untreated Ruptures of the Anterior Cruciate Ligament.** W. Jason McDaniel, Jr., and Thomas B. Dameron, Jr. (Raleigh Orthopaedic Clinic, N.C.) present a retrospective review of data on 50 patients (53 knees) with documented ruptures of the anterior cruciate ligament. Review was done an average of 10 years after injury. Preoperative diagnosis almost always was a torn meniscus. Arthrotomy showed that the anterior cruciate ligament was completely torn in 39 knees and partially torn or redundant in 14 knees; the medial meniscus was torn in 33 knees, and the lateral meniscus was torn in 10 knees. No treatment of the tear of the anterior cruciate ligament was provided

(4–83) J. Bone Joint Surg. [Am.] 62-A:696–705, July 1980.

in 18 knees; excision of loose tags of the ligament was done in 32 knees; direct repair with 1 suture was attempted in 3 knees; and 3 patients had pes anserinus transfers at the initial procedure. Subsequent operations in 9 knees included lateral and medial meniscectomies. Retrospective review was undertaken to learn the results when the ligament injury is treated conservatively.

Patients were evaluated according to symptoms, instability, a follow-up score, clinical examination, roentgenograms, degenerative arthritis, and recovery of thigh circumference. Only 1 patient complained of constant pain; 14 knees had no pain, and 23 had discomfort with certain activities or with giving way. Swelling did not occur in 22 knees but occurred in 25 knees with overuse or reinjury. Twenty knees were considered weaker than the normal knee. Forty-two knees had episodes of giving way. Strenuous sports were resumed by 72% of the patients, and 47% felt they had no restrictions. Twenty-four patients had atrophy of the thigh, and 18 had limited motion of the affected knee. There was a high incidence of anterior laxity, rotatory instability, and meniscal tears. Only 3 knees had frank osteoarthritis; 8 others had medial joint space narrowing, which can follow a meniscectomy. Findings suggest that the knee with rupture of a single cruciate ligament develops osteoarthritic changes more slowly than the knee with injuries to more than one ligament. Better results were found in patients whose thigh circumference on the involved side was normal, and best results were seen in 7 patients with hypertrophy of the thigh on the involved side.

Whether or not rupture of the anterior cruciate ligament occurs as an isolated injury is controversial. Only 8 knees had both menisci intact at follow-up. It seems that degenerative changes in the articular cartilage are more likely to be related to meniscal injuries and changes after meniscectomy than to the instability of the anterior cruciate ligament.

▶ [This article and the three preceding ones set the stage for a very interesting observation. Ivey et al. attempted to correct "severe anterior instability" by replacing the anterior cruciate ligament with either the meniscus or the central third of the patellar tendon, with additional extra-articular procedures as appropriate. Using the anterior drawer test and pivot shift test as objective parameters, they report 79% successful results in their group of 42 patients.

Ireland and Trickey reviewed data on 50 patients who have undergone the MacIntosh procedure for anterior lateral instability due to a torn anterior cruciate ligament. They reported that 42, or 84%, of the 50 patients had a negative jerk test postoperatively and 37, or 74%, of the patients returned to some form of active sport.

Teitge et al. reports a summary of 54 cases having the iliotibial band transfer for anterior lateral rotatory instability of the knee. Of these patients, 83% were considered objectively improved as determined by limitation or reduction of the jerk test.

McDaniel and Dameron reported on untreated ruptures of the anterior cruciate ligament, reviewing data on 53 knees an average of 10 years after injury. None of these patients had had surgery to attempt to deal with the completely torn anterior cruciate ligament. Of significance, particularly when reviewed in terms of the results presented in the preceding three papers, is that strenuous sports were resumed by 72% of the patients in this group with untreated ruptures of the anterior cruciate ligament. In view of these figures, the question is raised as to whether surgical attempts to compensate or improve for absent anterior cruciate ligament function actually accomplishes this goal.—J.S.T.] ◀

4–84 **Intra- and Extra-Articular Reconstructive Surgery for Anterior Cruciate Ligament Insufficiency in Athletes.** H. Nakajima, M. Kondo, T. Doi, K. Watarai, T. Mannoji, H. Kurosawa, and Y. Hoshikawa (Kawasaki, Japan) have reported results of procedures on 18 unstable knees caused by anterior cruciate ligament insufficiency, one of the most troublesome injuries in Japan.

As operative treatment for 11 fresh cases, the torn ligaments were sutured primarily and the iliotibial tract plasty by MacIntosh was added extra-articularly. In 7 chronic cases the intra-articular ligament plasty by Eriksson was combined with the extra-articular method.

In a follow-up study for 1 year, 14 (82%) of the 17 patients had good or excellent results and were participating in former sports activities. Among the 6 with excellent results were 4 patients with fresh injuries who had played American football or been a skier or gymnast, or had been a physical education instructor. One chronic case was in a female basketball player and another involved a student of physical education. Among the 8 cases with good results, patients with the fresh cases could return to former sporting activities, but there was complaint of mild pain or limitation of motion. When individual sporting activities (running, cutting, landing, twisting, stopping, and sidestep) were considered, fresh cases had far better results than chronic.

In the Japanese life-style of tatami mat, full flexion of the knee joint is needed. In this series, postoperative limitation of flexion was noticed in 6 cases (5–20 degrees).

It is concluded that in the treatment of fresh anterior cruciate ligament injury the best results can be obtained by primary repair and extra-articular iliotibial tract plasty. On the other hand, in chronic cases of this series, results of greater excellence were obtained than in former series in which only the extra-articular method was used.— Hiroyuki Nakajima

4–85 **Pes Anserinus Transfer and Medial Transplantation of the Tibial Tubercle in Treatment of Rotatory Instability of the Knee.** D. Goutallier, A. Barthélémy, and J. Debeyre (Paris) reviewed 23 of 28 treated cases, with an average follow-up of 5 years. The chronic anteromedial instability was the result of trauma during athletic endeavors in most cases and was noted on the average 1 year after the initial trauma. Five of these patients had submitted to medial meniscectomy with transient functional amelioration in only 2 instances. Before ligamentoplasty, 26 patients complained of significant instability despite satisfactory reeducation of the quadriceps.

Clinical examination most often revealed an anteromedial laxity of stage II; others noted 20 instances of quadriceps atrophy. Rupture of the anterior cruciate ligament was noted in all patients, with frequent medial meniscal lesions (14). Cartilagenous lesions were found

(4–84) Orthop. Traum. Surg. 23:1633–1639, 1980. (Jpn.)
(4–85) Rev. Chir. Orthop. 66:69–73, March, 1980. (Fre.)

in 10 of 20 knees in which the surgical report described the state of the articular cartilage—chondromalacia of edematous or fissural type.

Surgery always included medial transposition of the anterior tibial tubercle according to the Elmslie technique, a subcutaneous section of the external patellar plicae and external synovium, and a pes anserinum transfer. The knee was then immobilized at 30 degrees of flexion for 1 month. Hematoma, phlebitis, or sepsis never occurred.

Results were considered excellent when no functional difference existed between the knee operated on and the healthy knee; good, when former activities, including athletic endeavors, could be resumed with minimal to moderate pain, or only slight instability remained, for example, when descending stairs. Results were considered poor when significant pain necessitated analgesic treatment and persisting instability prohibited resumption of former activities. According to these criteria, results among the 26 interventions were considered very good in 13 patients, good in 11, and poor in 2. Although all knees seemed to be more stable, most showed some degree of effusion, quadriceps wasting, and some pain. It is concluded that this type of surgical procedure may provide a satisfactory knee for lighter athletic activities, but not for competitive sports.

▶ [A surgical procedure that provides "a satisfactory knee for lighter athletic activities, but not for competitive sports" is not impressive. Perhaps the same results would have been achieved in this group of patients by simply removing the deranged meniscus.— J.S.T.] ◀

4–86 **Pathomechanics and Treatment of Anterolateral Rotatory Instability of the Knee.** Konsei Shi, Norimitsu Nasu, Fumio Fukushima, Hitoshi Hirose, and Keiro Ono reviewed the findings in 24 patients who had surgery for anterolateral rotatory instability (ALRI) of the knee. The patients were classified into two groups based on the mechanism of the injuries: "noncontact" and "contact," with "contact" indicating direct trauma to the affected lower limb, such as that rendered in the tackle in rugby football. The anterior pull of the quadriceps femoris muscle was perhaps the major cause of ALRI, especially in the noncontact group.

The Nakajima test (N-test) as well as the pivot shift test were used in diagnosing ALRI.

Eleven cases of torn medial meniscus, 4 cases of torn lateral meniscus, 4 cases of tears in both menisci, and torn anterior cruciate ligaments in all cases were found at operation. In chronic cases, 5 patients were operated on by the Losee-Kennedy procedure initially, but the knee operated on was unstable 1 year after operation. In such cases, the increased anteromedial rotatory instability (AMRI) was thought to be the cause of the unsatisfactory results. The dual-sling operation was devised to control AMRI. This operative procedure involves the anterolateral sling of transplanted iliotibial band, same as the Losee-Kennedy procedure, and the intra-articular sling, which is

(4–86) Clin. Orthop. 15:1123–1129, 1980. (Jpn.)

the reconstructed anterior cruciate ligament, with the use of the iliotibial band through the over-the-top route. Seventeen patients were operated on by this procedure, and much better results were obtained.

It was concluded that the dual-sling operation was better, because both the primary and secondary restraints for ALRI were reconstructed at the same time.—Hiroyuki Nakajima

4–87 **Posterior Cruciate Ligament Injuries: Results of Early Surgical Repair.** Howard A. Moore (Dallas) and Robert L. Larson (Eugene, Ore.) have reviewed the reports of 19 men and 1 woman with a clinical diagnosis of posterior cruciate ligament injury, seen in 1969–1977. Eighteen had surgical repair an average of 2.6 days after injury. Average patient age was 23.5 years. Ten injuries were a result of sports activities, 6 resulted from motor vehicle accidents, and 3 were associated with logging. Four knees were dislocated and either reduced spontaneously or were reduced at the scene of injury. No neurovascular complications were observed. Tears of the posterior cruciate ligament were confirmed in all patients at surgery, and many associated ligament injuries were found; there were no truly isolated posterior cruciate injuries. Torn ligaments were repaired to bone where possible. Irreparable disruptions and unstable repairs were reinforced with dynamic tendon transfers. The medial third of the medial head of the gastrocnemius was preferred as a tendon transfer.

Average follow-up was 30.8 months. Residual instability in one or more planes was present in 83% of cases, but many of these patients had excellent or good functional results. Two of 3 patients having a medial gastrocnemius transfer had an excellent or good outcome. All 4 who had reinforcement of the medial collateral ligament with the sartorius muscle had excellent or good results. The overall functional results were excellent in 7 cases, good in 7, fair in 3, and poor in 1. The patient with a poor outcome developed disabling anterior and anteromedial rotatory instability postoperatively. Three patients had x-ray evidence of degenerative changes at follow-up; in 2 both the medial and lateral compartments were involved. One patient had a pin track infection. Two patients required further surgery.

Early surgical repair of the injured posterior cruciate ligament and other damaged structures can lead to an acceptable functional outcome in most cases. Excellent and good results have been obtained in repair of all categories of associated injuries. Early complete ligament repair with dynamic reinforcement or substitutions, as indicated, provides the best prognosis for long-term functional stability in these cases.

▶ [It is interesting to note that the authors state that at postoperative follow-up "The majority of patients (83%) in this series had residual instability in one or more planes. However, many of these same patients (61%) also rated excellent or good functionally. It is apparent that acceptable functional stability does not necessarily require absolute static stability." If this is so, the point legitimately may be made that if "functional stability does not require static stability," perhaps in the instance of posterior cruciate ligament tear, repair and/or reconstruction is not necessary. The fact that one of the patients in this series had a good result without operation suggests this. Comparison

(4–87) Am. J. Sports Med. 8:68–78, Mar.–Apr. 1980.

of the patients treated surgically with a similar group treated nonsurgically has not been done. It has been my experience that in instances of posterior cruciate disruption, if associated derangements are corrected the patients do well functionally even if the posterior cruciate ligament is neglected.—J.S.T.] ◄

4–88 **Acute Tears of the Posterior Cruciate Ligament: Results of Operative Treatment.** Jack C. Hughston, James A. Bowden, James R. Andrews, and Lyle A. Norwood reviewed 32 consecutive acute tears of the posterior cruciate ligament (PCL) associated with tears of the medial or lateral compartment ligaments, or both. The PCL is an intra-articular but extrasynovial, static stabilizer of the knee, which in its distal third is in apposition with the posterior capsule. The PCL is composed of two major bands that can be recognized more easily on flexion and extension of the knee (Fig 4–27). The anterolateral band (AL) progressively tightens as flexion of the knee increases and is less taut in full extension. The shorter, thicker posteromedial band (*PM*) becomes extremely tight when the knee is in hyperextension and is a little less taut when the knee is flexed more than 30 degrees.

The injury occurred during sports in 22 of the 29 patients for whom sufficient data were available for inclusion in the study. Preoperative diagnosis was based on abduction and adduction stress tests with the knee in full extension and in 30 degrees of flexion, an anterior drawer test with the knee in maximum internal and external rotation, a posterior drawer test, and a test of the passive stability of the patella with the knee in 45 degrees of flexion. Of the 29 knees, 23 demonstrated a 2+ to 3+ abduction or adduction stress test in maximum extension and a positive anterior drawer test in maximum internal rotation; only 9 had a definitely positive posterior drawer test. A positive abduction stress test in extension, a positive anterior drawer test in internal rotation, and, less frequently, a positive posterior drawer test are criteria for diagnosis of acute tear of the PCL associated with a tear of the medial or lateral ligament. All operations were performed within 5 days of injury.

For knees with tears of the medial ligaments and PCL, a medial hockey stick incision is used to facilitate exposure and repair of the PCL at its femoral or tibial attachment. For tears of the lateral ligaments associated with PCL injuries, a similar approach is used on the lateral side of the knee, with accessory incisions. The associated lesions in the 29 patients included 26 medial compartment injuries, 2 lateral compartment injuries, and 1 combined injury to both compartments. The anterior cruciate ligament was grossly normal in 7 and was torn in 22 knees: in the middle third in 13, near the femoral attachment in 7, and near the tibial attachment in 2. In 20 knees with mop end-type tears, the anterior cruciate ligament was excised; in 2 knees with tears near the tibia, repair was attempted. The medial meniscus was torn in 21 knees. Twelve had interstitial tears necessitating medial meniscectomy. The other 9 had peripheral tears; in 6 the torn meniscus was used as a PCL graft and in 3 the peripheral tear was repaired. The PCL was torn at the femoral attachment

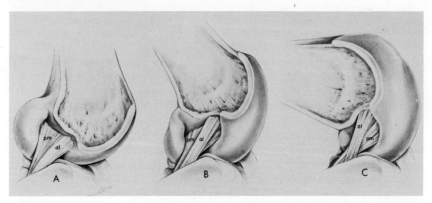

Fig 4–27.—Posterior cruciate ligament is composed of posteromedial and anteromedial bundles, and one of these bundles is more taut than the other in different positions of extension *(A)*, moderate flexion *(B)*, and full flexion *(C)*. Anterior inclination of PCL relative to long axis of tibia remains at about 30 degrees in all positions of knee flexion. (Courtesy of Hughston, J. C., et al.: J. Bone Joint Surg. [Am.] 62-A:438, April 1980.)

in 16 knees, at the tibial attachment or in the distal third in 8, and in the middle third in 5. The PCL was repaired or replaced by a graft in all 29 knees.

Objective, functional, and subjective follow-up evaluations were made of 20 patients. Eighteen subjective results were good, 2 fair, and none poor. Functional results in 16 patients were good; several others had limited activities secondary to other disabilities. Objective testing showed 13 good, 4 fair, and 3 poor results. The series provides sound evidence that acute tears of the PCL should be repaired surgically regardless of location. A medial meniscal graft is not recommended unless direct repair of the PCL fails. Only 1 result was poor on the basis of failure of the repair of the PCL; the other 2 poor results were due to failure of the medial ligament repair.

▶ [The authors' assertion that the posterior cruciate ligament is responsible for the basic stability of the knee and provides a central axis about which normal and abnormal internal and external rotations occur is not substantiated either by adequate documentation or biomechanical analysis or modeling. Therefore, this assertion cannot be considered valid. It would seem that the authors' observation that the posterior drawer test result was negative in 26 of the 29 knees described would be contrary to the experience of most knee surgeons. The conclusion that a positive abduction stress test in extension, a positive anterior drawer test in internal rotation, and also, but less often, a positive posterior drawer test are the criteria for diagnosis of acute tear of the posterior cruciate ligament in association with the tear of either the medial or lateral ligaments is not explained on a mechanical basis. As this is a rambling and rather confusing paper, it is understandable why, as the authors themselves complain, "In postgraduate courses and scientific meetings, our diagnostic criteria for associated tears of the posterior cruciate ligament have been criticized by discussors and other panelists."—J.S.T.] ◀

4–89 **Interstitial Tears of the Posterior Cruciate Ligament of the Knee.** Michael B. Clendenin, Jesse C. DeLee, and James D. Heckman (Univ. of Texas, San Antonio) describe a primary repair of midsub-

(4–89) Orthopedics 3:764–772, August 1980.

stance posterior cruciate injuries that uses the tendon of the medial head of the gastrocnemius as reinforcement. Early results in 10 patients are reported. The mechanism of injury in 9 patients was a blow to the anterior proximal part of the tibia with the knee flexed. All patients had knee pain when first evaluated. The most common physical finding was a posterior drawer sign. A posterior sag was present in 9 patients. An anterior drawer sign was present in 1 patient who had a hyperextension injury and knee dislocation. Stress roentgenograms in 5 patients confirmed posterior displacement of the tibia with respect to the femur. Examination under anesthesia in 8 patients confirmed the ligament tear, and arthroscopy in 8 patients revealed other injuries in 4. Associated injuries of posterior capsule and medial capsular ligament and meniscal detachment were treated with primary repair. Anterior cruciate tears were not repaired. Postoperative immobilization consisted of a long leg cast with the knee in flexion. In 9 cases, a pin was placed in the proximal tibia and incorporated into the cast.

PROCEDURE.—An anteromedial parapatellar incision is made with the patient's hip and knee flexed and hip externally rotated. If the posterior cruciate ligament has been torn near its femoral insertion it is repaired directly to this area with sutures into bone. If the tear is interstitial the leg is extended and a posterior S-shaped incision is made. Deep dissection exposes the origin of the medial head of the gastrocnemius, which is detached at the origin. The femoral and tibial insertions of the cruciate are identified, and beds are created for placement of the gastrocnemius tendon. A suture placed through the tendon is brought out through the bed in the medial femoral condyle and is tied securely over bone, and a second suture is placed in the gastrocnemius tendon proximal to the point at which it passes over the tibial insertion of the posterior cruciate. The suture is passed anteriorly and dis-

Fig 4–28.—Completed reinforcement using tendon of medial head of gastrocnemius. (Courtesy of Clendenin, M. B., et al.: Orthopedics 3:764–772, August 1980.)

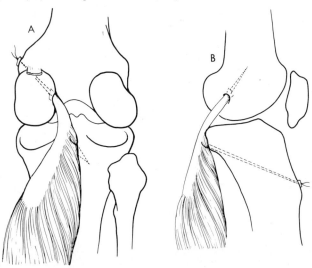

tally through drill holes and is tied over the tibia. This second suture creates a tenodesis of the tendon, but it eliminates any slack in the reinforcement, providing a tighter repair (Fig 4–28). After the capsular incision is repaired, a Bonnel pin is placed in the proximal part of the tibia, the leg is suspended by the skeletal pin, and a long leg cast is applied.

Seven of the 10 patients were followed-up an average of 22 months after operation. Four had no pain, 2 had mild pain after exercise, and 1 had constant pain. Two patients had no symptoms of instability, 4 had rare episodes, and 1 patient had occasional giving way at sport. All patients had a drawer sign. Measurement of thigh circumference showed residual muscle atrophy in 6 patients. No patient participated in formal rehabilitation because of lack of cooperation, and none was actively involved in sports. Roentgenograms revealed no degenerative changes.

Early operative treatment of interstitial tear of the posterior cruciate ligament is recommended. Reinforcement is advised. The importance of postoperative rehabilitation must be stressed to the patient.

▶ [It is interesting to note that all of the 10 patients in this study had a posterior drawer sign at follow-up examination.—J.S.T.] ◀

4–90 **The Meniscus: Can It Be Repaired? Experimental Investigation in Rabbits.** F. W. Heatley (St. Thomas' Hosp., London) exposed the menisci of 2.5-kg New Zealand white rabbits by a parapatellar incision and dislocated the patella either medially or laterally. After operation on the meniscus, the patella was repositioned, the wound closed in layers, and the knee splinted. The amount of meniscus excised, the interval between the meniscal incision and excision of the peripheral rim, and the type of material used to stabilize the meniscus were varied. After a suitable period, the rabbits were killed and the knees were examined. The experiments described by King in dogs were also duplicated in rabbits. Results were essentially the same, except that in the rabbit chondrocytes were clustered near the margin of the incision; in the dog the meniscus was unresponsive to incision.

In rabbits healing was likely to follow a small incision in the anterior horn that was extended as far as the synovium. A larger incision that reached back to the medial ligament was less likely to heal. Similarly with excision; when the amount of meniscus excised from the anterior horn was small, healing was reliable. It occurred more quickly and with less scarring when sutures were used. When large peripheral defects were created, sutures were necessary to provide stability and to reduce the size of the gap. They also appeared to act as bridges for passage of synovial cells to the meniscus. However, sutures also caused further areas of fibrocartilage cell death in the meniscus. Healing took place via a highly cellular but relatively avascular fibrous tissue stroma, which proliferated from the synovial margin and invaded along the cut edge of the meniscus. Presumably invading cells derive their nutrition largely from the synovial fluid. The proliferating synovial cells formed fibrous tissue that initially was highly cellular, but later became more fibrous and was occasionally transformed into fibrocartilage.

Excision of the meniscus in man is associated with the development of osteoarthritis some years later. These experiments in rabbits showed that cells derived from synovium can heal an incision in the substance of the meniscus, provided they can penetrate it. If such a healing mechanism exists in man, operations designed to allow ingrowth of synovial cells and to achieve initial stability could provide a more constructive approach to some longitudinal meniscal tears.

4-91   **The "Blind Side" of the Medial Meniscus.** Medial meniscectomy may be, at times, a difficult procedure because the posterior horn of the medial meniscus is inadequately visualized through an anteromedial incision. The surgeon with adequate knowledge of the poste-

Fig 4–29 (top).—The medial tibial plateau is viewed from behind while the posterior cruciate is retracted aside to reveal a deep recess *(arrow)* behind the intercondylar eminence. The medial meniscus inserts into this recess.

Fig 4–30 (bottom).—The meniscus fibers course over the edge of the medial tibial plateau and into the recess.

(Courtesy of Goldner, R. D., et al.: Am. J. Sports Med. 8:337–341, Sept.–Oct. 1980.)

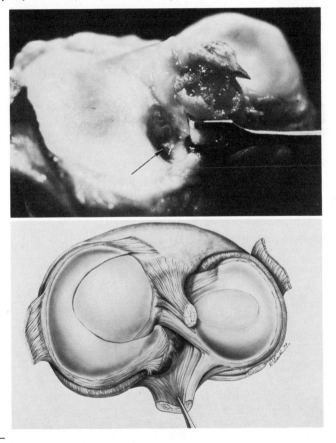

(4–91)   Am. J. Sports Med. 8:337–341, Sept.–Oct. 1980.

rior attachments of the medial meniscus should be able to perform medial meniscectomy more skillfully. Richard D. Goldner, Daniel N. Kulund, and Frank C. McCue III (Univ. of Virginia) evaluated the posterior attachments of the medial meniscus in 50 cadaver knees and performed medial meniscectomy on 10 recently amputated knee specimens.

Contrary to textbook illustrations, the major posterior insertion of the medial meniscus is not into the tibial plateau but into a deep recess behind the medial spine of the tibia (Fig 4–29). Dense peripheral meniscal fibers form a tough expansion into bone posterior to the tibial spine, proximal to the tibial insertion of the posterior cruciate ligament, and just lateral to the lateral edge of the medial tibial plateau. Some horizontally oriented meniscal fibers actually dive vertically as they attach posteriorly (Fig 4–30). If the meniscus adopts a vertical position when pulled anteriorly toward the middle of the notch, it indicates that the posterior capsular attachments have been freed. If the surgeon has any doubts whether or not an adequate meniscectomy has been performed, a posteromedial incision should be made. This incision enables the surgeon to visualize the posterior horn of the medial meniscus and to detect any bucket-handle tears or fragments of menisci. A review of 215 medial meniscectomies, 40 of which used the posteromedial approach, did not indicate increased perioperative morbidity as a result of posteromedial incision.

▶ [This excellent article is recommended for all who perform meniscal surgery.— J.S.T.] ◀

4-92 **Results After Meniscectomy in 147 Athletes.** Injury to a meniscus is the most common type of injury sustained by athletes, but the late results of meniscectomy have varied. Stig Sonne-Holm, Inger Fledelius and Niels C. N. Ahn (Copenhagen) studied the results of removing a meniscus from an otherwise normal knee in 147 subjects who had sustained injuries to one meniscus during athletic activities in 1964–1973. Of the 147, 142 were followed up after a median of 4.25 years. Median age at operation was 25 years. Ratio of male to female patients was about 6:3.

Postoperative complications included 1 case of pyarthrosis, 1 of deep thrombophlebitis, and 1 wound infection. Eleven patients (8%) had surgery on the knee during the follow-up interval because of further injuries. Twenty other patients (15%) had given up all athletic activities because of symptoms after meniscectomy, and 16 (12%) had restricted their activities. No symptoms were present in 60 of the 131 patients operated on only for the primary meniscal injury. Symptoms were not related to the length of follow-up. Most patients had had symptoms since the operation. Osteoarthrosis was observed on radiographic examination in 30 patients. Changes were significantly more frequent in the operated than in the unoperated knee. Radiologic changes were not related to the length of follow-up, and osteoarthrosis was not correlated with patients' symptoms.

(4–92) Acta Orthop. Scand. 51:303–309, April 1980.

Over half the patients in this series had symptoms following meniscectomy, the chief problems being instability and pain on weight-bearing. Collateral instability of the knee was increased in 14% of cases in this series after surgery for meniscal injury only. Meniscectomy appears to cause immediate functional changes in the knee which may produce symptoms. Symptoms were not correlated with radiologic findings of osteoarthrosis in the present series. It seems reasonable to advise resumption of sports activities following restitution of the quadriceps muscle when symptoms are not present.

▶ [The authors have made the usual error of relying on the classic anterior drawer test to determine the presence or absence of anterior cruciate ligament stability. Thus, they have failed to recognize the high association of anterior cruciate ligament disruption and lesions involving the medial or lateral meniscus. Simply put, a postmeniscectomy knee with an intact anterior cruciate ligament will do well. A patient with postmeniscectomy knee with a torn anterior cruciate ligament in many, if not most instances, will continue to have complaints, effusion, and instability.—J.S.T.] ◀

4–93 **Prognosis of Meniscectomy in Athletes: Simple Meniscus Lesions Without Ligamentous Instabilities.** Y. Hoshikawa, H. Kurosawa, H. Nakajima, and K. Watarai (Tokyo) have analyzed the influence of athletic activities on the results of meniscectomy. Cases of ligamentous instability, which makes the results worse, were excluded.

Seventy simple meniscus lesions without ligamentous insufficiency were studied by means of detailed questionnaires and clinical and radiologic examinations. These cases were classified into two groups, depending on the intensity of athletic activities. Group 1 consisted of international class athletes and group 2 consisted of some competitive athletes and some recreational athletes. None of those studied had quit sports following meniscectomy. Results were poorer in group 1 than in group 2 in both clinical and subjective evaluation. In group 1, volleyball players had worse results, particularly those who had lateral meniscectomies, compared with players of American football and wrestlers. Volleyball players returned to full sports activities in 3 months after operation and started training 49 hours per week, which was about three times the number of training hours of American football players and wrestlers. In group 2, there were no significant differences in results among the various sports athletes engaged in. Age at operation, preoperative duration, follow-up duration, and type of tear did not show any significant relation to the results. The results were worse in women and those with history of severe trauma.

In conclusion: The results of meniscectomy are strongly influenced by the quality and quantity of postoperative athletic activity, and they suggest that the meniscus is an extremely important structure for distributing the weight properly on the tibial plateau.—Hiroyuki Nakajima

4–94 **Occult Knee Ligament Injuries Associated With Femoral Shaft Fractures.** Diagnosis of ligamentous injuries of the knee in

(4–93) Orthop. Traum. Surg. 23:1625–1632, 1980. (Jpn.)
(4–94) Am. J. Sports Med. 8:172–174, May–June 1980.

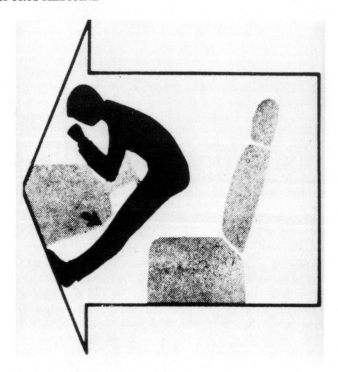

Fig 4–31.—Hyperextension-dashboard injury mechanism. Damage to the cruciate ligaments and capsule results when the knees are trapped beneath the dashboard and the trunk is carried up and over the top, thereby hyperextending the knee. (Courtesy of Walker, D. M., and Kennedy, J. C.: Am. J. Sports Med. 8:172–174, May–June 1980; reproduced from Clin. Orthop. 126:203, 1977.)

the acute phase in the multitraumatized patient with a fractured femur is essential for optimal treatment and prognosis. Dennis M. Walker (Lake Charles, La.) and J. C. Kennedy (London, Ont.) retrospectively reviewed the records of 52 patients with 54 midshaft fractures of the femur (2 had bilateral fractures); all patients had returned for follow-up examination. Average follow-up was 24.5 months. Motor vehicle accidents accounted for 48 of the fractures, athletic injuries for 4, and falls for 2.

At follow-up, 26 (48%) of the fractures were accompanied by ipsilateral knee ligament damage. Sixteen knees showed instability of grade II or more in at least one of the major ligaments or disabling instability unrelated to the patella, or both. The anterior cruciate was the most commonly injured ligament (16), followed by the medial collateral ligament (10), the lateral collateral ligament (4), and the posterior cruciate ligament (2). The average interval between injury and documentation of knee instability was 12.8 months. Most of the injuries were dashboard inpacts (Fig 4–31) and were treated by balanced traction with subsequent case bracing. Although most of the patients had regained full quadriceps and hamstring strength, 30 had an average decrease in flexion of 15 degrees.

Because hyperextension knee ligament injuries are associated with femoral shaft fractures, in such instances, a Lachman test, aspiration of the effusions, examinations during anesthesia including stress films, and arthroscopy are recommended. The presence of acute ipsilateral knee instability is a strong indication for primary rigid immobilization of the fractured femur to permit early ligamentous repair.

▶ [This is an important paper that would have been more appropriately titled "Major Knee Ligament Injuries Associated with Femoral Shaft Fractures." The analysis of the data is somewhat misleading. Actually, this report is of 26 cases of knee ligament damage from a pool of 162 patients, 52 of whom responded to a questionnaire. This represents approximately a 16% incidence of ipsilateral knee ligament injuries as documented by the authors. All other percentages should be scaled down appropriately.— J.S.T.] ◀

4–95 **Popliteal Artery Injury Associated With Knee Dislocation: Improved Outlook?** Injuries to the popliteal artery secondary to knee dislocation are being reported more often and are being treated more successfully. Robert Savage (Providence, R.I.) has reviewed data on 4 patients who were admitted to Rhode Island Hospital in a 1-year period in 1978–1979 with knee dislocation and documented popliteal artery injury. In 1974–1978, 40 new cases of arterial compromise secondary to knee dislocation were reported. Thirty-four of these patients had successful arterial reconstruction and did not require amputation, for a salvage rate of 85%. Previously, the salvage rate was 65%–70%.

Diagnosis of knee dislocation usually is obvious on inspection, and site of arterial injury usually is predictable from the area of dislocation or fracture. A dislocation should be reduced as soon as it is recognized, even before x-ray examination. The delay before vascular repair is the chief determinant of success in these cases. The site of vascular damage often can be accurately judged clinically. Arteriographic examination is indicated if signs of vascular compromise are ambiguous or if multiple fractures are present. Meticulous debridement and skin coverage are essential; sepsis has been a significant factor in late failures. Most surgeons prefer a medial approach, but posterior incisions have been used successfully. The usual treatment is excision and reversed saphenous vein grafting; the vein should be taken from the uninvolved extremity. Occasionally, excision and end-to-end anastomosis are possible. Any distal thrombus should be removed with a Fogarty catheter. Regional heparinization is recommended. Fasciotomy is favored by most workers. Popliteal vein reconstruction should also be done where possible. Only when excessive manipulation of bony instability threatens compromise of the vascular repair is orthopedic fixation indicated initially. Often internal fixation and ligament repair can be done at the same time as vascular repair.

(4–95) Am. Surg. 46:627–631, November 1980.

Methods of producing peripheral vasodilatation in these cases remain unproved. Anticoagulants have been recommended sporadically, but are of questionable value.

▶ [This report of 4 new cases of popliteal artery injury associated with knee dislocation and review of the recent literature emphasize the need for the awareness of potential arterial thrombosis with this injury. To be stressed is the necessity of early diagnosis and arterial repair performed within 6 to 8 hours after injury if the limb is to survive. This was vividly demonstrated by the Green and Allen (*J. Bone Joint Surg.* [*Am.*] 59-A:315, 1970) report of 51 cases of knee dislocation with popliteal artery injury. Of 19 extremities treated conservatively, 16 required amputation. Of 21 patients who underwent arterial repair within 8 hours of the injury, 18 regained normal circulation to the leg and only 3 patients required amputation. Another 11 patients had popliteal artery repair performed 8 hours after dislocation and all 11 later required amputation.—J.S.T.] ◀

4–96   **Fracture of Distal Medial Femoral Epiphysis With Subluxation of the Knee Joint.** Edward Abraham, Aftab Ansari, and Teng Liang Huang (Univ. of Illinois, Chicago) describe complete posterior displacement of a Salter-Harris type III distal medial femoral epiphyseal fracture, with posterior subluxation of the knee.

Boy, 16, was injured while playing football. At physical examination, the left knee was locked in 45 degrees of flexion and a fullness was felt over the posterior medial aspect of the popliteal fossa. Roentgenograms showed a fracture-dislocation.

Closed reduction was attempted by applying direct distal force over the fragment with the knee flexed and then in extension under general anesthesia, but reduction was not obtained. Reduction was accomplished only after the medial origin of the gastrocnemius was incised. The muscle was displaced posteriorly under tension by the medial femoral epiphysis, which had penetrated the substance of the muscle. There were no soft tissue interpositions between the fragments. Longitudinal traction on the leg and direct distal force on the fracture surface of the epiphyseal fragment were used to relocate the fragment and correct the posteriorly subluxated tibia. The fracture was stabilized by interfragment compression, and the gastrocnemius was sutured back to the periosteum at the site of origin. The leg was immobilized in a non-weight-bearing cast with the knee in 30 degrees of flexion for 6 weeks. Two weeks of daily quadriceps setting and range-of-motion exercises followed.

Arthroscopy was performed 2 months after operation, when no increase in knee motion had been obtained. Examination of the internal structures of the knee was unremarkable, except for adhesions in the suprapatellar pouch. A 60-degree increase in active knee flexion was observed at the end of the procedure, after the adhesions were broken by distention of the knee with saline and the arthroscope barrel.

Failure of closed reduction of this uncommon fracture was due mainly to invagination of the gastrocnemius by the displaced fragment. It was elected to fix the fracture rigidly to permit manipulation to determine ligamentous injury and minimize cast immobilization. Knee arthrotomy was not performed earlier for fear of further devitalization of the medial epiphysis and increase of soft tissue injury

(4–96)   J. Trauma 20:339–341, April 1980.

and scarring about the knee, and because no joint instability was demonstrated by manipulation.

▶ [Salter-Harris type III fracture of the medial femoral condyle requiring open reduction is indeed a rare lesion. Rogers et al. (*Am. J. Roentgenol.* 121:69–78, 1974) had recently reported seven undisplaced fractures and we have reported 6 (*J. Bone Joint Surg.* [*Am.*] 63-A:586–591, 1981), all of which were satisfactorily managed with closed treatment. Lombardo and Harvey (ibid. 59-A:742–751, 1977) have reported 5 Salter-Harris type III fractures, all of which were displaced, and 3 required open reduction and internal fixation. In those fractures that reduced spontaneously, it has been postulated that the medial condylar fragment is held in relationship to the proximal part of the tibia by the medial collateral and posterior cruciate ligaments. The lateral femoral condylar fragment rotates on the lateral tibial condyle, but because of the restraining effect of the anterior cruciate and lateral cancellous ligaments, spontaneous reduction occurs. The question raised is whether or not in those fractures requiring open reduction there is associated disruption of one or more of the restraining ligamentous structures.—J.S.T.] ◀

4–97 **Developmental Defects of the Distal Femoral Metaphysis.** William K. Dunham, Neal W. Marcus, William F. Enneking, and Cosmo Haun discuss a developmental defect in the posteromedial aspect of the distal end of the femur, in the area of insertion of the adductor magnus, which may have the roentgenographic characteristics of a malignant bone tumor. The defect is asymptomatic and thus almost always is an incidental finding. Histologically the lesion has been mistaken for osteosarcoma because of the immature reactive bone and fibrous tissue present. Nine case histories were reviewed, and the material from 8 biopsies was studied. The diagnoses in cases 1 through 9 were: nonossifying fibroma, chronic periostitis at tendon insertion, mature fibrous tissue and bone compatible with adductor magnus avulsive lesion, fibrous cortical defect, fibrosis of segment of femoral condyle, periosteal desmoid, mature fibrous tissue compatible with desmoplastic fibroma or subperiosteal cortical defect, reparative fibrous tissue, and bilateral lesions (no biopsy).

These cystlike defects are reported to be present in 7%–22% of all children aged 2–12 years. They are most commonly located on the posteromedial aspect of the distal end of the femur and are more common in boys. As one gains familiarity with this variant, there is less likelihood of performing an unnecessary biopsy. Tomograms will confirm the lesion's presence and lend assurance to the diagnosis, whereas interpretation of a particular roentgenogram as a normal variant depends on the clinical situation, the degree of cortical irregularity, the roentgenographic projection, and the experience of radiologist and orthopedist. If a bone scan demonstrates more than a minimal increase in uptake, a biopsy is indicated. The variability of the diagnoses in these 9 cases demonstrates the difficulty in histologic diagnosis of these lesions. The developmental defect under discussion differs roentgenographically from nonossifying fibroma and fibrous cortical defect in that bone margins of the defect are less sharply defined or are absent. The lesion is probably due to either trauma or

(4–97)   J. Bone Joint Surg. [Am.] 62-A:801–806, July 1980.

muscle avulsions of small bits of bone at the insertion of the adductor magnus tendon. The avulsed bone elicits a vascular response in the area, further weakening the bone. A cycle of microavulsion followed by vascular fibroblastic response and further avulsions stops as the bone strengthens at maturity. The proliferation of fibrous tissue and periosteum occurs in an area undergoing marked remodeling. These lesions probably represent developmental variations rather than true neoplastic processes.

▶ [The recognition and management of this lesion are totally dependent on familiarity. The clinical situation often does not aid in the diagnosis because, although reportedly asymptomatic, a child requiring an x-ray study is having complaints, even if vague. The degree of cortical irregularity, the x-ray projection, and tomography do not aid in the diagnosis.—J.S.T.] ◀

4–98 **The Patellofemoral Joint: 30, 60, and 90-Degree Views.** Arthur H. Newberg and David Seligson (Univ. of Vermont) have found that dynamic radiography with axial projections at 30, 60, and 90 degrees (Ficat views) yields diagnostic information on the patellofemoral joint that is not obtainable from single static radiographs. The method of examination is illustrated in Figure 4–32. The central beam is directed from the feet and inclined about 10 degrees toward the tibia, with the cassette held on the distal thighs, perpendicular to the beam. The 30-degree view may not be possible in very obese patients or those with a prominent tibial tubercle. This view is most likely to show a tendency toward subluxation. The 60-degree view

Fig 4–32.—Radiographic technique and patient position for the 30-degree view. Note goniometer, used to assist in the accurate measurement of knee flexion. The patient holds the cassette on the thighs, and the radiographic tube is low enough to be tangential to the patellofemoral joint. (Courtesy of Newberg, A. H., and Seligson, D.: Radiology 137:57–61, October 1980.)

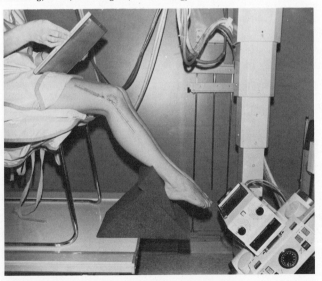

shows the patellar morphology and is best for demonstrating the central contact area.

Studies were done in 70 patients with an average age of 28 years. The most common presenting conditions were chondromalacia, knee pain, subluxation-dislocation, and trauma. The Ficat views proved useful after the technical difficulties were overcome. The study was abnormal in 19 patients. Six had evidence of prior dislocation with osteochondral fragments, 4 showed patellar subluxation, and 3 had posttraumatic changes. Two patients had signs of excessive lateral pressure, and 4 showed advanced patellofemoral arthritis. Two of 7 patients who underwent knee arthrography had a torn meniscus. One patient had evidence of patellar subluxation on the Ficat study, which had not been suspected clinically.

The Ficat views are helpful in studying the morphology and dynamics of the patellofemoral joint. The patella may contain fairly marked cartilaginous changes that are not apparent on radiographs. Subluxation probably is the most common and most frequently missed cause of chondromalacia, and dynamic views of the patellofemoral joint can help in diagnosing this condition in selected cases.

▶ [These views demonstrate a low yield of positive findings related to dynamic function. Of the 70 patellofemoral joints, only 19 had abnormalities and 15 of these had bony changes (osteochondral fractures, 6; posttraumatic changes, 3; excessive lateral pressure, 2; and advanced patellofemoral arthritis, 4). The use of these views should be restricted to patients with patellofemoral pain who do not have osseous changes on a single Ficat view of the patella performed at 60 degrees or on a Merchant view. Similarly, these three dynamic views should be performed after arthrography only if arthrogram is otherwise normal and the 60-degree Ficat view or Merchant view is normal.—J.S.T.] ◀

4–99 **Anterior Displacement of the Tibial Tuberosity in the Treatment of Chondromalacia Patellae.** Chondromalacia patellae usually affects young, healthy persons, reducing their ability to do heavy work. Recent studies indicate that anterior displacement of the tibial tuberosity, including distal anchorage of the patellar tendon, considerably reduces the mechanical load on the patellofemoral joint, and relieves pain in chondromalacia patellae. Einar Sudmann and Berndt Salkowitsch (Univ. of Tromsø, Tromsø, Norway) used this method to treat 29 consecutive patients with presumed chondromalacia patellae in 33 knees in 1976–1978. The 17 men and 12 women had a median age of 30 years. All were unfit for work or in 1 case, for competitive sports. Median duration of symptoms was 3 years. The chief complaint was pain located either ventrally or medially in the knee, or both, on exertion. Muscle wasting in the thigh was noted in 18 cases and intra-articular fluid in 15.

All diseased cartilage was removed before displacing the tibial tuberosity, using a triangular bone block from the anterior iliac crest and an AO screw. Full weight-bearing was delayed until the tuberosity had healed, about 2 months postoperatively. Median follow-up was 22 months, and the minimum was 8 months.

(4–99) Acta Orthop. Scand. 51:171–174, February 1980.

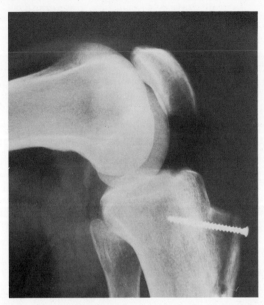

Fig 4–33.—Lateral radiograph of right knee. Anterior displacement of the tibial tuberosity is maintained by a triangular bone block and a screw. (Courtesy of Sudmann, E., and Salkowitsch, B.: Acta Orthop. Scand. 51:171–174, February 1980.)

Chondromalacia was confirmed at operation in all knees but 1. In 1 case, anterior displacement was not maintained because the graft was pressed into the tibial metaphysis, but symptoms resolved. The median anterior displacement of the tibial tuberosity in the other cases was 15 mm (Fig 4–33). No joint effusion was noted at follow-up. All knees were relieved of pain on exertion and at rest except 3, which were unchanged. Three patients changed their jobs. Two knees had postoperative extra-articular wound infection by staphylococci. Three had deep venous thrombosis in the leg. Surgery for bleeding from the donor site was necessary in 1 patient on streptokinase-warfarin therapy.

Postoperative complications were frequent in this series, but no permanent sequelae resulted. Thrombosis can be reduced by avoiding compression bandaging of the knee and by early mobilization. The short-term results of this operation have been encouraging, and it appears to be a promising operative method for chondromalacia patellae in carefully selected patients who are unfit for work or competitive sports.

▶ [The authors have not noted whether an appropriate conservative treatment regimen was instituted prior to operation. The indications for surgery have not been clearly defined. Most worrisome is the reported postoperative complication rate of 18%. It has been our experience that most persons with chondromalacia patellae respond to isometric quadriceps exercises. Rarely, if ever, does a staphylococcal infection or a deep vein thrombosis result from such a regimen.—J.S.T.] ◄

4–100   **Efficacy of Various Forms of Fixation of Transverse Fractures of the Patella.** Michael J. Weber, Chet J. Janecki, Paul McLeod, Carl L. Nelson, and James A. Thompson (Univ. of Arkansas) fractured the patellae of 25 fresh cadaver knees transversely and then fixed them using the following techniques: circumferential wiring, tension-band wiring, Magnusson wiring, and a modification of tension-band wiring. The object was to determine whether any of the commonly used wiring techniques is rigid enough to allow early motion in the treatment of transverse fracture of the patella. The knees were mounted in a machine capable of measuring quadriceps force, flexion angle, and fracture separation simultaneously. They were extended from 90 to 0 degrees by applying tension to the quadriceps tendon with the force of gravity as the only resistance, and separation

Fig 4–34.—The four wiring techniques: **A,** circumferential; **B,** Magnusson; **C,** tension-band; **D,** modified tension-band. (Courtesy of Weber, M. J., et al.: J. Bone Joint Surg. [Am.] 62-A:215–220, March 1980.)

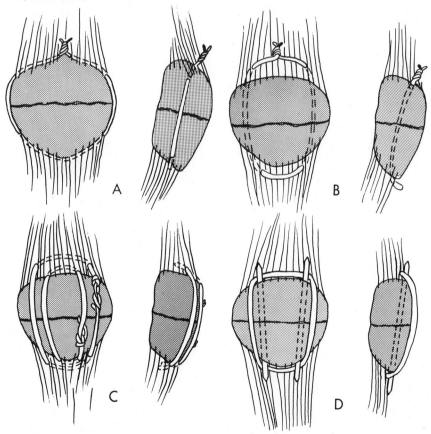

of the fracture fragments was measured first with the retinaculum unrepaired and then with the retinaculum repaired.

TECHNIQUE.—Standard circumferential wiring (Fig 4–34,A) was done with an 18-gauge wire pursestringed around the periphery of the patella, with the wire as close to the bone as possible. The wires were tightened and twisted. Magnusson wiring (Fig 4–34,B) was also performed with 18-gauge wire. Drill holes were made through the proximal fragment, beginning at the medial and lateral borders of the quadriceps tendon and progressing distally to exit on the fracture face posterior to a point midway between the anterior and posterior surfaces of the patella. Holes in the distal fragment were made opposite to those in the proximal fragment, and the wire was passed in a loop and tightened. With standard tension-band wiring (Fig 4–34,C), one 18-gauge wire was passed deep to the insertion of the quadriceps and patellar tendons and tightened in a loop over the anterior surface of the patella. A second wire was passed through the Sharpey fibers of the proximal and distal poles of the patella and tightened. Both wires were then tightened until the articular edges on the posterior surface of the patellar fragments were slightly separated. Modified tension-band wiring (Fig 4–34,D) was performed with two Kirschner wires introduced longitudinally across the fracture; the wire loop was passed behind the tips of the Kirschner wires and over the anterior surface of the patella.

Separation of the fracture fragments was much less with the Magnusson and modified tension-band wiring than with circumferential or standard tension-band wiring. The retinacular repair was found to contribute to stability; however, this seemed most important in the less rigid repairs.

If early motion is to be used in treating transverse fractures of the patella, techniques in which the wire is anchored directly in bone should be used, and the retinaculum should be repaired. In this study, tension-band wiring, advocated by others, did not prevent separation of the fragments' articular surfaces in early postoperative motion. The excellent fixation provided by Magnusson and by modified tension-band wiring was attributed to the stability of the interface between the wire loop and the bone. Magnusson wiring was found to fix the fracture fragments rigidly through an arc of motion from 90 degrees of flexion through 10 degrees. Minimal separation of fracture fragments occurred from 10 to 0 degrees. In modified tension-band wiring, there was no separation of fragments throughout the entire 90-degree arc of motion.

► [The conclusion of the authors that techniques in which wire is anchored directly in bone should be done if early motion is to be used in treating transverse fractures of the patella is well founded.—J.S.T.] ◄

4–101 **Surgical Injury to the Lateral Aspect of the Knee: A Comparison of Transverse and Vertical Knee Incisions.** A number of incisions have been recommended for lateral meniscectomy following athletic injury. J. S. Keene, J. N. Amalfitano, W. G. Clancy, Jr., A. A. McBeath and R. G. Narechania (Univ. of Wisconsin, Madison) compared knees of patients having transverse (Bruser) capsular incisions with those of patients having vertical (parapatellar) lateral cap-

(4–101) Am. J. Sports Med. 8:93–96, Mar.–Apr. 1980.

sular incisions, which require sectioning of the anterior third of the lateral capsule and the lateral patellar retinaculum. The incision in Bruser approach must parallel the fibers of the iliotibial band but cut transversely the anterior and middle thirds of the lateral capsule. Twenty patients having each type of incision for lateral meniscectomy were reviewed a year or more after surgery. All were reported to have normal stability at the time of operation. All patients but 1 were men. The average age of the Bruser group was 43 years and of the parapatellar group, 24 years. The respective average follow-up times were 5 and 1.5 years, respectively.

Patients with an intact anterior cruciate ligament showed less than 1 degree of difference in average varus or valgus measurements in the normal and operated knees. Average mechanical values were slightly greater for both knees in the Bruser group. Average values for anterior drawer testing differed by less than 1 mm when the two incision groups were compared. No patient had more than 1+ laxity in any plane. In patients with a deficient anterior cruciate ligament, the knee operated on had more than a 1-mm increase in the anterior drawer after each incision. This displacement was 50% greater in the Bruser group than in the parapatellar group, and increased clinical laxity was noted in all patients with Bruser incisions. No patient with a vertical incision had a positive pivot shift test.

A transverse or vertical lateral capsular incision for lateral meniscectomy does not lead to measurable lateral or anterolateral rotatory instability in patients with intact anterior cruciate ligaments. Where these ligaments are deficient, a lateral transverse capsular incision may contribute to subsequent anterolateral rotatory instability. A vertical lateral capsular incision aids examination of the knee joint.

4–102   **Lipohemarthrosis: Its Occurrence With Occult Cortical Fracture of the Knee.** John S. Train and George Hermann (Mt. Sinai School of Medicine, New York) report fat fluid levels in the knees of 3 patients following trauma associated with small, subtle cortical fractures. None of the fractures was visible in routine roentgenograms. Because of fat fluid levels in the area of the suprapatellar pouch, additional roentgenograms were taken until the small cortical fractures could be seen. A cross-table lateral roentgenogram of the knee reveals a great fat fluid level in the suprapatellar bursa (Fig 4–35, A). A slight oblique view of the same knee reveals a small cortical fracture of the medial femoral condyle (Fig 4–35, B).

Visualization of fat in the knee, shoulder, and elbow has been described as an indication of intra-articular injuries, but it has been assumed that these injuries always coexist with obvious fractures. There are no descriptions of subtle fractures associated with fat fluid levels in the English-language literature. The use of cross-table lateral roentgenograms for patients with initially negative roentgenograms but with significant clinical findings is therefore suggested, al-

(4–102)   Orthopedics 3:416–418, May 1980.

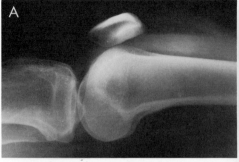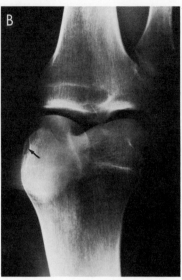

Fig 4–35.—A, a cross-table lateral roentgenogram of the knee shows a great fat fluid level in the suprapatellar bursa. Routine anteroposterior, lateral, and tunnel views demonstrated no fracture. **B,** a slight oblique view of the same knee reveals a small cortical fracture of the medial femoral condyle *(arrow)*. (Courtesy of Train, J. S., and Hermann, G.: Orthopedics 3:416–418, May 1980.)

though such films should not replace the standard vertical-beam lateral film.

▶ [The value of this article is to illustrate the usefulness of the cross-table lateral roentgenogram to demonstrate the fat fluid level seen in lipohemarthrosis. It appears that the value of this projection is not commonly appreciated by the orthopedic surgeon.—J.S.T.] ◀

4–103 **O'Donoghue's Triad Plus Patellar Tendon Rupture.** Bruce E. Baker (SUNY, Upstate Med. Center) presents a case of disruption of the medial aspect of the knee resulting in O'Donoghue's triad and rupture of the patellar tendon.

Man, 24, while playing basketball came down from a rebound attempt with the knee in a flexed, externally rotated position as the foot struck the floor. The injury found at surgery was disruption of the superficial medial collateral ligament, deep collateral ligament, and medial meniscus, and a tear of the anterior cruciate ligament in the middle third (Fig 4–37). There was also total rupture of the patellar tendon at its origin on the inferior pole of the patella. The anterior cruciate ligament and medial meniscus were deemed not to be repairable and were excised. Repair of the patellar tendon was carried out with multiple sutures through the tendon and reinsertion through drill holes on a roughened inferior pole of the patella. A figure-of-eight tension band wire was used to protect the repair. The medial tibial attachment of the capsule was reinserted through drill holes around the tibial plateau from the patellar tendon to the posterior medial corner. The superficial part of the medial collateral ligament was reattached to the tibia with a staple, and a primary pes anserinus transfer was done (Fig 4–38). The knee was placed in a bent knee cast, and after 6 weeks of immobilization the patient was started on a rehabilitation program. The metal was removed 4 months later. One year postoperatively, the patient had full extension and 135 degrees of flexion, 1+ anteroposterior laxity, no medial laxity to valgus stress,

(4–103) N. Y. State J. Med. 80:1436–1437, August 1980.

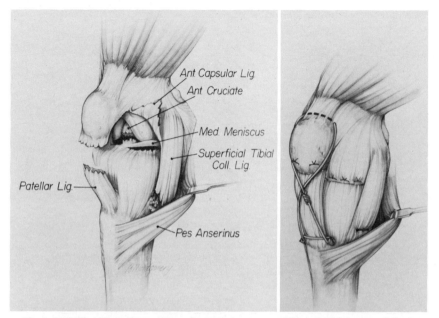

Fig 4–37 (left).—Disruptions at time of surgery in man, aged 24, included rupture of the deep and superficial tibial collateral ligaments, the anterior cruciate ligament, the peripheral attachment of the medial meniscus, and the patellar tendon.

Fig 4–38 (right).—Repair of O'Donoghue's triad with patellar tendon rupture. A tension band wire is used to protect the patellar tendon repair.

(Courtesy of Baker, B. E.: N. Y. State J. Med. 80:1436–1437, August 1980.)

and no anteromedial laxity. He was able to perform such activities as bicycle riding, jogging, and tennis.

The combination of a triad plus patellar tendon rupture is infrequently seen. The conflicting positions of immobilization associated with the repair of complete patellar tendon rupture and disruption of medial supporting structures are resolved by the use of a tension band wire, producing relief of the stresses across the patellar tendon while the knee is flexed and internally rotated for immobilization.

▶ [This is an interesting and unusual lesion obviously designed to tax the skill of the surgeon. Personal experience with a similar problem treated in a like manner revealed that postoperatively the patient had patella baja and 15-degree limitation of knee flexion.—J.S.T.] ◀

4–104 **A Modified Cast Brace: Its Use in Nonoperative and Postoperative Management of Serious Knee Ligament Injuries.** Frank H. Bassett III, John L. Beck, and Garron Weiker have treated 94 patients with major knee trauma by early protected motion since prolonged immobilization has been shown to be detrimental to synovial joints. A hinged long leg cast was used on patients with a variety of knee problems. Knees with acute ligament injuries not requiring surgery were placed in the cast brace immediately, while operative cases

(4–104) Am. J. Sports Med. 8:63–67, Mar.–Apr. 1980.

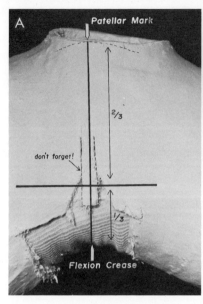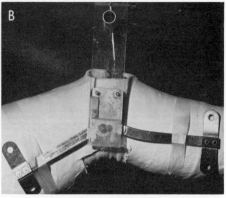

Fig 4–39.—A, the orthotic center is determined by the intersection of the vertical axis from patellar mark to flexion crease, and the horizontal axis is two-thirds the distance from the anterior surface of the patella to the posterior surface of the knee. **B,** joints are positioned over the center marks, with the arms parallel but posterior to the axes of the femur and tibia. The jig assures parallel alignment of the joints. (Courtesy of Bassett, F. H., III, et al.: Am. J. Sports Med. 8:63–67, Mar.–Apr. 1980.)

were started about the 10th postoperative day. The method stresses proper alignment of joints, security of limb position, prevention of swelling complications, and economy of physician time. A special feature is a modified single axis joint that restricts the arc of motion to safe limits, generally 30–90 degrees.

TECHNIQUE.—The long leg cast is applied, preferably over an elastic support. In application of the joints, the necessary landmarks are the patella anteriorly and the flexion crease posteriorly. The patellar bump is windowed. The orthotic center of the knee is determined by marking a point on the patella 0.25-in. proximal to the midpoint. With a piece of string as a guide, a straight line is drawn around each side of the cast from this point to the flexion crease posteriorly. A point on each side is then determined with a ruler that lies two-thirds the distance from the anterior surface of the patella, one-third from the back of the knee. These points of intersection are reasonable determinations of the center of rotation for that knee (Fig 4–39, A). The joints are positioned over center marks with arms parallel but posterior to the axes of the femur and tibia. The alignment jig ensures parallel alignment of the joints (Fig 4–39, B).

Functionally, results compared favorably with results obtained using traditional methods in four categories of cases: acute, moderate ligament tears treated only with the brace (22 knees); acute, severe injuries, with immediate surgical repair (19 knees); chronic instability in patients who had never undergone surgery (28 knees); and chronic instability with previous surgery (25 knees). Rehabilitation times were markedly shortened, patient acceptance was high, and complications were rare. Early motion was extremely well tolerated, with only one cast removed because of discomfort. Postoperative effusion rapidly disappeared with beginning of motion. Rapid return of motion did not correlate with a poor result, and the stability of operated knees did not loosen with time. Although lack of controls precludes definite comparisons, it is concluded that early protected motion is safe and provides significant benefits. The knees of the patients were ready for active exercises the day the cast was removed.

▶ [The failure of the authors to establish definite criteria with regard to specific anatomical instabilities suitable for treatment with this device is noteworthy.—J.S.T.] ◀

4–105 **Runner's Knee.** Benjamin D. Rubin and H. Royer Collins describe a differential diagnostic approach to knee pain in runners and treatments for selected conditions. The history is obtained with a questionnaire. Changes in workout schedule, flexibility exercises, and location and duration of pain must be considered. Both legs must be examined. Body habitus, leg lengths, alignment of hips, knees, and tibias, and patellar mechanics are assessed. The knee is examined systematically to determine the site of pain and tenderness, ligamentous laxity, and quadriceps atrophy. X-ray evaluation is helpful in many cases. Standard views include standing anteroposterior, lateral, tunnel, and bilateral modified Hughston views. Arthrography or a therapeutic test may be necessary. In the latter, running may be resumed with a corrective heel lift or arch pad; alleviation of symptoms is indicative.

Differential diagnosis is best approached by anatomical location of symptoms. Patellar pain may be caused by tendinitis at the quadriceps insertion at the proximal end of the patella or at the patellar tendon origin at the inferior pole of the patella. These conditions and Osgood-Schlatter disease require rest, ice, and salicylates. Chondromalacia patellae denotes patellar symptoms secondary to the patellar compression syndrome and is the most common cause of knee pain. Treatment involves rest, ice, and isometric, progressive resistance exercises for the quadriceps. Orthotics may be useful to correct misalignment. Transarthroscopic patellar shaving and lateral retinaculum release may be useful if conservative measures fail. Medial knee pain may be caused by pes anserinus or Voschel bursitis or by proximal tibial stress fracture. Bursitis occurs most frequently in beginning runners or in runners who are increasing their mileage. Rest and oral treatment with anti-inflammatory agents are useful, besides corticosteroid and local anesthetic injection in the acute stage. Stress fractures are almost always on the medial side and appear as a sclerotic line on x-ray films (Fig 4–41). Lateral knee pain, caused by bursitis, popliteal tendinitis or tenosynovitis, or iliotibial band syndrome, responds to conservative measures. Intra-articular changes include torn or degenerated meniscus (medial or lateral) or degenerative joint disease, especially if ligamentous laxity is present, consistent with an old ligament tear. Degenerative arthritis, rheumatoid diseases, osteochondral fractures, and osseous or cartilaginous loose bodies must

(4–105) Physician Sportsmed. 8:49–58, June 1980.

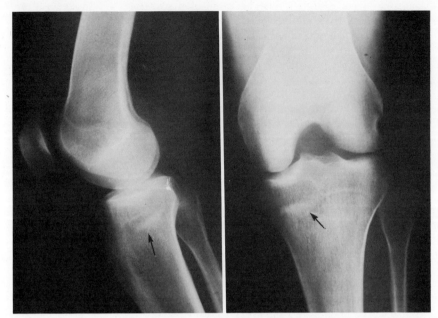

Fig 4–41.—Stress fracture of proximal portion of tibia appears as sclerotic line *(arrows)* on x-ray films. (Courtesy of Rubin, B. D., and Collins, H. R.: Physician Sportsmed. 8:49–58, June 1980.)

also be considered. Surgical removal is required for obvious meniscal tears or loose body. Discoid lateral and cystic meniscus may also necessitate meniscectomy. The medial synovial plica, seen in 50% of patients, may become thickened and fibrotic causing pain on walking up stairs and other symptoms of chondromalacia patellae. However, patients have no signs of an abnormal quadriceps mechanism such as an underdeveloped vastus medialis obliquus, an increased Q angle, patella alta, or subluxing patella. Conservative treatment may be useful in true pathologic synovial plica, but in some cases the plica must be excised. Differential diagnosis of knee pain must include consideration of tumors, which are found most often in young adult patients.

▶ [A complete, concise, and well-illustrated essay on the subject of knee pain in runners is presented here. The reader is referred to the original article.—J.S.T.] ◀

4–106 **Foot-Related Knee Problems in the Long-Distance Runner.** Lowell D. Lutter (St. Anthony Orthopaedic Clinic, St. Paul) reviewed the data on and followed 213 runners with knee injuries for 9 months to 4 years after injury. Of these injuries, 164 were associated with abnormal foot configuration such as pronation or cavus configuration (43% and 34%, respectively, 77% total). Chondromalacia patellae constituted 28% of knee pain; iliotibial band pain was 25%; medial joint pain, 15%, and lateral joint pain, 9%. Knee injuries were mostly non-

(4–106) Foot Ankle 1:112–116, September 1980.

meniscal, generally involved soft tissues, and responded to definite periods of nonrunning, depending on location or cause. The program of treatment in these knee problems should entail activity attenuation, acute pain management, a stretch and strengthening program, and shoe control or orthotic foot control.

Not all runners' knee problems can be treated with an orthosis; however, an orthosis can be an important adjunct in managing pronation problems. A semiflexible cork and leather longitudinal arch support is used as the first mode of treatment in the minimally to moderately pronating foot. A more rigid orthosis is made of Orthoplast, which is heated in a water bath and is then molded around the foot to place the heel in neutral and support the longitudinal arch. Molding may also provide metatarsal support. Use time is about a year. The most recalcitrant problem associated with cavus configuration is iliotibial band pain. Cold/heat application and quadriceps exercises are appropriate. Soft heel pads may be useful. An orthosis has been constructed with a lateral heel buildup in an attempt to compensate for the cavus configuration. This is designed to pronate the foot slightly and place a varus heel in a more neutral position.

The cavus configuration foot has a rigid longitudinal arch that does not pronate down to the weight-bearing surface. There may also be varus configuration of the heel. The mechanics of the pain are partially explained on the basis of stress dissipation at heel strike. The individual strikes with the heel in excessive varus. Midtarsal joints remain rigid. Varus movement is also produced at the knee.

Pronation and tibial torsion are normally present. When these events are disrupted, deviation in the normal amount of pronation produces secondary deviation in the internal tibial torsion. With pronation, increased internal tibial torsion causes dissipation of this additional stress into the medial part of the knee.

In this series, periods of recovery to full running were 86 days for cavus-related iliotibial band pain and 49 days for pronation-related chondromalacia.

▶ [The author has presented valid clinical observations regarding knee problems seen in the runner. However, he describes definite "correlation" between knee problems and foot abnormalities without offering statistically verifiable data. Also, we should not delude ourselves into thinking that "biomechanics" is simply the description of postural changes that occur during the gait cycle. The biomechanics of function should entail measurement, data analysis, and statistical substantiation. We have recently witnessed many observers who use this term inappropriately to describe simple clinical observations.—J.S.T.] ◀

4–107 **Breaststroker's Knee: Pathology, Etiology, and Treatment.** S. David Stulberg, Keith Shulman, Steven Stuart, and Peggy Culp (Univ. of Chicago) observed that most competitive breaststrokers with knee problems have pain under the medial patellar facet, in place of or in addition to pain along the tibial collateral ligament. Twenty-three competitive breaststroke swimmers with painful knees, aged 6–30 years, were evaluated. Four breaststroke swimmers who

(4–107) Am. J. Sports Med. 8:164–171, May–June 1980.

used the whipkick but were asymptomatic also were examined. Underwater movies of these swimmers were taken. Ten swimmers had had knee pain during the first year of participation, and all but 4 had knee pain within 3 years of starting the breaststroke. Most had pain only while performing the breaststroke.

Ligamentous laxity was not more frequent in the swimmers than in other age-matched swimmers or nonswimming athletes. Eighteen swimmers had local tenderness under the medial patellar facet and over the opposing surface of the medial femoral intercondylar ridge, 12 unilaterally. All 18 had bilateral tenderness under the patella and over the medial femoral condyle. Five swimmers also had tenderness along the tibial collateral ligament, and 5 others had tenderness only at this site. None of the knees was unstable. Symptoms were more marked in 4 swimmers who had done the breaststroke for more than 8 years. Tenderness persisted 2–6 months after the end of the swimming season. No definite abnormalities were found on x-ray films. Arthroscopic studies in 2 swimmers showed extreme fibrillation of the medial patellar facet and also fibrillation of the medial femoral intercondylar ridge, flakes of articular cartilage within the joint, and moderate synovitis.

The swimmers without knee pain kept their heels and knees quite close together during the recovery phase of the whipkick, and the thighs were internally rotated and brought or held together as the hips and knees extended. Swimmers with patellar tenderness had widely abducted legs as the hips and knees were flexed, and the legs often were thrust down into the water as the hips and knees were extended. Close evaluation of the whipkick technique of a young swimmer and correction of any abnormalities of the kick can eliminate or prevent knee pain. Patellofemoral tenderness in young swimmers may be the forerunner of serious patellofemoral disease in adulthood.

▶ [The observations made by the authors should be considered in light of the observations and conclusions of Kennedy and Hawkins (*Am. J. Sports Med.* 6:309–322, 1978). The latter authors believe that injury or strain to the tibial collateral ligament is the primary cause of knee pain in breaststrokers.

The photographic analysis of the various peculiarities in executing the whipkick with correlation of symptoms and clinical findings are noteworthy. However, the data do not support the contention that correction of any abnormalities of kick can eliminate or prevent knee pain, or that patellofemoral tenderness in young swimmers may be the forerunner of serious patellofemoral disease in adulthood.—J.S.T.] ◀

FOOT AND ANKLE INJURIES

4–108 **Disabling Sports Injury of the Great Toe.** Donald L. Mullis and Wallace E. Miller (Univ. of Miami) report an athletic injury of 3 months' duration, an isolated tear of the adductor hallucis tendon to the right big toe.

Man, 18, while playing basketball, came down on the right foot after a jump and began to pivot and externally rotate on the fixed right foot. Swell-

(4–108) Foot Ankle 1:22–25, July 1980.

ing and a knot appeared in the first web space on the dorsum of the foot; this persisted, along with pain on the plantar aspect of the right big toe. The injury became disabling; placing a varus stress on the big toe caused a popping sensation and a feeling that the toe was dislocating.

Three months after a private physician misdiagnosed the injury, the patient was referred. Physical examination revealed significant instability on a varus stress to the metatarsophalangeal joint of the right big toe, which was confirmed on x-ray examination. The joint gapped open laterally; there was fullness in the first web space. The diagnosis was a torn conjoined tendon, capsule, and collateral ligaments to the metatarsophalangeal joint. Three months after injury, with the use of a tourniquet, the dissection was carried down to this joint with care not to injure the neurovascular structures. The adductor hallucis tendon was avulsed from the base of the proximal phalanx and had retracted. This was in a ball of scar. Both transverse and oblique heads of the adductor hallucis were torn from the base of the proximal phalanx of the toe, which, along with the capsule and collateral ligament tears, caused instability on the lateral aspect of the joint. The tendon was replaced at the base of the proximal phalanx of the big toe by 2–0 silk Polydek and chromic suture, and 12–15 minutes of traction permitted stretching of the muscle bellies of the adductor to normal and placement of the tendon back to its original insertion site. No tendon graft replacement was necessary. The suture was taken through drill holes made in the base of the proximal phalanx, and the tendon was placed down to periosteum and bone. Steinmann pins were placed through the first metatarsal into the second metatarsal in a parallel fashion to prevent splaying, to protect the soft tissue repair, and to keep the tendinous insertion to bone intact. The patient was placed in a short leg cast, and after 3 weeks the pins were removed. Weight-bearing was resumed during the seventh and eighth weeks, and after 6 months the patient had resumed sports activities.

The case demonstrates that this injury lends itself to primary repair even at a late date, because the muscle can stretch, permitting resuturing of the tendon to its former insertion site. Any salvage procedure such as tendon graft cannot substitute for the demands that an athlete places on the foot.

▶ [On the basis of one case report, the authors have suggested surgical intervention for disruption of the lateral conjoined tendon, capsule, and collateral ligaments to the metatarsophalangeal joint. They describe the patient presented as having been "treated conservatively." However, they fail to elaborate on the nature of the treatment. The question raised is: "Would adequate immobilization for a sufficient period immediately after the injury result in adequate healing, thus precluding the necessity for surgical intervention?"—J.S.T.] ◀

4–109   **Traumatic Dislocations of the First Metatarsophalangeal Joint.** Melvin H. Jahss (Mt. Sinai Hosp., New York) presents two cases of dislocations of the first metatarsophalangeal joint and discusses the mechanics, anatomy, and pathomechanics of this injury. The injury usually is caused by vehicular accidents or by a fall from a great height. At the moment of impact the hallux is forcefully hyperextended, causing acute pain at the base of the toe with painful limitation of motion. The most important clinical finding is prominence of the first metatarsal head under the plantar aspect of the foot.

(4–109)   Foot Ankle 1:15–21, July 1980.

Roentgenologic findings in both patients showed a complete dislocation of the base of the proximal phalanx dorsally over the first metatarsal head. Frank separation of the sesamoids to either side of the metatarsal head in the first patient indicated complete disruption of the intersesamoid ligament, which was readily reduced. The second patient showed transverse fracture of the medial sesamoid with ragged fracture margins. An offending fragment was subsequently excised.

Proximally, the sesamoid mass is continuous with a thick plantar capsule, which is attached proximally to the plantar aspect of the neck of the first metatarsal (Fig 4–42,A). As the hallux is dorsiflexed, this capsule is stretched, and the sesamoids are drawn forward by their strong insertions on either side of the plantar aspect of the base of the proximal phalanx. Further pathologic dorsiflexion ruptures the plantar capsule at its attachment under the metatarsal neck. The hallux rides over the dorsum of the metatarsal head or neck and locks the head plantarward. The medial and lateral conjoined tendons lie tautly to either side of the metatarsal neck (Fig 4–42,B, type I dislocation). Such dislocations are usually irreducible on closed reduction, since the metatarsal head is incarcerated by the conjoined tendons with their intact sesamoids. Further dorsiflexion force either ruptures

Fig 4–42.—A, normal relationship of sesamoid mass. **B,** simple dorsal dislocation of metatarsophalangeal joint with sesamoids lying on the dorsum of the metatarsal neck, maintaining their attachment to the base of the proximal phalanx, with the metatarsal head incarcerated plantarward (type I). **C,** dorsal dislocation with rupture of intersesamoid ligament, usually reducible on closed manipulation (type IIA). **D,** dorsal dislocation with transverse fracture of medial sesamoid; the distal fragment is drawn distally, while the proximal fragment is in normal relationship with the lateral sesamoid, usually reducible on closed manipulation (type IIB). (Courtesy of Jahss, M. H.: Foot Ankle 1:15–21, July 1980.)

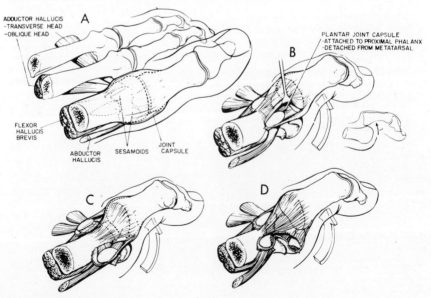

the intersesamoid ligament, resulting in wide separation of the sesamoids (Fig 4–42,C, type IIA dislocation), or transversely fractures one of the sesamoids (Fig 4–42,D, type IIB dislocation). In more common pure hyperextension injuries, fractures are avulsion in type. In cases of falls from a height, sesamoid fractures also may be due to crushing against metatarsal condyles. The more proximal fragment remains in normal position relative to its adjacent sesamoid via the remnant of the intact intersesamoid ligament; the distal fragment separates from its proximal portion, because it is separated from its attachment to the ligament and is drawn distally into the joint space by its peripheral attachment at the base of the proximal phalanx. This fragment requires excision. In rupture of the volar plate, reduction usually is readily accomplished.

▶ [The authors have provided a worthy clinical observation.—J.S.T.] ◀

4–110 **Running Footwear: Examination of the Training Shoe, the Foot, and Functional Orthotic Devices** is reported by David Drez (Lake Charles, La.). About 160 models of running shoe presently are available. A good training shoe should provide cushioning, support, and stability yet be adequately flexible, soft, and light. The studded outer sole probably provides more traction and shock absorption than does the solid sole. A flexible sole is important to allow adequate dorsiflexion at the metatarsophalangeal joint level at toeoff. A straight-last shoe should be used to prevent gait alterations that might occur with the inflare that most shoes have built in to them. The heel should be elevated about 0.5 in. to relieve stress on the gastrocnemius-soleus area. A heel more than 3 in. wide causes too rapid pronation of the foot at heelstrike. A firm heel cup or heel counter stabilizes the foot and also prevents shoe breakdown. The Achilles pad and tongue should be well padded and soft to prevent irritation. A round toe box at least 1–1½ in. high will prevent crowding of the toes. Inside supports may help support the foot despite their soft construction. A nylon mesh outer construction is probably best.

Anatomical abnormalities that produce symptoms in runners may be subtle because of the high stresses encountered in running. The "neutral position of the subtalar joint" is assumed to be the position where the foot functions most efficiently with the least amount of stress exerted on the joints, ligaments, and tendons. Abnormalities of foot alignment are sought with the foot in this neutral position. When abnormalities in the neutral position of the subtalar joint exist, the foot undergoes compensatory motions, and a functional orthotic device may be helpful. Posts or wedges are added to an orthosis in the heel or forefoot area as required. Soft orthotic devices may be used on a trial basis. Rigid orthotic devices are made by obtaining a neutral-position cast of the foot and sending it to an orthotic laboratory, where appropriate posts or wedges are added.

▶ [The original article is recommended for those physicians who feel uncomfortable in dealing with the complaints and problems of the runner.—J.S.T.] ◀

(4–110) Am. J. Sports Med. 8:140–141, Mar.–Apr. 1980.

4–111 **Metatarsal Stress Fractures.** David Drez, Jr., John C. Young, Roy D. Johnston, and William D. Parker (Lake Charles, La.) have evaluated metatarsal lengths from roentgenograms in a group of patients with metatarsal stress fractures and compared them with those of a control group having no foot symptoms to determine if a short first metatarsal could be implicated as a cause for metatarsal stress fractures. The 65 roentgenograms showing metatarsal stress fractures were made with patients in both the weight-bearing and non-weight-bearing positions. A control group consisted of 50 roentgenograms in both positions, in the anteroposterior projection of the feet of randomly selected persons with no record of foot problems. Absolute lengths of the first and second metatarsals in millimeters were obtained by measuring the distance from the lateral aspect (first metatarsal) and medial aspect (second metatarsal) of the base at the metatarsocuneiform articulation to the highest point on the metatarsal head. Relative lengths were determined by measuring the distance from the highest point on the talar head to the highest point on the metatarsal head.

Statistical analysis (*F* tests) showed that the absolute lengths of the first and second metatarsals in the group with stress fractures did not differ from those in the control group. The ratios of the relative lengths of the first and second metatarsals also did not differ significantly. Analysis of metatarsal lengths in the control group showed no statistical difference in weight-bearing and non-weight-bearing measurements.

The data of the two groups were combined, and the ratio of the

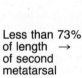

Less than 73% of length → of second metatarsal

Fig 4–43.—A short first metatarsal. (Courtesy of Drez, David, Jr.: Am. J. Sports Med. 8:123–125, Mar.–Apr. 1980.)

(4–111) Am. J. Sports Med. 8:123–125, Mar.–Apr. 1980.

absolute length of the first metatarsal to that of the second was calculated. The average ratio was 0.833565, with a SD of 0.0564. If that ratio is normally distributed, about 95% of all observations should fall within 2 SD of the mean. Hence, a short first metatarsal would be one that is less than 73% of the length of the second metatarsal (Fig 4–43), and a long first metatarsal would be one that is over 94% of the second metatarsal.

Hypermobility of the first metatarsal segment could not be evaluated. This factor may be important, and further study is suggested.

▶ [It is not appropriate for the authors to express their findings to six significant figures when their measurements were made to no better than three. The following are critical questions that the authors fail to answer: Which metatarsals were fractured? Were these injuries sports related? Was there commonality as to the injury mechanism? What was the activity level of the control group? The authors use ANOVA (analysis of variance) for their statistical analysis. Their handling of its formatting requisites in both data tables is incorrect. For the level of utility needed in their application, ANOVA actually defaults to a simple unpaired *t* test. The authors bring up a third conclusion regarding weight-bearing and non-weight-bearing measurements. None of these data is explicitly given, nor is this question in the original statement of purpose.— J.S.T.] ◀

4–112 **Stress Fracture of the Cuneiform Bones.** K. O. A. Meurman and S. Elfving (Helsinki) report 2 cases of stress fracture of the cuneiform bones in nonathletic military recruits. Stress fractures are fairly common among military recruits. The most common sites are the tibia, the calcaneus, and the metatarsal bones.

CASE 1.—Man, 20, felt pain in the left leg after a 12-minute running test. Swelling, tenderness, and local pain were present over the bases of the second and third metatarsals. Roentgenograms revealed no abnormalities, but a bone scan showed increased activity dorsolaterally in the tarsometatarsal region. Three weeks later a transverse sclerotic zone across the long axis of the third cuneiform bone was observed (Figs 4–44 and 4–45). Clinical symptoms were resolving since painful activities had been avoided. Three months later the sclerotic zone persisted but was disappearing.

CASE 2.—Man, 18, felt pain on the dorsal aspect of the right foot several weeks after beginning military service and later had pain in the right knee. An x-ray film revealed a stress fracture with periosteal and internal callus in the upper third of the tibial diaphysis, and a bone scan showed increased activity in the upper tibial area and in the right foot dorsomedially in the tarsometatarsal region. A roentgenogram of the foot showed a delicate sclerotic zone perpendicular to the trabecular structure of the bone in the first cuneiform. Tomography revealed internal callus formation.

Two repeated forces cause stress fractures: bending forces and compression forces. Roentgenographic signs are periosteal new bone formation and a cortical break or medullary sclerosis. The base of the first metatarsal is especially liable to stress fracture of the compression type, since a large proportion of body weight passes through this bone, which is opposed by strong muscular contraction. Perhaps the same can be attributed to the first and biggest cuneiform. The third cuneiform occupies a central position in the vault of the distal tarsals and may be affected by compressive forces.

(4–112) Br. J. Radiol. 53:157–160, February 1980.

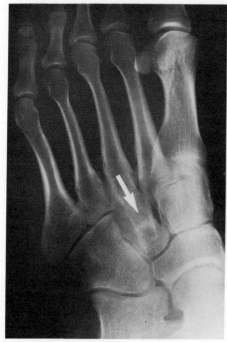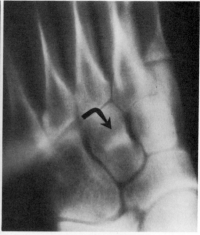

Fig 4–44 (left).—Transverse sclerotic band perpendicular to long axis of third cuneiform: callus of stress fracture.
Fig 4–45 (above).—Tomogram of same foot. Callus zone is evident.
(Courtesy of Meurman, K. O. A., and Elfving, S.: Br. J. Radiol. 53:157–160, February 1980.)

X-ray films are invaluable in diagnosis. Radiologic findings depend on callus formation. An x-ray film is usually normal during the first posttrauma weeks. Scintigraphy is useful for early screening, and if the scan is abnormal, x-ray follow-up some weeks later should confirm the diagnosis. The scan itself does not permit exact localization.

Stress injuries in the cuneiform region may not be so extremely rare as has been assumed. These case reports demonstrate the usefulness of scintigraphy combined with x-ray techniques in doubtful cases of stress fracture.

▶ [A cuneiform fracture can be better located on a radionuclide bone scan with a "lightened" scan and a plantar view. A "lightened" scan is one that limits the scan time according to the maximum area of nuclide augmentation. The plantar view optimally demonstrates the midfoot. The "anteroposterior views" presented in this report are anterior views that limit midfoot evaluation because of overlap nuclide interaction from the hindfoot and ankle.—J.S.T.] ◀

4–113 **Fracture of the Lateral Cuneiform Bone in the Absence of Severe Direct Trauma: Diagnosis by Radionuclide Bone Scan.** Jesse H. Marymont, Jr., George Q. Mills, and W. Davis Merritt, III (Wesley Med. Center, Wichita, Kan.) present a case of fracture of the lateral cuneiform bone.

Boy, 17, with no history of trauma, consulted an orthopedic surgeon after 9 days of pain in the lateral aspect of the left foot. The pain was first noted during a basketball game and increased in intensity over the 9-day period.

(4–113) Am. J. Sports Med. 8:135–136, Mar.–Apr. 1980.

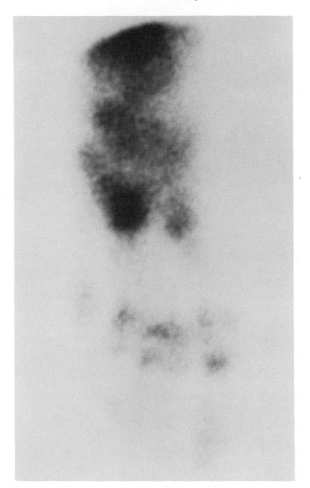

Fig 4–46.—Radionuclide bone scan of left foot in boy, aged 17, with unexplained pain in the lateral aspect of the foot. An area of greatly increased concentration in the region of the lateral cuneiform bone is consistent with a recent fracture. The scan was done 5 weeks after injury. (Courtesy of Marymont, J. H., Jr., et al.: Am. J. Sports Med. 8:135–136, Mar.–Apr. 1980.)

Physical examination revealed no significant swelling or deformity, and a radiogram was considered within normal limits. After 1 month of no improvement, a bone scan was performed (Fig 4–46), which showed an area of greatly increased radiotracer concentration in the region of the lateral cuneiform bone.

The authors propose that the fracture was sustained while the patient was playing basketball. Unfortunately, the resolution obtainable in the scan does not permit clear visualization of the base of the metatarsal. A possible fracture of the base of the third metatarsal cannot be refuted. However, the fact that a fracture was made apparent on the bone scan and not demonstrated on a conventional radiogram cannot be disputed. This alone establishes the value of bone scanning in differential diagnosis of pain that could be skeletal in origin and also illustrates its usefulness in athletes with pain of unknown etiology. Whereas fractures of the cuneiform bones are considered to be rare and the result of severe direct trauma, it may well be that such fractures are more common than previously believed.

▶ [The value of radionuclide bone scan for ill-defined foot pain in the absence of specific trauma is worthy of emphasis. The question raised by this case report is why an attempt was not made to demonstrate the fracture by tomography.—J.S.T.] ◀

4–114 **Stress Lesions of the Talus** are described by K. A. Meurman (Helsinki). Motorizing the army has not decreased the occurrence of fractures among soldiers. Stress fractures in healthy bones are also found among civilians, especially athletes and weekend outdoor enthusiasts. In military recruits, stress lesions appear in almost all bones of the lower extremities, with the majority in the tibia. Although stress fractures of the calcaneus are common in the armed forces, damage seldom appears in the ankle bone.

Man, 20, at the beginning of military service, experienced pain in front of the right ankle joint after a 3-minute running test (Cooper test). After 1½ months, he had pain mainly when running, but also to a lesser degree when resting after strenuous training. He visited the doctor 11 times and usually was excused from marching. He was moved to the central military hospital for examination. On palpation, he had a definite circumscribed, painful pressure sensitivity on the dorsum of the right foot somewhat distal to the upper ankle bone. There was no considerable swelling. Roentgen examination of the right foot revealed an 8-mm wide, transversal, sclerotic band in the anterior

Fig 4–47 (left).—Increased radiodensity in the anterosuperior aspect of the distal part of the talus, corresponding with the point of sensitivity to pressure.

Fig 4–48 (right).—Pathologic accumulation of isotope in the right talus, corresponding with roentgenographic finding in Figure 4–48.

(Courtesy of Meurman, K. A.: Fortschr. Geb. Roentgenstr. Nuklearmed. 132:469–471, April 1980.)

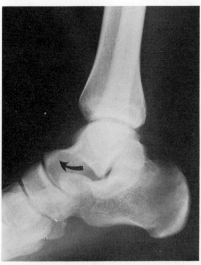 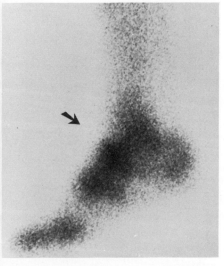

(4–114) Fortschr. Geb. Roentgenstr. Nuklearmed. 132:469–471, April 1980. (Ger.)

distal corner of the talus (Fig 4–47). The same could be found with tomography. Scintigraphy (10 mCi of ^{99m}Tc-methylenediphosphonate) of the lower extremities showed pathologic isotope accumulation on the right in the distal talus region (Fig 4–48). In addition, there was a pathologic accumulation on the left in the neck of the heel bone as well as on the right in the inner condyle of the tibia. Control x-ray films of the heels and knees showed typical stress fracture on the left in the neck of the calcaneus and normal knees. After the patient was questioned, it became apparent that the left heel was painful for a longer time, although only moderately, and he had never mentioned this to the doctor. In addition, the pain on the right side had become increasingly more severe. There was no pain or pressure sensitivity in the tibial condyle at any time.

Stress lesions are often bilateral. However, frequently the symptoms in one region become so dominant that lesions in other areas remain unnoticed.

The following conclusions can be drawn: The possibility of a stress lesion exists not only in the talus and the heel, but also in the other tarsal bones. A stress fracture may deviate from the classic picture. The subjective and clinical reports may reveal intense symptoms and the x-ray findings may remain moderate, doubtful, or even negative; or the x-ray examination may show typical changes with only mild complaints and clinical findings or no symptoms at all. Doubtful cases should give reason for an isotopic examination.

▶ [We have recently reported 17 stress fractures of the tarsal navicular characterized by negative findings on routine roentgenograms (Annual Meeting American Orthopaedic Society for Sports Medicine, Las Vegas, Nev., 1981). The lesions were demonstrated by radionuclide bone scanning and anteroposterior planograms. Apparently, stress fractures of the talus may present similarly.—J.S.T.] ◀

4–115 **The Anterior Impingement Syndrome of the Ankle.** Osteophytes on the anterior aspect of the tibia and talus are fairly common in athletes who run and jump. The spur on the anterior aspect of the dorsum of the talus can impinge on the tibia during ankle dorsiflexion, causing pain and limiting motion. J. C. Parkes II, W. G. Hamilton, A. H. Patterson, and J. G. Rawles, Jr. (Roosevelt Hosp., New York) report four cases of anterior impingement syndrome of the ankle in baseball, basketball, and tennis players and in a ballet dancer.

Man, 27, a professional baseball outfielder, incurred a fracture of the middle third of the right tibia and fibula and was treated with plaster immobilization. A malunion resulted, and the patient also had pain and limited motion on dorsiflexion of the right ankle. Bone spurs were seen on the dorsum of the talus and on the anterior lip of the tibia (Fig 4–49). The ankle joint itself showed no arthritic changes. Limited dorsiflexion interfered with the patient's playing ability. The spurs were therefore excised from the talus and tibia, and the patient recovered uneventfully and returned to playing professional baseball.

The repetitive pull of the anterior ankle joint capsule and impingement of the talus against the tibia on running and jumping can lead to calcific deposits along the lines of the capsular fibers. The joint itself is usually free of degenerative changes. An anterior spur may

(4–115) J. Trauma 20:895, October 1980.

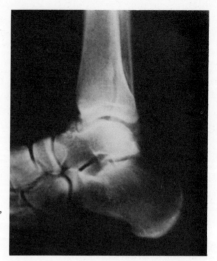

Fig 4–49.—X-ray film of baseball player, aged 27 years, showing typical anterior bone spurs on the tibia and talus. (Courtesy of Parkes, J. C., II, et al.: J. Trauma 20:895, October 1980.)

occur on the talus or the tibia, or both, in any activity involving running or jumping. If pain and reduced motion interfere with athletic ability, removal of the spur or spurs most likely will give satisfactory results. Several subjects have returned to professional competition after this procedure. The procedure is not of great magnitude and should not make the situation worse.

▶ [Recent experience indicates that the painful foot associated with anterior talus impingement spurs may have an associated stress fracture of the tarsal navicular. In addition to routine radiograms, a radionuclide bone scan is recommended, and if it is positive, anteroposterior tomograms are indicated.—J.S.T.] ◀

4–116 **Air Stirrup Management of Ankle Injuries in the Athlete.** Cornelius N. Stover (Flemington, N.J.) discusses some of the factors in joint immobilization techniques that led to the development of an air stirrup support system and describes results in two patients with injury to the lateral ligament of the ankle who were successfully treated with this system. The air stirrup is a prefabricated, universal-fitting plastic brace composed of an outer shell lined with self-sealing air bags inflatable by mouth. The device limits inversion while protecting ankle function. Designed for use with a regular athletic shoe, the device allows an early return to activity.

The splint is especially useful in patients with acute ligament injuries, stable malleolar fractures, and posterior tibial tendinitis, and as an adjunct to internal fixation following early removal of plaster casts. It is also helpful during assessment of ankle injuries. The system was used to treat a tennis player who sustained an inversion injury to the ankle; results were dramatic in that within 1 week the patient resumed playing tennis while wearing the splint. In another instance, when a high school basketball player sustained a severe ankle sprain, a plaster cast was applied. Upon removal of the cast after

(4–116) Am. J. Sports Med. 8:360–365, Sept.–Oct. 1980.

4 days, extensive swelling and ecchymosis were evident. Three days after an air stirrup was applied, the ecchymosis began to resolve and the swelling decreased. Two days later, the boy was able to participate competitively, playing well. In addition to the applications described, the air stirrup has been used to treat os calcis fractures and subtalar synovitis, and in open reduction.

The air stirrup support system is durable and highly versatile. A major advantage of the air stirrup over plaster casts is that it provides an early return to ankle function without sacrificing protection.

▶ [It is impossible to draw a meaningful conclusion from an inadequately documented series of two patients. Presentation of a new treatment device and method without supporting data from a controlled evaluation of its efficacy verges on being irresponsible.—J.S.T.] ◀

4–117 **Instability of the Ankle After Injury to the Lateral Ligament.** Malcolm Glasgow, Andrew Jackson, and Angus M. Jamieson (London) emphasize the importance of the lateral view in assessment of instability of the ankle and relate the radiologic findings to the anatomy of injuries to the lateral ligament. The place of the anteroposterior varus stress view (Fig 4–50) when acute or chronic instability is suspected is established, but the lateral view, which shows anterior subluxation of the talus (Fig 4–51), is frequently omitted.

Twenty cadaver ankles were examined to determine the functional instability resulting from division of the different components of the

Fig 4–50 (left).—Standard varus stress view with talar tilt.
Fig 4–51 (right).—Lateral stress view demonstrating anterior subluxation of talus. Gap of more than 6 mm between posterior articular margin of tibia and dome of talus was significant.
(Courtesy of Glasgow, M., et al.: J. Bone Joint Surg. [Br.] 62-B:196–200, May 1980.)

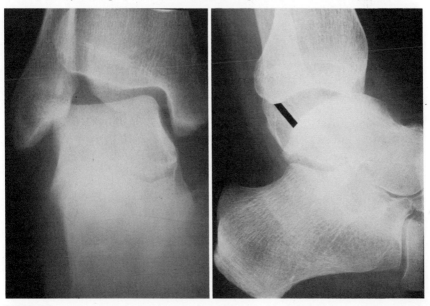

lateral ligament. Division of the anterior talofibular ligament alone allowed anterior subluxation, the talus rotating medially. The ankle remained stable to varus stress except at the extreme of plantar flexion. When the calcaneofibular ligament was divided in isolation, minor varus instability could be demonstrated, but anterior subluxation did not occur. In forced inversion of the plantar-flexed foot, the anterior talofibular ligament is the first to rupture, and only anterior instability can be demonstrated at this stage. With increasing force the rupture is extended, and both varus and anterior instability are apparent.

Forty-six patients (54 ankles) with radiologic evidence of instability of the ankles were studied to assess the importance of the anterior stress view. Anterior subluxation alone was seen in 26 ankles, and varus instability alone was seen in 6. With varus stress views alone, 48% of cases of ligamentous instability would have been missed, and with anterior stress views alone, 11% would have been missed. Roentgenograms made in two planes are particularly important in chronic instability, the long-term consequence of which is degenerative arthritis of the ankle. Anterior subluxation was demonstrated more frequently than varus laxity after acute injury to a ligament and with chronic instability of the ankle. The anatomical observations explain why anterior subluxation was found clinically so much more commonly than varus instability in these patients. A talar tilt of more than 6 degrees was considered to be excessive and to contribute to the instability. If a higher figure had been accepted, dependence on the lateral view for diagnosis of ligamentous instability would have been even greater.

▶ [This excellent article demonstrates anterior subluxation to be considerably more common than varus tilt in injury to the lateral ligaments of the ankle. The point is well taken that the lateral stress view is an essential part of the evaluation of the sprained ankle.—J.S.T.] ◀

4–118 **Arthrographic Diagnosis of Ruptured Calcaneofibular Ligament: II. Clinical Evaluation of a New Method.** M. Vuust and B. Niedermann have introduced the use of an oblique axial projection in arthrography and have proposed criteria for distinction between ruptures of the anterior talofibular ligament and rupture of both lateral ligaments. These criteria were assessed in a clinical series of 19 patients with ankle distortions who were operated on for ruptured lateral ligaments of the talocrural joint. All patients with sprained ankles admitted to the hospital in a 4-month period were clinically evaluated. If rupture of the lateral ligaments was suggested, an arthrography was performed within 24 hours after the trauma. An oblique axial film was included if the arthrography revealed a leakage of contrast medium on the anterolateral aspect of the talocrural joint. Surgery was done if there was suggested rupture of both lateral ligaments. The projections used in arthrography were anteroposterior, lateral, and anteroposterior, with the foot rotated 20 degrees laterally and medially, and oblique axial exposure when indicated. The

(4–118) Acta Radiol. [Diagn.] (Stockh.) 21:231–234, 1980.

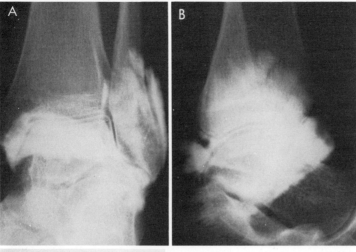

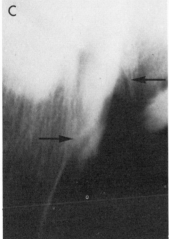

Fig 4–52.—Partial rupture of the calcaneofibular ligament (Percy type III). Contrast medium is mainly situated lateral to the malleolus, and there is no peroneal sheath filling. **C,** two tongues of contrast medium are shown on the oblique axial film; the medial one indicates the ruptured calcaneofibular ligament, which is positioned between the arrows. (Courtesy of Vuust, M., and Niedermann, B.: Acta Radiol. [Diagn.] (Stockh.) 21:231–234, 1980.)

validity of the criteria defined in part I of the authors' study for diagnosing rupture of the calcaneofibular ligament was compared to that of Percy and colleagues (type III arthrographic finding) (Fig 4–52). Filling of the peroneal sheath was not used in this series as an indicator of rupture but was compared retrospectively.

The new criteria permitted correct diagnosis of rupture in all 19 cases. Rupture of both the anterior talofibular ligament and the calcaneofibular ligament was found in all patients. The appearance of the leakage, described in part I, corresponded to clinical findings. It is possible to distinguish the contrast medium that extends around the lateral aspect of the malleolus from that situated beneath and medial to the tip of the fibula in the malleolar fossa. Only the latter indicates a rupture of the calcaneofibular ligament. Filling of the per-

oneal sheath was a better criterion for rupture of the lateral ligaments than was the extension of contrast medium on the anteroposterior and lateral films; the correct diagnosis was 74%. In this series,
no filling of the peroneal sheath occurred in 5 cases, despite rupture
of the sheath found at operation. The criteria of Percy suggested rupture of both lateral ligaments in 10 ankles.

▶ [The number of patients in this study is limited (19) and all had tears of both the
calcaneofibular and the anterior talofibular ligaments. A larger series will be necessary
to establish if this view has clinical application and can make a distinction between
ruptures of these two ligaments.—J.S.T.] ◀

4–119 **Ankle Sprains: Surgical Treatment for Recurrent Sprains.**
Chronic instability of the ankle is commonly associated with a history
of recurrent inversion sprains of the ankle. A. A. Savastano and Ernest B. Lowe, Jr. (Providence, R.I.) report their experience with the
Chrisman-Snook procedure, a modification of the Elmslie procedure,
in the surgical repair of chronic ankle instability. Ten patients, 3 female and 7 male athletes, with a mean age of 21 years, who participated in bicycling, boxing, tennis, hockey, basketball, football, soccer,
or a combination of sports, were evaluated before and after surgery.
Each had a history of numerous ankle sprains. The Chrisman-Snook
modification of the Elmslie procedure involves the use of one half of
the tendinous portion of the peroneus brevis ligament, instead of the
fascia lata, to reconstruct the anterior talofibular and the calcaneofibular ligaments.

The procedure yielded satisfactory results in 9 ankles with minimal
symptoms even though physical examination revealed limited inversion and stress x-ray films showed a decrease in talar tilt (average,
12.4 degrees preoperatively; 5.6 degrees postoperatively). These 9 patients, including a former boxer aged 57 years, returned to active participation in sports without symptoms. Two of the patients lost to follow-up are known to be actively engaged in intercollegiate varsity
sports.

It is concluded that the Chrisman-Snook modification of the Elmslie procedure is simpler to perform than the Watson-Jones procedure
and yielded satisfactory results in most of the patients in this study.

▶ [A well-documented account of the results of the Chrisman-Snook modification of
the Elmslie procedure is presented here.—J.S.T.] ◀

4–120 **Lateral Instability of the Ankle and Results When Treated by
the Evans Procedure.** The anterior talofibular ligament prevents
lateral instability of the ankle. Evans has described a procedure for
correcting posttraumatic lateral instability, which is illustrated in
Figure 4–53. Seppo Vainionpää, Pekka Kirves, and Erkki Läike
(Kotka, Finland) evaluated the Evans procedure carried out at Kotka
Central Hospital in 81 ankles of 77 patients with lateral ankle instability in 1968–1976.

In this procedure, the peroneus brevis is sectioned and its belly sutured to the peroneus longus. The distal end is drawn down through

(4–119) Am. J. Sports Med. 8:208–211, May–June 1980.
(4–120) Ibid. 8:437–439, Nov.–Dec. 1980.

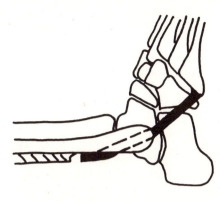

Fig 4–53.—Completed Evans operation. (Courtesy of Vainionpää, S., et al.: Am. J. Sports Med. 8:437–439, Nov.–Dec. 1980.)

the proximal retinaculum, brought up through a tunnel drilled in the lateral malleolus, and sutured to the fibular periosteum at either end of the tunnel. Patients are placed in a below-knee walking cast for about 5 weeks.

Sixty patients with 62 operated ankles were followed up an average of 5.2 years after surgery. Most injuries were sports related. Average time from injury to surgery was 3.2 years. Mean patient age was 28.3 years.

Excellent or good results were obtained in 87% of ankles, satisfactory results in 8%, and poor results in 5%. Limited supination was not harmful. All but 1 of 6 patients with slight osteoarthritis had good results. Ten of 16 athletes remained active at follow-up. One poor result was in a so-called insurance-judicial case. Two patients had superficial wound infection after surgery, but no osteomyelitis was observed.

In this series, the Evans procedure prevented talar tilting and provided good stability in the anteroposterior plane.

▶ [This is another well-documented study indicating that there is more than one way of "skinning a cat."—J.S.T.] ◀

4–121　**Rupture of the Lateral Ligaments of the Ankle: A Controlled Clinical Trial.** Tore Grønmark, Odd Johnsen and Odd Kogstad (Skien, Norway) compared three different principles used in treating ruptured lateral ligaments of the ankle in 67 men and 28 women with an average age of 26.2 years. Sports injuries were responsible in 41 subjects; a fall on the level was responsible in 39. Initial treatment included ice, compression, and elevation. Thirty-two patients were then treated with primary suture, 33 with plaster of Paris casts, and 30 with strapping. The cast was changed after 2 weeks, and walking plasters were used for 4 weeks more. Nonelastic zinc oxide strapping was used for 6 weeks.

Fifty-eight patients were treated immediately after injury. Rehabilitation time averaged 8 weeks for each of the three groups. Average follow-up was 17 months. In the operative group there were 18

(4–121)　Injury 11:215–218, February 1980.

ruptures of the anterior talofibular ligament and 14 of the anterior talofibular and calcaneofibular ligaments. One patient developed deep vein thrombosis. Eighty percent of patients were free of symptoms at follow-up, but 19 had moderate pain on prolonged weight-bearing and a slight tendency of the ankle to tilt. Only 1 patient who had primary repair had residual symptoms, as did 7 patients having strapping, and 11 treated in plaster. Four patients had substantial symptoms.

Patients who were operated on had the best results in this trial. Among conservatively treated patients, those having strapping had better results than those treated with a plaster of Paris cast. Radiologic examination with forced supination and comparison with the other ankle is strongly recommended in all cases. Younger, more active persons, especially sportsmen and women, should be offered primary suture of the ligaments. If conservative therapy is elected, immobilization should be for at least 6 weeks; strapping is preferable. Local cooling, pressure bandaging, and elevation should be started as soon as possible after injury.

▶ [The authors have failed to indicate the range and average duration of follow-up on many of the patients. Also, the parameter of posttreatment evaluation was simply whether the patient was free of symptoms or had symptoms remaining. Use of subjective parameter does not provide an adequate basis for comparison among the three methods of treatment.—J.S.T.] ◀

4–122 **Early and Late Repair of the Lateral Ligament of the Ankle.** Nathaniel Gould, David Seligson, and Jeffrey Gassman (Univ. of Vermont) describe an apparatus for separately testing the status of the anterior talofibular and calcaneofibular ligaments of the ankle in 25 healthy subjects aged 15–30 years. They also describe operative and nonoperative protocols for treatment of injuries to the lateral ligament of the ankle. It was found that ankle stability depends primarily on the integrity of the anterior talofibular ligament. When the fore-and-aft stress measurement exceeds 4 mm, a positive anterior drawer test is elicited, and the ankle ligaments require surgical repair. Normal tibial talar tilt values range up to 18 degrees, but one ankle should not vary too much in tilt from the other.

Compression bandaging and crutches are used if swelling is minimal and the fore-and-aft shift is less than 3 mm. Where avulsion is suspected, an ambulatory short cast is used for 4 weeks. A small number of casted patients have later been operated on.

Repair (early and late) is carried out by suturing what is found (there is always some ligament present) and reinforcing the anterior talofibular ligament repair by overlapping the nearby lateral talocalcaneal ligament plus the marginal ankle retinaculum. After 4 weeks in a plaster walking cast, the patient uses Ace bandages for 2 weeks. Light activity is begun 6 weeks after surgery, with normal activity at 8 weeks. Stress testing is repeated 3 months postoperatively.

This surgery has been performed in about 165 patients in the past 19 years. Fifty patients were reevaluated at least a year after surgery. The average time from initial injury to late repair was 2–3

(4–122) Foot Ankle 1:84–89, September 1980.

years. At follow-up, 47 of the 50 patients were engaging in some athletic activity. All patients felt that the operation had improved the ankle, and none complained of instability. In all cases the fore-and-aft shift was reduced to 2 mm or less, and in 32 cases there was no shift. Tibiotalar tilt was reduced to less than 12 degrees in all cases and to less than 6 degrees in most. One patient required neurolysis for compression of the anterior branch of the sural nerve. No infections occurred. Four patients were seen in the subsequent year with mild sprains from new trauma; all recovered within a few days.

This repair method, used early or late after ankle injury, appears to be adequate. There is no need for more radical surgery involving other muscles.

4–123 **The Role of Flexible Carbon-Fiber Implants as Tendon and Ligament Substitutes in Clinical Practice: A Preliminary Report.** Experimental work indicates that implants of flexible carbon fiber may develop into satisfactory substitutes for tendons and ligaments. The material acts to induce formation of a living substitute for the original structure. In contrast to simple prosthetic replacements, the implant can adapt physiologically and grows stronger with age. Long-term animal studies have shown no late adverse tissue reactions. D. H. R. Jenkins and B. McKibbin (Cardiff Royal Infirm., Cardiff, Wales) studied flexible carbon fiber implants in 102 patients aged 14–86 years in the past 3 years and have followed 60 patients for 1 year or longer. Only patients with substantial disability were treated. Thirty-six patients were reexamined by one of these authors. Generally one continuous strand of material was used and was passed through drill holes made through very limited incisions. Repairs were protected by a plaster cast for 5–6 weeks.

Most repairs involve the knee and ankle, and most repairs of collateral ligaments of the knee were successful. Loss of 10–20 degrees of flexion was usual in successful cases. Similar results were obtained in cruciate and combined ligament repairs. Some patients reported vague discomfort within the knee. Ankle repairs were particularly successful; all provided complete restoration of stability. Subtalar movements were not compromised. There were surprisingly few complications. Two patients with late wound breakdown at the ankle and sinus formation required removal of the implant; in both cases the implant was very close to the surface. No mechanical implant failures were observed. There was no evidence of node enlargement, although work in sheep indicated that carbon fragments can be found in the regional lymph nodes a year or more after implantation.

At present the use of carbon fiber implants should be confined to severe cases of disabling instability where possible residual symptoms are more acceptable in light of a great improvement in stability. Late mechanical failure of these implants has not been a problem, and the new ligament is likely to become stronger in time in response to functional stress.

(4–123) J. Bone Joint Surg. [Br.] 62-B:497–499, November 1980.

4-124 **Long-Term Treatment Results in Malleolar Fractures.** P. Joz-Roland, N. Kritsikis, and J.-M. Cyprien (Geneva) reviewed 116 malleolar fractures after an average follow-up of 8 years, in an effort to ascertain what factors may possibly influence the quality of results.

Most often used for surgical treatment (93 cases) was metallic fixation of the syndesmosis with two parallel Kirschner wires, transfixation at an angle of about 60 degrees and injected into the internal cortex of the tibia. The wires, while allowing good fixation, have the advantage over transverse tibiofibular screws because of greater flexibility and the fact that they may be removed at the same time as the rest of the material. Orthopedic treatment (23 cases) followed Böhler's (1943–1957) principles, consisting of reduction followed by immobilization for 4–12 weeks. Results were similar for both types of treatment: 51% good, 29% satisfactory, 20% poor. In 31%, reduction was not complete (28% after surgical treatment); 37% had posttraumatic arthrosis (34% after surgery). The latter was particularly apt to occur in poorly reduced fractures, but was generally well tolerated. The severity of fractures situated at a high level in the fibula (type C of Weber) is stressed.

Of primary importance for good results is perfect restoration of articular anatomy. Surgical treatment is indicated in most cases, since it alone allows repair of the entire osteoligamentous damage. Conservative treatment should be reserved for the rare fracture without displacement, for elderly patients with marked osteoporosis or restricted motor function, and for inoperable fractures based on local or general contraindications.

4-125 **Treatment of Acute and Chronic Luxations of the Peroneal Tendons.** Dislocation of the peroneal tendon from the retromalleolar groove is more prevalent than previously thought. Such injuries are seen in various sports, particularly skiing, soccer, and ice skating, and most are caused by sudden forceful and passive dorsiflexion of the inverted foot with contraction of the peroneal muscles. Occasionally, x-ray films may show an avulsion fracture of the rim or lateral ridge of the lateral malleolus. Jon G. McLennan (Northern Inyo Hosp., Bishop, Calif.) reviewed data on 16 patients seen in 1974–1977 with dislocating or subluxing peroneal tendons in 19 ankles. All but 2 injuries were a result of trauma. Five patients had acute injuries. Half the patients with chronic injuries were seen within 1 month of injury; the others were first seen up to 2 years after initial injury. Fourteen of the patients were younger than age 30 years.

Most patients were taped with crescent-shaped pads. All but 2 ambulated on crutches for the first 3 weeks. Good to excellent results were obtained in 14 of 16 patients. Seven had surgery. The modified Kelly method was used in 3 cases of chronically dislocating peroneal tendons. Two patients had open reduction and internal fixation of avulsion fractures of the lateral malleolar ridge. One patient had osteoperiosteal flap reconstruction and one had primary repair of the

(4–124) Rev. Chir. Orthop. 66:173–182, May, 1980. (Fre.)
(4–125) Am. J. Sports Med. 8:432–436, Nov.–Dec. 1980.

superior peroneal retinaculum. All operative procedures gave good to excellent results. Three patients treated nonoperatively had evidence of resubluxation, but the functional outcome was good to excellent, with little if any disability. No resubluxation was noted in patients treated surgically. One patient required secondary surgery for loose bodies in the ankle joint from another injury.

Conservative treatment of subluxation or dislocation of the peroneal tendons gives satisfactory results in most cases. Surgery is indicated in athletically active patients who have acute injuries of the peroneal tendons, especially if a rim fracture is present. Resubluxation of these tendons is minimally disabling, but surgical reconstruction is necessary if instability occurs, particularly in the athlete.

5. Pediatric Sports Medicine

5–1 **Physiologic Problems Associated With the "Making of Weight"** in scholastic wrestling are discussed by Charles M. Tipton (Iowa City, Ia.). Specific weight classes have been established for scholastic wrestling. Athletes who lose the most weight to be certified are the youngest. Most lose the majority of weight in a short time by water loss and compete in a dehydrated state. Most wrestlers believe that they can "make weight" for a lower weight class with no loss in performance capacity. The more successful wrestlers appear to lose 9% to 15% of their preseason body weight to compete in a specific weight class. They dehydrate by exercising in rubber suits or by sitting in a sauna or whirlpool. Some have used laxatives and diuretics to make weight, and induced vomiting has also been used. Food deprivation has been observed, resulting in decreased muscle strength and endurance and lower maximal oxygen consumption. Renal ischemia is a possibility.

One immediate solution would be acceptance of a minimum body weight that contains 5% fat. Subjects with a fat content below 5% of certified body weight several weeks before the competitive season should receive medical clearance before being allowed to compete. A balanced diet should be encouraged for wrestlers. Fluid deprivation and dehydration should be discouraged. Coaches and wrestlers could be educated in the physiologic consequences and medical complications that can result from these practices. Regulations might be standardized so that wrestlers may only participate in those weight classes in which they had the highest frequencies of matches throughout the season. Data should be collected on the hydration state of wrestlers and its relation to growth and development. More knowledge is needed about the acute or chronic effects of fluid and food restriction practices on growing persons.

▶ [There are few sports that cause as many health problems as scholastic wrestling. Some of the reasons are enumerated in the summary. The medical profession and the coaching fraternity are not unaware of these problems. Yet, the situation is not likely to change, for simple reasons of peer pressure, coaching incentive, and the fact that in this sport, as much as most, the premium for winning is considered higher than that of graceful participation.—L.J.K.] ◀

5–2 **The Uniqueness of the Young Athlete: Medical Considerations.** William B. Strong (Med. College of Georgia, Augusta) reviewed the literature (21 references) in a discussion of various acute and chronic illnesses that can affect a youth's participation in sports. Acute conditions discussed include fever, respiratory tract infections,

(5–1)   Am. J. Sports Med. 8:449–450, Nov.–Dec. 1980.
(5–2)   Ibid. 8:372–376, Sept.–Oct. 1980.

infectious mononucleosis, and dermatoses caused by viral agents, bacteria, fungi, parasites, and trauma. The chronic diseases reviewed were epilepsy, diabetes mellitus, asthma and other respiratory difficulties, and cardiovascular abnormalities. The cardiac evaluation of the sports participant with regard to heart murmurs, hypertension, or arrhythmias is outlined in detail. It is recommended that when a disease contraindicates strenuous contact sports, the individual should be tailored to a less demanding sport.

▶ [This is a good summary article of the problem of surveying the health difficulties of the young. It is particularly good in its description of the cardiac workup. However, I think a much overlooked area of health screening in the young athlete, particularly now that increasing numbers of girls are participating in sports, is the simple test of a hemoglobin count, which is usually omitted in the sports physical examination. The presence of anemia in 40% of an adolescent female population is very real, and it is very easily corrected when due to the usual cause of iron deficiency.—L.J.K.] ◀

5–3 **Cardiologic Assessment in Participants of Pop Warner Junior League Football.** To determine the cardiovascular and ECG variations that might occur in the young, untrained athlete, Grace S. Wolff, Matthew Farina, and Robert Rinaldi (Albany Med. Center Hosp., Albany, N.Y.) performed physical examinations and ECG studies on 50 boys, aged 9.8–15 years (mean, 12.3 years), who were engaged in preseason training for a junior football league. One boy was excluded because of mild pulmonic stenosis.

The remaining 48 boys were 130–173 cm tall (mean, 152 cm), weighed 29–60 kg (mean, 43 kg), and had systolic blood pressure readings of 90–130 mm Hg (mean, 113 mm Hg) and diastolic pressure readings of 40–80 mm Hg (mean, 67 mm Hg). None of the boys had cardiac pathology, but 52% had a functional cardiac murmur best heard at the second left interspace. It initiated after the first heart sound and terminated before the second and was of grade 2/6 or less in intensity. Such a murmur should not be a deterrent to participation in competitive sports.

Bradycardia, a recognized adaptation to physical training that reflects a state of physical fitness in the athlete, was found in only 8% of the boys. When compared to ECGs of sedentary persons, those of athletes may show right ventricular hypertrophy, left ventricular hypertrophy, myocardial repolarization changes, and conduction disturbances, but these findings are not pathologic, and few were present in the 48 boys. However, the incidence of rsr' pattern was 13%, which exceeds that in reported normal series for this age group, and 25% of the boys had slurring of the S wave in V_1. The higher incidences of these two findings may reflect some degree of physical training. They should be considered normal variants.

Most participants in junior football leagues are untrained athletes and exhibit clinical and ECG findings not unlike those of sedentary persons. However, some are better trained, and they present findings known to occur in trained athletes.

▶ [The point made is that there will be a group of young athletes who present with the cardiac and ECG abnormalities that are seen in older athletes. This group should not be judged by the standards for sedentary persons; there should be an awareness that occasional evidence for right ventricular hypertrophy, left ventricular hypertrophy, repolarization changes, and conduction disturbances may exist but may not necessarily reflect pathology. For example, the right ventricular hypertrophy pattern in 69% of professional basketball players, the left ventricular hypertrophy pattern in 26%, and the abnormal T waves seen in 30% may have a reflection in the screening of younger athletes as well.—L.J.K.] ◄

5–4 **Two Years' Follow-up of Asthmatic Boys Participating in Physical Activity Program.** Many children with asthma are limited in physical activities through fear of the development of exercise-induced asthma. Physical inactivity in adolescence can lead to reduced work capacity and ultimately to social isolation and a loss of self-confidence. V. Graff-Lonnevig, S. Bevegård, B. O. Eriksson, S. Kraepelien, and B. Saltin (Stockholm) evaluated various activities that permit asthmatic children to participate safely in physical education at school and in sports activities outside of school. Eleven boys with asthma participated in a training program for 20 months; 9 others formed a nontraining group. The study group had a mean age of 11.2 years at the start of the study. Most had severe asthma, experiencing over 10 attacks a year. Four were taking long-term hormone therapy. Training was performed in a gymnasium for 1 hour twice a week. Ability in cross-country skiing was evaluated at a winter camp after 5 months of training.

The 2 boys who experienced exercise-induced asthma more often than the others trained the most. When present, these attacks nearly always subsided within 5–10 minutes without medical treatment. Inhalation of β_2-receptor stimulators was necessary only occasionally. Team games (e.g., basketball and soccer) were the most common causes of exercise-induced asthma. Cardiorespiratory function increased with maximal exercise, and both groups adapted well to heavy physical work. Total ventilation capacity rose substantially more in the trained group. The maximal work load rose 39% in this group and 29% in the nontrained group. Lowering of the forced expiratory volume in 1 second was observed after exercise in a ski race. Boys having more severe asthma had the most marked reductions in expiratory flow after exercise.

Asthmatic boys can participate in a physical training program similar to the physical education offered at school without premedication if minor modifications are made. The use of cromolyn or sympathomimetic agents before training sessions permits the children to participate more fully in activities without experiencing the development of exercise-induced asthma. Premedication is necessary if work capacity and aerobic power are to be increased.

► [The sense of this study is fairly straightforward to me. Separating an asthmatic group into a training group and a control group seems to make very little difference in terms of the appropriate parameters of function. Nevertheless, the asthmatic group with the appropriate concern of exercise-induced asthma, can be protected by the use of cromolyn sodium as premedication so that the usual physical activities of nonasthmatics are not contraindicated.—L.J.K.] ◄

(5–4) Acta Paediatr. Scand. 69:347–352, May 1980.

5-5 **Baseball Elbow.** A field survey for the Little Leaguer's elbow was performed by Akira Kuge. The study comprised 1,486 children who belonged to Little League baseball. The method of the survey consisted of the following items: (1) a questionnaire about the constitution, age at the start of play, fielding position, pitching style, duration of playing, and clinical symptoms; (2) function of the elbow joints in 398 players; and (3) the radiologic examination in 260 players (players who had any sign or symptom and pitchers and catchers).

Overall, pain in the elbow joints was present in 44.1% of the players. The frequency was noted in the pitchers. Restrictions of flexion and extension in the elbow joint of the arm used in playing were noticed in 45.6% and 56.5%, respectively. The increased and decreased carrying angles of the joint were observed with equal frequency, 34.6% and 34.7%, respectively.

Abnormal radiographic findings were noticed in 60.0% of the children. The segmentation and separation of the medial epicondyle, the most characteristic findings in the Little League elbow, were found in 45.0%. These findings were mostly noted in players with a slender constitution, pitchers, and players who started at an earlier age. It was noteworthy that aseptic necrosis of the capitulum of the humerus was found in 4.6%.

In conclusion, symptoms in Little Leaguer's elbow seemed to be affected by various factors such as age at the start of play, duration of playing, fielding position, and constitution of the players.—Hiroyuki Nakajima

5-6 **The Relative Merits of Cromolyn Sodium and High-Dose Theophylline Therapy in Childhood Asthma** are discussed by S. Godfrey (Hadassah Univ., Jerusalem). High-dose theophylline is preferred for the management of chronic childhood asthma in the United States, whereas sodium is preferred in Europe. Differences in the types of patients treated can produce conflicting results. Both treatments appear to be most appropriate for children who have symptoms on most days which are not controlled by sympathomimetic agents. Cromolyn sodium appears to act by stabilizing mast cell membranes and possibly the membranes of other cells with mediators capable of evoking bronchoconstriction. Theophylline and its derivatives have bronchodilator effects. Recently, there has been interest in giving cromolyn sodium to younger children by means of nebulization. Studies have failed to confirm a carryover effect of cromolyn sodium (Fig 5-1). The half-life of theophylline is shorter in children than in adults and considerably longer in newborn infants; great individual variation is seen in response to its use. Results with slow-release formulations have been encouraging.

Short-term studies indicate that both cromolyn sodium and high-dose theophylline can control the symptoms of chronic perennial childhood asthma. However, neither drug permits cessation of steroid therapy in truly steroid-dependent asthmatics. Cromolyn sodium

(5–5) Orthop. Traum. Surg. 23:1609–1615, 1980. (Jpn.)

(5–6) J. Allergy Clin. Immunol. 65:97–104, February 1980.

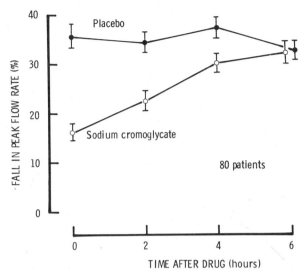

Fig 5–1.—Rate of loss of protection against exercise-induced asthma by cromolyn sodium in 80 patients. Postexercise fall in peak flow rate remained relatively constant after placebo. The reduction in this decrease after cromolyn administration wore off steadily over 6 hours. (Courtesy of Godfrey, S.: J. Allergy Clin. Immunol. 65:97–104, February 1980. From Anderson, S.D., et al.: Br. J. Dis. Chest 69:1, 1975.)

should be used shortly before planned exercise or sport. No formal studies of the long-term effects of theophylline are available. One third of children taking long-term cromolyn sodium treatment have been able to stop using the drug. Adverse effects from cromolyn sodium are uncommon, but some young children cannot use the Spinhaler adequately or regularly. The common side effects of theophylline are rare when blood levels of 10–20 μg/ml are maintained. Cromolyn sodium is more expensive than theophylline. Oral theophylline is preferable for younger children because of its simplicity of administration. Older children may be given cromolyn sodium because of its freedom from side effects and the lack of a need to monitor blood levels. With either agent, close follow-up is essential to insure that treatment remains necessary and effective.

▶ [It seems that either high-dose theophylline or cromolyn sodium is capable of controlling a large percentage of children with chronic perennial asthma. Theophylline is preferable for younger children because of the simplicity of administration, whereas the freedom from side effects and the need to monitor theophylline blood levels would make cromolyn sodium preferable for older children. Steroids are necessary for children when theophylline and cromolyn sodium are not effective, and neither of these drugs seems to have much impact on the group that requires steroids. Both of these drugs appear reasonably safe, and their use should be encouraged if they permit relatively normal function.—L.J.K.] ◀

5–7 **Oral and Inhaled Salbutamol in the Prevention of Exercise-Induced Bronchospasm.** Paul W. J. Francis, Inese R. B. Krastins, and Henry Levison (Hosp. for Sick Children, Toronto) compared the

(5–7) Pediatrics 66:103–108, July 1980.

effectiveness of oral salbutamol (0.15 mg/kg of body weight) and salbutamol aerosol (0.2 mg, total dose) in promoting bronchodilation and in preventing exercise-induced bronchospasm (EIB) in a single-blind crossover study of 16 asthmatic children. The 10 boys and 6 girls had a mean age of 12 years. The subjects exercised on a standardized treadmill 40 minutes after administration of the aerosol and 120 minutes after taking the oral preparation. Pulmonary function was assessed by measurement of peak expiratory flow (PEF), forced vital capacity (FVC), forced expiratory volume in 1 second (FEV_1), forced expiratory flow during the middle half of the FVC ($FEF_{25\%-75\%}$), and maximum expiratory flow after 75% of the FVC had been expired ($\dot{V}_{25}$).

Based on changes in all variables of pulmonary function, oral salbutamol and salbutamol aerosol were equally effective in promoting bronchodilation. Changes in PEF and FEV_1 indicated that both forms of treatment were equally effective in preventing EIB after treadmill exercising. However, based on postexercise changes in $FEF_{25\%-75\%}$ and $\dot{V}_{25}$, the aerosol was slightly, but significantly, more effective than oral salbutamol in preventing EIB. Oral salbutamol was clinically effective in preventing EIB for 4.9 hours with respect to changes in FEV_1 and for 5.8 hours as reflected by changes in PEF.

The results show that salbutamol aerosol has a faster onset of action, fewer side effects, and offers greater protection against EIB with respect to small airways function. However, oral salbutamol is a useful substitute for patients who are unable to use a metered aerosol.

▶ [The comparison of oral vs. aerosol salbutamol is made in a single-blind crossover study. The aerosol route has the advantage of faster onset of action, fewer side effects and apparently greater protection against exercise-induced bronchospasm with respect to small airway function. The oral preparation is a reasonable alternative, but only for those who cannot use a metered aerosol. I think the preference is clear.—L.J.K.] ◀

5-8 **Total Daily Energy Expenditure of Healthy, Free-Ranging Schoolchildren.** Daily energy expenditure is difficult to measure, particularly in children. D. W. Spady (Univ. of Alberta) estimated the energy expenditure of a group of healthy schoolchildren living and playing under the normal conditions of a home and school environment. Twenty-two boys and 15 girls aged 7.9 to 11.6 years were studied. Heart rates were measured with a counter worn on the subject's belt and oxygen consumption by an open circuit technique with an oxygen analyzer during treadmill exercise. The heart rate counter was worn for 48 hours during usual daily activities, excluding those such as gymnastics, in which a fall might lead to injury from the instrument.

Maintenance energy expenditure (MEE) was estimated from the resting energy expenditure and basal metabolic rate (BMR). Total daily energy expenditure (TDEE) was estimated from the estimated energy expenditure while awake (EEA) and the BMR. The difference between the TDEE and the MEE represented energy for activity

(5–8) Am. J. Clin. Nutr. 33:766–775, April 1980.

(EAc). The mean TDEE for boys was 2,164 kcal and that for girls, 1,716 kcal. The respective mean MEE values were 1,503 and 1,263 kcal per day. The mean EAc for boys was 673 kcal per day and that for girls, 434 kcal per day. All the differences were significant and, except for EAc, remained significant when expressed in terms of lean body mass.

The estimates of MEE in this study were close to theoretical estimates for MEE of 105 kcal/kg. The lower TDEE in girls suggests that their recommended dietary allowance for energy should be less than that for boys and less than that presently recommended.

▶ [The data collected serve as a benchmark, of sorts, for possible dietary consideration. I think it is important not to accept these data without reservation for at least two reasons: The sample of 22 boys and 15 girls is a very small one on which to make far-ranging conclusions, and there might be a very significant differential if the factors of endomorphy, mesomorphy, and ectomorphy were considered in the population group. One could go further and say that there might be an extremely critical change in the pubertal years. A final question might be whether there were racial differences as well. I find the total caloric expenditure surprisingly low.—L.J.K.] ◀

5–9 **Cardiac and Respiratory Responses to Exercise in Adolescent Idiopathic Scoliosis.** J. M. Shneerson (Bromptom Hosp., London) used lung function tests and a standardized progressive exercise test with a bicycle ergometer in a study of 20 consecutive girls, aged 11–15 years (mean, 13.7 years), with adolescent idiopathic scoliosis requiring spinal fusion. None had any cardiac or respiratory disease.

Resting lung function tests showed reduced peak flow rates, lung volumes, and maximum voluntary ventilation. Maximum oxygen uptake was slightly reduced, but maximum exercise ventilation was normal. The latter was achieved by the use of a greater than normal fraction of the vital capacity in tidal breathing while exercising. Mild hyperventilation during submaximal exercise and a trend toward exercise tachycardia with increasing body weight were also observed.

▶ [These scoliotic adolescent girls, studied within a few years of onset of their deformity, have acquired the same type of restrictive ventilatory defect and pattern of breathing during exercise as adults with scoliosis. Their maximum oxygen uptake is slightly diminished, but much less so than in adults with scoliosis. Their maximum exercise ventilation is still normal, and none had any symptoms of limitation of exercise tolerance. A longitudinal study would be required to determine at what later stage in their development the full picture of the abnormalities of the adult with scoliosis would develop.—L.J.K.] ◀

(5–9) Thorax 35:347–350, May 1980.

6. Women In Sports

6-1 **Differences in Attitude Toward the Concepts "Male," "Female," "Male Athlete," and "Female Athlete."** Traditionally, the masculine role has been identified as large, strong, self-reliant, outgoing, independent, assertive, and active, whereas the feminine role has been characterized as small, weak, passive, dependent, understanding, moderate, sincere, and accepting of others. When sport and physical activity are considered in light of sex role expectations, "masculine" characteristics are used to describe appropriate athletic behavior. There is evidence that sex role patterns are changing in our society, but it is not clear whether there is acceptance of a wider sex role model that encourages athletic participation by women. Joan Vickers, Michael Lashuk, and Terry Taerum (Univ. of Calgary) examined the attitudes of 264 seventh-and tenth-grade and university students of both sexes toward these concepts, using a semantic differential technique. The test, developed by Osgood et al., measures the meaning of concepts and consists of the concepts, adjective pairs, and semantic space or scalar positions.

Factor analysis of variance, with repeated measures over the four concepts of the evaluative dimension, indicated that the subjects were more positive in attitude toward those concepts identified as athletic and female. Multifactor analysis of variance indicated a hierarchy of approval that placed the concept of the female athlete in the most favored position, followed by female, male athlete, and male. The interaction of these concepts in influencing attitudes is shown in Figure 6-1. Post hoc analysis showed significant differences between all concepts, except for female athlete-female and female-male athlete. Perceptions of activity-potency established the male athlete as most active-potent, followed by male, female athlete, and female.

Both male and female subjects in this study were more positive in attitude toward concepts identified as female and athletic. Precedence of the concept of the female athlete over that of the male athlete may have resulted from increased participation by female athletes in sports activities in the past decade. Their emergence has not yet been accompanied by substantial instances of public criticism or disrepute, as has often been the case with males' involvement in sports. Findings in the activity-potency dimension were in contrast to those in the evaluative dimension, reflecting societal expectations and readily observable biologic realities.

▶ [It should not be surprising to any of us who have been involved with children in the United States that a hierarchy of approval would place "male athlete" above "male"

(6–1) Res. Q. Exerc. Sport 51:407–416, May 1980.

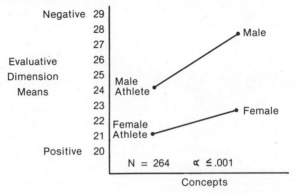

Fig 6–1.—Multifactor analysis of variance (evaluative dimension). Effect due to interaction of concept of sex and concept of athlete. (Courtesy of Vickers, J., et al.: Res. Q. Exerc. Sport 51:407–416, 1980.)

and "female athlete" above "female." However, the results of this study surprised me when the same hierarchy listed both "female athlete" and "female" in more favored positions than "male athlete" and "male." I wonder whether this is a result of increased participation in sports by women over the past decade, as suggested by the authors of the study, or whether that positive approval has always been there but has been misunderstood. My intuitive judgment is that it has always been there, at least for most, if not all, sports. The bad publicity that male athletes at all levels have received over the past decade has, no doubt, not been helpful—J.L.A.] ◀

6–2 **Women on Annapurna.** Piro Kramar and Barbara L. Drinkwater report observations on women who climbed Annapurna, the tenth highest mountain in the world, in 1978, after at least 18 months of intense preparation. Eight team members were evaluated to prescribe training programs. All were experienced mountaineers, and they all were capable of performing maximal exercise at sea level and also at a simulated altitude of 14,000 ft. None of the changes usually associated with aging, such as an increase in percent body fat, was noted. The highest aerobic power values were in women in their 40s. The average reduction in maximal aerobic power at a simulated 14,100 ft was 26.8%. The heart rate and ventilatory volumes followed patterns observed for men at altitude. Strength characteristics are given in the table.

General health was good during a 12-day, 80-mile hike to the base camp. One subject experienced pneumonitis and pleurisy while at 14,000 ft. Climbers gained in strength up to 18,200 ft, but easy fatigue was noted at 20,000 ft, and mild headaches occurred. Diamox was used after base camp, but was associated with severe calf and foot cramps. Subjects who did not take Diamox had no particular trouble sleeping. Prepresbyopic subjects had problems with accommodation and reading at altitude. An episode of frostbite of a finger occurred during presummit preparations. The first summit attempt succeeded, but a second attempt resulted in 2 deaths. At least 1 en-

(6–2) Physician Sportsmed. 8:93–99, March 1980.

STRENGTH CHARACTERISTICS OF FEMALE CLIMBERS

VARIABLE	CLIMBERS	NORM
Handgrip (kg)		
Right	40.9 ± 1.8	—
Left	37.9 ± 1.0	—
Both	78.8 ± 1.5	63.3*
Grip Endurance (sec at 30% maximum voluntary contraction)		
Right	233.1 ± 41.1	230.1† (preferred
Left	230.1 ± 20.1	hand
Bent-Arm Hang (sec)	58.0 ± 12.7	25.5‡
Wall Sit (sec)	103.1 ± 12.0	NA§
Harvard Step Test With pack + 30% of body weight (sec)	109 ± 24	NA

*Means.
†College-age women.
‡U.S. Service Academy women.
§Norms not available.

teric infection occurred on the trek out, but generally health remained good. The surviving climbers experienced an acute sense of displacement, feelings of unreality, and depression in the months at home after the expedition, but none has stopped climbing.

▶ [This is an interesting report on a group of women climbers who made an historic assault on Annapurna. It would be interesting to know the measures of their aerobic power after their training programs—both as a gauge of the effectiveness of the programs and as part of the historic record of their remarkable feat. I have noticed that although the preconditioning aerobic power values are significantly higher than age-group norms, the mean value for the eight climbers was about equal to the mean of a typical class of young women when they arrive at West Point to begin their freshman year. Not terribly remarkable.—J.L.A.] ◀

6–3 **Effects of Endurance Training on Thermoregulation in Females.** Many studies have shown lower sweat rates and greater rises in core temperature on heat exposure in women than in man, but some recent studies have found that fit women can achieve work tasks as well as men in hot environments with lower body temperatures. Yoshio Kobayashi, Yoshiro Ando, Noriaki Okuda, Shozo Takaba, and Kokichi Ohara (Nagoya, Japan) compared the thermal and cardiovascular responses of physically trained women with those of nonathletic men and women during rest in a hot environment. Eleven women athletes, 8 nonathletic women, and 8 nonathletic men, all university students, were studied. The study subjects had participated in endurance-type sports for many years, usually for 2 hours a day. Subjects were placed in a climatic chamber at 32 C with the lower legs immersed in water at 42 C for 2 hours.

The female athletes had higher sweat rates than the control women but lower rates than the male subjects. The core temperature thresh-

(6–3) Med. Sci. Sports 12:361–364, 1980.

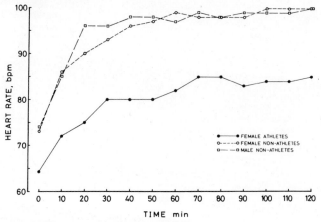

Fig 6–2.—Means of heart rates of three groups during two hours of rest in heat. (Courtesy of Kobayashi, Y., et al.: Med. Sci. Sports 12:361–364, 1980; copyright 1980, the American College of Sports Medicine. Reprinted by permission.)

old for sweating was significantly lower in the women athletes than in the two control groups. The slope of the sweat rate-core temperature curve of the female athletes was nearly parallel to that of the female nonathletes. The slope for male subjects was significantly steeper. Total sweat loss was greatest for the men and least for the female nonathletes. Heart rate changes are shown in Figure 6–2.

Differences in thermoregulation between athletic and nonathletic women were found. The athletes had lower core temperature thresholds for sweating during resting exposure to heat. The view that female thermoregulatory mechanisms are inferior to those of men may be contested by correcting for differences in body size and metabolic rate. Women who are physically trained for a long period become more adapted to heat than untreated women, and even untrained men with their increased sweat rate and lower threshold core temperature for sweating.

▶ [This adds something to the understanding of physiologic differences between men and women. It is too bad that a group of trained male athletes were not included in the study.—J.L.A.] ◀

6–4 **Relative Endurance of High- and Low-Strength Women.** Static strength of men appears to be inversely related to relative endurance time, and it has been suggested that the relative endurance ability of men varies with muscle strength because of morphological and physiologic changes associated with muscle hypertrophy and strength training. Vivian Heyward (Univ. of New Mexico, Albuquerque) analyzed the relative endurance ability of women in terms of muscle mass, static muscle strength, and critical occluding tension level (COTL). Studies were done in 56 women physical education majors, 28 in a high-strength and 28 in a low-strength group. One fourth of

(6–4) Res. Q. Exerc. Sport 51:486–493, October 1980.

the subjects in each group were assigned to relative endurance testing at 30%, 45%, 60%, and 75% maximal tension, with the local circulation to the forearm muscles intact and occluded by a pressure cuff.

No significant difference in endurance times was found between the high- and low-strength women. The relation between grip strength and relative endurance time was insignificant at each tension level. The COTL was the same for high- and low-strength women.

Strength training does not result in substantial gains in muscle mass in women, and the problem of a reduction in capillary-to-fiber size ratio associated with hypertrophy would be relatively insignificant for high-strength women. Since high- and low-strength women perform with the same degree of circulatory impairment in relative endurance tests, their endurance times should not differ significantly. In contrast to men, the relative endurance of women does not vary as a function of strength. This may be explained in part by the relatively small difference in muscle mass between high- and low-strength women and their similarities in COTL.

▶ [Muscle mass and strength are legitimate physiologic differences between men and women, so the findings of this study should not come as a surprise to us.—J.L.A.] ◀

6–5 **Relationships Between Selected Blood Indices and Competitive Performance in College Women Cross-Country Runners.** Lower maximal oxygen consumption and relatively poorer performances of female participants in endurance events may be attributed in part to a lower oxygen transport capacity. This in turn may be limited by the red blood cell number and hemoglobin concentration, both normally lower in women then in men. Further, iron deficiency anemia is more frequent in women after menarche. The ability of dietary iron supplementation to increase hemoglobin concentrations above individual norms is debatable. William S. Runyan and Jacqueline Puhl (Iowa State Univ.) examined the possible relationship between oxygen transport-related blood indices and competitive performance in 14 highly-trained young women runners.

The runners had normal mean hematologic values, but the ranges were wide and, except for hematocrit, exceeded normal ranges. The mean hemoglobin concentration was above the mean normal value. Red blood cell indices were also above mean normal values. None of the hematologic indices correlated significantly with performance in a cross-country championship race. When the subjects were divided into two groups on the basis of performance in the race, no significant differences in any of the blood indices were observed. A significant negative correlation was found between red blood cell count and red blood cell size, and this could explain the lack of relationship between hematocrit and red blood cell count or size.

The lack of relationship between competitive performance on cross-country running and hematologic indices in this study does not exclude such a relation in less well-trained or more heterogenous

(6–5)   J. Sports Med. 20:207–212, June 1980.

groups of subjects. Other factors influence oxygen delivery to the tissues. Studies are continuing on a possible relationship between maximal oxygen consumption and competitive performance.

▶ [The authors rightfully stated that the lack of relationship between actual competitive performance and hematologic indices in this study does not rule out the possibility that such a relationship might exist among groups of subjects who are less well trained or more heterogeneous. I feel certain that there are psychologic variables that are much more powerful in determining the outcome of an actual competitive performance. However, these individual athletes might have, and probably would have, performed better had the hematologic indices been at the optimum level—if we knew what the optimum level should be.—J.L.A.] ◀

6-6 **Hematologic Variations During Aerobic Training of College Women.** Decreased levels of some iron-related hematologic indices have been noted with training, but have not been established beyond doubt. Most of these studies have been done in men and have involved infrequent blood sampling during training. Jacqueline L. Puhl and William S. Runyan (Iowa State Univ.) followed hematologic changes in 19 healthy women aged 19–21 years who participated in a 9-week aerobic training program consisting of jogging 3 times a week at increasing distances, as well as some muscle strength muscle endurance, and flexibility exercises. The mean training heart rate was 173 beats per minute.

Significant positive changes in maximal aerobic power were noted with training. The relative maximal aerobic power increased 7.8%. The step-test heart rate decreased 11.3% after training. All blood variables except the mean corpuscular hemoglobin were significantly altered. There were significant decreasing quadratic trends for hemoglobin level, hematocrit reading, and red blood cell count and a significant cubic trend for mean corpuscular volume. All the parameters remained within normal ranges throughout the study, and tended to return to near pretraining levels by the end of the training program.

Although aerobic training of increasing intensity may be accompanied initially by decreases in hemoglobin level and red blood cell count and an increased mean corpuscular volume in young women, the changes are transient. If the changes result from red blood cell destruction rather than hemodilution, the return to hematopoietic balance could impose a draw on body iron stores. Additional draws on iron stores in persons with low iron reserves might be more deleterious than in those with adequate reserves.

▶ [Our findings at West Point Military Academy generally agree with these. I wonder what will happen when the training period lasts considerably longer than 9 weeks at an increased intensity level—similar to the program of some of our elite swimmers?— J.L.A.] ◀

6-7 **Effect of a Controlled Exercise Program on Serum Lipoprotein Levels in Women on Oral Contraceptives.** Oral contraceptives (OC) have been implicated in coronary heart disease and other cardiovascular diseases and are associated with elevated plasma tri-

(6–6) Res. Q. Exerc. Sport 51:533–541, October 1980.
(6–7) Metabolism 29:1267–1271, December 1980.

glyceride concentrations. Estrogen is directly and progestins are inversely related to both triglyceride and high-density lipoprotein cholesterol (C-HDL) values. Marathon runners have higher plasma C-HDL concentrations than do sedentary controls. Terrance P. Wynne, Mary Anne Bassett Frey, Lloyd L. Laubach, and Charles J. Glueck determined whether a regular exercise program could alter serum lipoprotein values among 19 women aged 19 to 30 years, who had taken an OC containing 50 μg of mestranol and 1 mg of norethisterone for at least 2 months. Thirteen participated in a 10-week bicycle exercise training program at an average of 70% of the maximum heart rate reserve. All subjects were nonsmokers and were free from cardiovascular disease.

Training produced significant changes in relative and absolute aerobic power and resting heart rate. No significant pretraining to posttraining changes in lipid or lipoprotein concentrations were found in either the trained or the control group. Plasma triglyceride values fell about 15% in the exercise group, but total cholesterol concentrations were essentially unchanged, as were those of the C-HDL and low-density lipoprotein fractions. Food habits were quite consistent during the study. Changes in aerobic power were weakly correlated with changes in triglyceride values.

Exercise training produced an increase in maximum oxygen uptake in this study of female OC users but no significant changes in plasma C-HDL or triglyceride concentrations. Changes in covariables associated with initiation of exercise programs may themselves be responsible for changes in C-HDL. These may include weight loss, cessation of smoking, and increased alcohol intake. Whether the duration of exercise is a determinant is unknown. The relative amounts of aerobic and anaerobic exercise may influence the findings in various studies. The present findings are consistent with preliminary evidence that exercise has more consistent and marked effects in men than in women.

▶ [It is strange that this study did not find any significant change in C-HDL. Maybe the exercise program was not intensive enough and did not last long enough. Whatever the reason, this is a fruitful area for further investigation. Maybe the study should be replicated using both men and women as subjects.—J.L.A.] ◀

6–8 **Cardiovascular, Metabolic, and Ventilatory Responses of Women to Equivalent Cycle Ergometer and Treadmill Exercise.** Different cardiovascular, respiratory, and metabolic responses have been observed in comparisons of exercise at the same metabolic rate on the cycle ergometer and on the treadmill. Daniel S. Miles, Jerry B. Critz, and Ronald G. Knowlton (Southern Illinois Univ.) compared the cardiovascular responses of 18 female subjects, aged 17 to 40 years, to cycling and treadmill exercise at levels approximating 30%, 60%, and 80% of maximal aerobic power capacity. The subjects were sedentary or moderately active; all were medically fit for exercise testing.

The mean maximal aerobic power was 1.93 L per minute maximal

(6–8) Med. Sci. Sports 12:14–19, Spring, 1980.

treadmill exercise and it was 1.78 L per minute on maximal cycle exercise. The mean difference in individual values was 7.8% greater for treadmill walking, but 5 subjects had greater values on cycle exercise. Maximal heart rates were significantly higher by 5 beats per minute on treadmill walking. Respiratory exchange ratios and lactate values were significantly higher on cycle exercise, but there were no differences in pulmonary ventilation. Lower stroke volume and higher heart rate were not observed on submaximal cycling compared with treadmill walking. At exercise intensities above 30% of maximal power, plasma bicarbonate and pH values were consistently lower after cycle exercise. Respiratory compensation was independent of the type of exercise, but it was linearly related to the resultant metabolic acidosis.

Cardiovascular responses to equivalent cycle ergometer and treadmill exercise are similar in women, but a greater metabolic acidosis is observed during cycle exercise, suggesting that a smaller muscle mass is used than in equivalent treadmill exercise. Contrary to previous findings in men, women do not exhibit a lower stroke volume or a higher heart rate during submaximal cycling than during treadmill walking.

▶ [We have seen enough now to make us realize that almost any research protocol that previously has been validated using men as subjects should be revalidated before assuming it will apply equally to women.—J.L.A.] ◀

6-9 **Effect of a Walking-Jogging Program on Personality Characteristics of Middle-Aged Females.** Some have suggested that middle-aged women participate in physical activity programs. Guy D. Penny and James O. Rust (Middle Tennessee State Univ.) examined the personalities of women aged 40 to 50 years before and just after a 15-week walking-jogging program to determine whether such exercise benefits women during the climacteric. The Minnesota Multiphasic Personality Inventory (MMPI) was used to assess the subjects' personalities. Fourteen women with an average age of 43.2 years in the exercise group were compared with 10 controls whose average age was 43.9. Exercise subjects met twice a week for 10 minutes of calisthenics, walking-jogging for $1^{1}/_{2}$ miles, and a cooling-down period of 10 minutes. Most subjects jogged the entire distance within 5 weeks.

Both groups showed significant improvement in self-confidence, acceptance, and contentment. No significant differences were found between the exercise and control groups, and none of the interactions reached significance. The sample in general appeared to be mentally alert and healthy.

Although a walking-jogging program significantly improves physiologic variables in middle-aged women, it does not necessarily lead to significant improvement in personality scales on the MMPI. This investigation emphasizes the importance of using a control group in studies of the effects of physical exercise on personality factors. If a control group had not been used in this study, gains in self-confidence and contentment might have been attributed to the walking-jogging program.

▶ [My major concern with this study is one I have with most psychologic studies, and that is the requirement to use volunteers as subjects. Regardless of the outcome of the study, it is impossible to tell whether the change or lack of change was a result of the experimental treatment or was due to the people who volunteered for the study being predisposed to react the way they did despite the treatment.—J.L.A.] ◀

6–10 **Fetal Heart Rate Response to Maternal Exercise Testing.** Dynamic muscular activity may cause fetal bradycardia or tachycardia, possibly through reduced uterine blood flow, and these observations have raised concern for the safety of the fetus during voluntary maternal exercise. However, well-trained pregnant women have remained active in sports without complications resulting, and women are becoming increasingly interested in maintaining fitness throughout pregnancy. Rudolph H. Dressendorfer and Robert C. Goodlin examined fetal heart rate responses to graded bicycle ergometer exercise in 5 healthy women aged 26–30 years to continued moderate endurance training during gestation. They swam laps for 30–45 minutes at least 3 times a week. All were gravida 1 with singleton pregnancies, and were in excellent health, with above-average cardiorespiratory fitness. Each subject was studied at least twice over 2 weeks at 32–39 weeks' gestation.

Fig 6–3.—Mean fetal *(triangles)* and maternal *(circles)* heart rates of 5 subjects and directly measured oxygen consumption at rest and at 4 submaximal cycling work loads (150, 300, 450, and 600 kg-m · minute^{-1}, respectively) performed in a semirecumbent position. Although maternal heart rate increased by 70 beats · minute^{-1} during exercise, baseline fetal heart rate increased by only 7 beats · minute^{-1}. (Courtesy of Dressendorfer, R. H., and Goodlin, R. C.: Physician Sportsmed. 8:91–94, November 1980.)

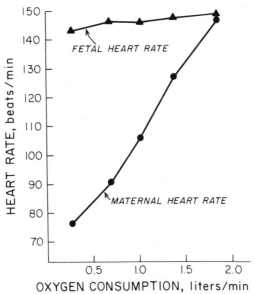

The resting maternal heart rate averaged 76 beats per minute and the blood pressure, 110/72 mm Hg. Oxygen consumption rose from 0.27 to 1.85 L/minute at a maternal heart rate of 146 beats per minute. The systolic blood pressure rose to 160 mm Hg at peak submaximal exercise. No abnormal maternal ECG changes were observed. The baseline fetal heart rate averaged 142 beats per minute and rose to 149 at peak exercise. The fetal heart rate rose much less than the maternal rate with increased aerobic energy production (Fig 6–3). Variability in fetal heart rate at rest and on exercise ranged from 5 to 20 beats per minute. Cyclic variability in fetal heart rate of 10–20 beats per minute was noted in all subjects.

These preliminary findings indicate that fetal heart responses to exercise by the healthy mother are within the normal range. Submaximal exercise stress testing could provide the obstetrician with guidance for approving regular exercise in trained women who wish to remain active in later pregnancy. However, further studies are necessary to determine the sensitivity and specificity of the maternal exercise test for identifying uteroplacental insufficiency.

▶ [It is good to see that this study confirms prior conclusions that exercise during pregnancy is not harmful to either the mother or the fetus. Although all is not yet known, these positive findings are helpful.—J.L.A.] ◀

6–11   **The Effects of Exercise on Pubertal Progression and Reproductive Function in Girls.** The initiation of menses now is thought to depend on attainment of a critical body weight and composition, especially body fat, and increasing interest by women in fitness and endurance sports has raised the possibility that a large energy drain may delay menarche and affect reproductive function. Michelle P. Warren (Columbia Univ.) examined this possibility in 15 ballet dancers ages 13–15 years who maintained a high level of physical activity from early adolescence and had follow-up for a mean of 4 years. Twenty music students aged 15–18 years who had similar goal-oriented life-styles and 20 women with secondary amenorrhea and a history of dieting and weight loss also were reviewed. The study subjects spent a mean maximum of 30 hours a week dancing at age 17 and older. Control subjects did not exercise for more than 5 hours a week, the mean being 3.2 hours.

Menarche was remarkably delayed in the young ballet dancers (Fig 6–4). It occurred at a mean age of 15.4 years, compared with 12.5 years for age-matched controls subjects and 12.4 years for the subjects with secondary amenorrhea and the music students. The dancers remained lighter than control subjects and had less body fat at all intervals. Some delay in height growth also was observed, but normal height was reached 1–2 years after the menarche. Weight gain declined rapidly after menarche in all groups. Breast development was associated with periods of relative inactivity in the study subjects. Eleven of the 13 dancers who reached menarche during the study developed amenorrhea lasting 6 months or longer. Suppression of lu-

(6–11)   J. Clin. Endocrinol. Metab. 51:1150, November 1980.

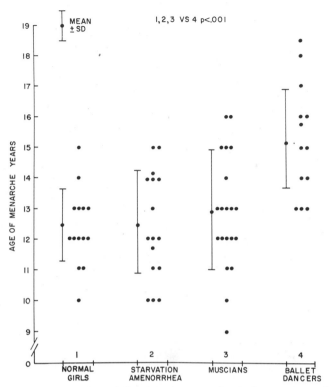

Fig 6–4.—Ages of menarche in ballet dancers compared with those in three other groups. (Courtesy of Warren, M. P.: J. Clin. Endocrinol. Metab. 51:1150, November 1980.)

teinizing hormone was more marked than that of follicle-stimulating hormone in the subjects who became amenorrheic.

An energy drain may have a significant modulating effect on the hypothalamic pituitary set point at puberty and, combined with low body fat, may prolong the prepubertal state and induce amenorrhea. This response may represent a natural form of reversible fertility control. It has been observed in some primitive cultures whose life-styles exhibit cyclic changes in nutrition, weight, and activity. Exercise may transiently affect the fertility of malnourished and underweight populations far more than has been realized.

▶ [It has been stated that the onset of menses appears to be occurring at an earlier age within our society now than 100 years ago. If heavy exercise delays the onset of menarche, could this evolutionary change be a result of the less physically demanding life-style of young women today? I doubt that percent body fat has a significant impact on secondary amenorrhea. At West Point, we have found no relationship between secondary amenorrhea and body weight or percent body fat. It appears that total stress, physical as well as psychologic, may be the cause of secondary amenorrhea among our freshman women.—J.L.A.] ◀

6–12 **Influence of Physical Exercise on Sex Hormone Metabolism.** Increased plasma estradiol concentrations have been reported in

(6–12) J. Appl. Physiol. 48:765–769, May 1980.

young, healthy women during bicycle ergometer exercise. H. A. Keizer, J. Poortman, and G. S. J. Bunnik (State Univ. of Utrecht) used a continuous infusion technique to determine the acute effects of submaximal exercise on the metabolic clearance rate (MCR) of estradiol (E_2) in 6 women with a mean age of 20.7 years, all of whom had regular menstrual cycles. Four subjects had never used oral contraceptives. Three subjects were fairly active physical education students, and 3 were highly trained middle- and long-distance runners. All subjects were in good health. The MCR of E_2 was determined 7 to 10 days after the start of menstruation. Exercise began about $2^1/_4$ hours after the priming dose of ^3H-E_2 at 70% of maximal oxygen uptake and was followed by a 30-minute recovery period at 25% of maximal oxygen uptake.

The mean baseline MCR of E_2 was 1,144 L/24 hours. A sharp, consistent decrease in MCR occurred during exercise at 70% of maximal oxygen uptake. The mean reduction at the end of the work load was 36%. The MCR tended to increase in some subjects during exercise at 25% of maximal oxygen uptake, whereas others showed a further reduction. The MCR remained below baseline in all subjects at the end of the study.

Even short-term physical exercise at a submaximal work load can cause a marked reduction in the MCR of E_2 in healthy young women. The underlying mechanism is unknown.

▶ [This excellent pilot study hopefully will stimulate additional research to answer the question on the underlying mechanism that explains why and how short-term submaximal physical exercise can induce a marked decrease in the metabolic clearance rate of estradiol in healthy young women.—J.L.A.] ◀

6-13 **Sports and Menstrual Function** are discussed by Mona M. Shangold (Albert Einstein College of Medicine, New York). Although the reported incidence of menstrual dysfunction is higher in athletes than in nonathletes, most reports do not include the subjects' pretraining menstrual patterns. Hypoestrogenic amenorrhea is the most common problem in amenorrheic athletes. It often occurs in women with low weight, low body fat, or both. Both hypogonadotropic and eugonadotropic hypoestrogenic athletes should be screened for hyperprolactinemia and pituitary tumor, and, when these are excluded, estrogen should be offered for its protective effects, with cyclic progesterone to guard the endometrium. Ovarian failure occurs in athletes as well as nonathletes, and athletes require equally thorough evaluation. Euestrogenic anovulation may be somewhat analogous to polycystic ovary syndrome. Affected athletes generally have normal weight and body fat. Clomiphene should be given for infertility and progesterone monthly for endometrial protection to women who do not desire immediate fertility.

Besides the apparent effects of estrogen and progesterone on performance, dysmenorrhea can adversely affect an athlete's ability to function. Many athletes, however, report less dysmenorrhea during inten-

(6–13) Physician Sportsmed. 8:66–70, August 1980.

sive training. Women with functional dysmenorrhea are best treated with prostaglandin inhibitors. Athletic women seem to be less incapacitated than sedentary women by pain. There is no reason to avoid athletic participation during menstruation. There is no evidence that running leads to prolapse.

No evidence suggests that exercise causes amenorrhea. A menstrual interval of 20 to 60 days probably requires no attention unless infertility is a problem. Medical attention is indicated if menstrual irregularity develops in association with increased training. Menstrual dysfunction in athletes should be evaluated as thoroughly as that in nonathletes; it is dangerous to assume that a problem is caused by strenuous exercise. The lengthening list of benefits of regular exercise justifies its encouragement.

▶ [Shangold has stated that the association, observed by other writers, between intensive training and later menarcheal age does not imply a causal relationship. She also states that there is no evidence that exercise causes amenorrhea. From my observations at West Point Military Academy, I am more in agreement than disagreement. I am convinced that psychologic stress plays a major role in the secondary amenorrhea that we find. The physical activity that the young women experience at West Point is not nearly so intense as that experienced by women training for a marathon.—J.L.A.] ◀

6–14 **Exercise and Menstrual Function.** There is growing awareness that women who compete in sports or participate in strenuous activities such as ballet and modern dance have a high rate of menstrual irregularity and amenorrhea. Leon Speroff and David B. Redwine (Univ. of Oregon) obtained questionnaire responses regarding menstrual function from 859 respondents. About 7% of respondents were pregnant and running, 3% were breast-feeding and running, and 14% had run during a pregnancy. Nearly half the subjects had never been pregnant. Of 115 women who had aborted or had a premature delivery, 18% had done so while they were running. Nearly 30% of the women were dieting. About 10% were taking birth control pills. The women reported having somewhat longer menstrual cycles after they started to run; most had cycle lengths of 28 to 30 days. A slight increase in menstrual irregularity and amenorrhea was apparent in women who had run for an extended period, but amenorrhea was not related to the number of miles run per week. Most women who became amenorrheic weighed less than 120 lb. Menstrual irregularity showed little correlation with weight loss except with losses of over 25 lb.

The chief factors in the development of menstrual irregularity and amenorrhea in this series were weight and weight loss. Young women who weigh less than 115 lb and who lose more than 10 lb after starting to run are most likely to develop menstrual irregularity and amenorrhea. One third of women who lost more than 10 lb while running developed secondary amenorrhea. There was no correlation with number of miles run, but only 18.6% of the respondents ran more than 20 miles a week. More needs to be known of the relations among exercise, menstrual function, fertility problems, and hormonal status

(6–14) Physician Sportsmed. 8:42–52, May 1980.

before physicians can properly advise amenorrheic hypoestrogenic women engaged in strenuous exercise.

▶ [Our experiences at West Point showed no relation between body weight or body composition and incidences of secondary amenorrhea. The mean percent body fat for those women who experienced secondary amenorrhea was 19.3%. This corresponds with the mean of the total population of women. There was also no evidence that those who experienced secondary amenorrhea the longest—20% for 12 months or longer—were the lightest women or those with the lowest percent body fat.—J.L.A.] ◀

6–15 **Delayed Menarche and Amenorrhea in Ballet Dancers.** Young female ballet dancers often restrict their food intake and are highly active. Amenorrhea and late menarche in females with average activity levels appear to be associated with undernutrition and weight loss on the order of 10% to 15% of normal weight for height. Such weight loss apparently reduces the fat-lean ratio to below a critical level. Rose E. Frisch, Grace Wyshak, and Larry Vincent reviewed the findings in 89 young dancers involved in highly competitive programs at professional ballet schools.

Nine subjects reported primary amenorrhea occurring at a mean age of 18.5 years; 6 were over age 18 years. Twelve percent of the subjects reported not having undergone menarche at a mean age of 14.3 years; 5 were in their fifteenth year. Secondary amenorrhea was reported by 13 subjects and irregular cycles by 27. Mean age at menarche in 67 postmenarcheal subjects was 13.7 years, significantly later than the mean of 12.8 years for American girls. Dancers with amenorrhea and irregular cycles were significantly leaner than those with regular cycles. Those with no menarche were leaner than the other dancers. Even subjects with regular cycles were in the very low range of weight for height and relative fatness for age. The mean height of dancers reporting no menarche at a mean age of 14.3 years was similar to that of well-nourished nondancers with menarche at a mean age of 12.9 years, but the mean weight of the dancers was significantly less than that of the well-nourished girls.

Either late maturers choose to be ballet dancers, or hard training and low food intake are related to excessive thinness and delayed puberty. The observation of menarche occurring after injury that prevents dancing supports the view that a change in the fat-lean ratio and accompanying changes in metabolic and hormone levels with hard exercise may be involved in delayed menarche and menstrual disturbances in ballet dancers. A change in the fat-lean ratio may result from an increase in leanness, besides a decrease in fatness, without weight loss or even with weight gain, as is observed in many athletes.

▶ [Another possibility is that serious students of ballet are subjected to such psychologic stress in striving to succeed that this, rather than the physical exertion, leads them to not eat and to lose weight and also contributes to the causes of secondary amenorrhea. Other young athletes train hard but (except for gymnasts) do not have the pressure to stay slim. Swimmers train hard but often carry a normal percent body fat, and they also experience delayed menarche. I agree that more study is needed.— J.L.A.] ◀

(6–15) N. Engl. J. Med. 303:17–19, July 3, 1980.

6–16 **Association of Somatotype and Body Composition With Physical Performance in 7- to 12-Year-Old Girls.** More needs to be known of the physical capacities of girls and women because of their increasing involvement in athletics and new federal guidelines requiring institutions to provide equal opportunity to women in intramural sports, physical education, and athletic activities. M. H. Slaughter, T. G. Lohman, and J. E. Misner (Univ. of Illinois, Champaign) sought to relate body composition, somatotype, and size to physical performance in 50 girls, aged 7 to 12 years, in a summer sports-fitness program. The girls were chiefly from middle and upper socioeconomic backgrounds. Data were collected from 1973 to 1976. Body composition was assessed by whole body ^{40}K counting. The physical performance tests included mile and 600-yd runs, a 50-yd dash, the standing broad jump, and the vertical jump.

Moderate relationships were observed between somatotype components, measures of body size, and measures of body composition, on the one hand, and running and jumping, on the other. Relative fatness and relative linearity were more closely related to physical performance than was relative musculoskeletal development in relation to height. Percent fat and relative fatness, combined with age, height, and weight, each accounted for a similar amount of the variability in running and jumping performance. Lean body mass, combined with age, height, and weight, accounted for more of the variation in performance than did relative musculoskeletal development related to height.

The findings closely parallel those obtained in boys and indicate that body fatness and linearity are significant in predictors of performance scores in both girls and boys. The magnitude and direction of relationships of these indices in active, prepubescent females are similar to those found for boys. Different combinations of anthropometric measurements, derived from multiple regression analysis, may replace the standardized deviation from height approach used by Heath and Carter to relate muscular composition to physical performance in children.

▶ [We know that prepubescent girls and boys are more nearly equal in physical performance variables and anthropometric measures than they will be after puberty. This excellent study should be repeated using postpubescent subjects.—J.L.A.] ◀

6–17 **The Underweight Female.** Little is known of the body composition and nutritional status of underweight females, but for many the expression is synonymous with frail and malnourished. Frank I. Katch, Victor L. Katch, and Albert R. Behnke studied 45 underweight college women, including 4 with less than 10% body fat, 15 with 10% to 15% body fat, and 26 with 15% to 20% body fat. Forty-one women with 20% to 30% body fat and 17 with over 30% fat also were studied. Only 1 of the study subjects was a serious distance runner.

All five groups had higher lean weights than Behnke's reference

(6–16) J. Sports Med. 20:189–198, June 1980.
(6–17) Physician Sportsmed. 8:55–60, December 1980.

woman, who is aged 20 to 24 years, weighs 125 lb, has 25% body fat, and is 64.5 in. tall. Controls with over 30% body fat had larger abdomen and buttocks girths than the other groups. The groups showed no significant differences in forearm and wrist girths or in knee, calf, and ankle measurements. The fattest group had larger biceps. Biacromial, chest, and bi-iliac widths were similar in the various groups. Subjects with 15% or less body fat had smaller bitrochanteric diameters. Overall skeletal dimensions were similar in all groups.

Women with a low percentage of body fat have physiques and dimensional characteristics similar to those of average and obese women. The concept of a small frame is incorrect. It is questioned whether a given low percentage of body fat automatically triggers a hormonal response that results in menstrual dysfunction or irregularity. A classification system has been devised that includes type 1 women with a lean body weight of 35 to 45 kg; type 2 women with a lean weight of 42 to 50 kg; and type 3 women who are athletic and typically have a lean weight of 50 kg and more. Type 1 women have physical features similar to those of preanorectic women and usually are nutritionally deficient. Type 2 women are physically active but are not high-level athletes. Their menstrual function and nutritional status are usually normal. Type 3 women often have menstrual irregularities; their nutritional status is normal.

▶ [We still do not agree on what precent body fat is healthy for men or women. Our literature usually reports what is normal, but that makes the assumption that our population is now healthy. I agree with the authors that more research is needed in this area. At West Point, we have set upper limits on percent body fat for men and women at 15% and 22%, respectively.—J.L.A.] ◀

6-18 **Generalized Equations for Predicting Body Density of Women.** Previous studies of women have shown that body composition regression equations derived from anthropometric variables are population specific. Andrew S. Jackson, Michael L. Pollock, and Ann Ward undertook to derive generalized equations for women differing in age and body composition. A total of 331 women aged 18 to 55 years served as subjects. They varied widely in body structure, body composition, and exercise habits. The sample was divided into a validation group of 249 subjects and a cross-validation group of 82. The hydrostatic method was used to determine body density and percent fat. Skin fold fat, gluteal circumference, and age were independent variables.

The quadratic form of the sum of 3, 4, and 7 S (skin fold fat), combined with age and gluteal circumference, produced multiple correlations ranging from 0.842 to 0.867, with standard errors of 3.6% to 3.8% fat. In cross-validating the equations on a sample of women of similar age and percent fat, correlations between predicted and hydrostatically determined percent fat ranged from 0.815 to 0.820, with standard errors of 3.7% to 4.0% fat.

Valid generalized body composition equations can be derived for women varying in age and body composition, although care must be

(6–18) Med. Sci. Sports 12:175–182, 1980.

taken with women over age 40 years. The multiple correlations found for the generalized equations in this study are high and compare favorably with results reported in the literature. These results and those reported in a similar study of men support the concept of generalized body composition regression equations for adults of varying age and body composition.

▶ [The requirement to use equations designed for specific populations has often been a drawback in determining body composition. It is generally agreed that body composition is more valuable as a classification tool than is height/weight. However, it has always been too cumbersome for the lay person to measure body composition. This move toward generalized equations is one move toward removing some of the complications in the determination of body composition.—J.L.A.] ◀

6–19 **Epidemiology of Women's Gymnastics Injuries.** Participation in women's sports has increased markedly in the past decade, and gymnastics is among the most popular of these sports. James G. Garrick (San Francisco) and Ralph K. Requa (Phoenix, Ariz.) obtained injury information from 98 participants in 2 years of interscholastic women's gymnastics competition in 4 Seattle-area high schools, collected by certified athletic trainers. A 12-team high school league, 2 college teams, and 3 private clubs also were surveyed in the second year of data collection because of the high injury rate found in the first year of the survey—56 injuries per 100 participants.

In the interscholastic study, a total of 39 injuries occurred in 98 participants, for an overall injury rate of 39 per 100 participants per season. More than one third of the injuries resulted from floor exercise and/or tumbling activities (table). In the first year, trampoline routines and floor exercise-tumbling each caused nearly one third of injuries. Sprains were the most common injury, accounting for 43% of all medical problems. Contusions and strains followed. There were no fractures. Injuries were distributed throughout the body, few anatomical areas being spared. The head, spine, and trunk were particularly affected. More than one third of injuries involved the legs. Only 5% of injuries occurred during competition, but the risk per unit of time was greater during competition than during workouts. In the mixed study, 317 gymnasts aged 6–21 years incurred 106 injuries, for a rate of 33 per 100 participants per season. Floor exercise and tumbling again caused the most injuries. Sprains were the most common injury, followed by strains, fractures, and contusions. The legs were involved in about half the cases, and the arms in nearly a third.

As in most sports, ankle sprains are among the most common injuries in women's gymnastics. Gymnastics is a "burst" activity as well as a highly sophisticated and skill-demanding sport. Thigh and leg strains and overuse problems of the leg also are common, suggesting that there may well be room for improvement in conditioning and other preventive programs in women's gymnastics.

▶ [Injury data collection is always complicated, and reports are often misleading. One should always look for the definition of "injury" that the authors used. In this study, the authors defined an injury as "a sport-related incident that resulted in an athlete

(6–19) Am. J. Sports Med. 8:261–264, July–Aug. 1980.

FEMALE GYMNASTICS INJURIES PER EVENT

Event	Interscholastic study		Mixed study								
	High school[a]		High school[b]		Club		College		Total	
	%	(n)	%	(n)	%	(n)	%	(n)	%	(n)
Balance beam	21	(8)	12	(9)	19	(3)	6	(1)	12	(13)
Floor exercise/tumbling	38	(15)	49	(36)	37	(6)	47	(8)	47	(50)
Uneven parallel bars	18	(7)	10	(7)	6	(1)	12	(2)	9	(10)
Vaulting	5	(2)	11	(8)	13	(2)	12	(2)	11	(12)
Other			18	(13)	25	(4)	23	(4)	20	(21)
Trampoline[c]	18	(7)								
Total	100	(39)	100	(73)	100	(16)	100	(17)	99	(106)

[a] Gymnastics portion of All-Sports Study 1973–1975.
[b] High School League, 1974–1975.
[c] All-Sports Study, 1973–1974.

missing any portion of a workout or competitive event." With this definition, a blister counts as much as a broken leg if one looks only at injury rates. In the following two articles, the authors used the same definition as above to define a reportable injury; however, they added another classification, called a "significant injury," which was any injury that prevents effective participation for at least 7 days. As you can see, definitions are important in injury statistics.—J.L.A.] ◄

6–20 **Men's and Women's Injuries in Comparable Sports.** Studies of womens' sports injuries are relatively new, and few studies have dealt specifically with the epidemiology of sports injuries. Patricia A. Whiteside (Pennsylvania State Univ., University Park) analyzed men's and women's injuries in college sports from data in the National Athletic Injury/Illness Reporting System records for the 1975–1976 and 1976–1977 seasons. Only sports conducted for women and men that had five or more schools reporting were included in the study.

The relative frequency of reportable injuries in men and women is given in the table. Basketball had the highest rate of reportable injuries for game- and practice-related situations for both men and women, followed by gymnastics and baseball-softball. The relative frequency of significant injuries was highest in men's and women's gymnastics in game-related situations, followed by basketball. In practice situations, basketball had the highest rate of significant injuries. The number of practice injuries was proportional to the time at risk. Sprains were the most common reportable injury for women in game situations. Fractures and neurologic problems were infrequent in all sports. Sprains also were the leading reportable game-related injury for men. The pattern of reportable injuries by body part was similar for men and women, but women had a higher relative frequency of ankle injuries.

Basketball caused the highest number of sports-related injuries in this survey, followed by gymnastics and baseball-softball. Both women and men have a higher rate of injury in contact sports. Injuries generally are more numerous in practice than in game situations, but are proportional to the time the athlete is at risk. The

NUMBER AND RELATIVE FREQUENCY (R) OF MEN'S AND
WOMEN'S REPORTABLE INJURIES
1975–1977

	No.	R*
Women		
Basketball	383	19.5
Gymnastics	95	9.4
Softball	76	3.1
Men		
Basketball	566	15.9
Gymnastics	95	7.7
Baseball	133	2.9

*Cases per 1,000 exposures.

(6–20) Physician Sportsmed. 8:130–140, March 1980.

relative frequency of injuries is higher in game situations for both women and men. In this survey, men had a higher relative frequency of game-related strains and fractures in basketball and gymnastics than did women.

6–21 **Women's Injuries in Collegiate Sports: A Preliminary Comparative Overview of Three Seasons.** Kenneth S. Clarke and William E. Buckley reviewed data reported on injuries of collegiate women athletes to the National Athletic Injury/Illness Reporting System (NAIRS) in its first 3 years of operation, 1975–1978. More dissimilarities in injury patterns were observed between women's sports than between comparable men and women's sports. The findings are presented in the table. Only sports followed by an average of at least 5 college teams per year were included. Significant injuries are those causing the athlete to miss at least 1 week of participation.

The coupled sports exhibited quite comparable patterns by sex, although women in basketball, gymnastics, and track and field had more leg injuries, men in track and field had more strains, whereas women had more fractures. Women ballplayers had more knee injuries than men; the men had more strains, and the women more fractures. Women softball players had more major injuries. Male baseball players required more surgical repairs of their injuries. In gymnastics, women had more leg injuries and more sprains. Matched sports exhibited similar patterns of game- and practice-related injuries for women and men; the differences were between different sports.

NAIRS DATA: AVERAGE ANNUAL RELATIVE FREQUENCY OF SIGNIFICANT
INJURIES IN SELECTED COLLEGIATE SPORTS, 1975–1978

	Sport	Average annual teams followed	Significant injuries per	
			1000 Athlete exposures	100 Athletes
I.	Spring football (M)[a]	26	6.3	12.6
II.	Wrestling (M)	20	4.2	35.7
	Fall football (M)	49	3.0	25.0
	Gymnastics (W)	9	2.7	28.4
	Ice hockey (M)	8	2.5	26.9
	Basketball (W)	21	2.5	20.3
	Lacrosse (M)	5	2.5	11.7
III.	Soccer (M)	13	2.3	13.2
	Track and field (W)	8	2.2	12.0
	Basketball (M)	31	2.1	20.7
	Volleyball (W)	16	2.1	10.9
	Track and Field (M)	14	1.9	10.0
	Softball (W)	10	1.8	8.7
IV.	Gymnastics (M)	6	1.5	16.4
	Baseball (M)	13	1.3	9.2
	Field hockey (W)	16	1.0	5.5
V.	Tennis (W)	5	0.6	5.7
	Swimming/diving (M)	7	0.6	4.0
	Swimming/diving (W)	7	0.2	2.3

[a]M indicates men; W indicates women.

(6–21) Am. J. Sports Med. 8:187, May–June 1980.

More dissimilarities are evident between women's sports than between comparable men's and women's sports, and it is of little value to consider the nature of women's or men's sports injuries without delimiting attention to a particular sport. With respect to the continuing surge of interest in athletic opportunities for women, injuries are sport related, not sex related. Future investigative reports should focus on a particular sport, with attention given to the patterns of injury within that sport under competitive and practice conditions so that potential preventive measures can be recognized.

▶ [These data are interesting in that they may tell us something about the injury mechanism when men and women are preparing for and participating in their own sport. However, it should not be accepted that under nearly identical conditions, the injury rates will be the same if men and women are playing together. At West Point, we found that when men and women took part in the same physical activity over an extended period (7 weeks), the injury rate of the men leveled off somewhere between 3% to 5%, but injury rate of the women after 1 week was 7.5% and gradually climbed to about 26% during the seventh week. As reported by Clarke and Buckley, the women at West Point had more leg injuries. The women had a stress fracture rate of 10%, compared to less than 1% for the men.—J.L.A.] ◀

6–22 **Nature and Causes of Injuries in Women Resulting From an Endurance Training Program.** More knowledge is needed about the response of women to physical training because of the increasing recruitment of women into the armed forces. Dennis M. Kowal (U.S. Army Res. Inst. of Environmental Medicine, Natick, Mass.) examined the occurrence of injuries in 400 women, aged 18 to 29 years, who completed an 8-week basic training cycle as recruits. They participated in an integrated endurance training and conditioning program for 1 hour a day, five or six times a week. The program included calisthenics and a run of 1 to 2 miles at an initial 10-minute-per-mile pace.

Self-report questionnaires indicated that 54% of 347 women sustained injuries requiring medical attention during the training period. The rate for men undergoing the same training was 26%. Injuries resulted in an average loss of 13 training days, and 41% of injuries prevented participation in all physical activity. Injuries usually resulted from a combination of continued hard training after onset of symptoms, inherent structural weakness, or biomechanical anomaly. Tibial and femoral stress fractures constituted one third of all injuries. Factors correlated with injuries included body composition, leg muscle strength, previous athletic participation, self-perception of fitness, and psychosomatic predisposition.

Major factors in injuries in women undergoing training include lack of previous conditioning, greater body weight and percent fat, and limited leg strength. These factors probably operate in conjunction with such inherent physiologic characteristics of women as wide pelvis, less strength, and greater joint flexibility to produce an increased risk of injury during training. Susceptibility to injuries can be identified before training begins and minimized through proper remedial measures. Lower limb disorders are costly in terms of medical care, hospitalization, and training time lost, and preventive programs could reduce the occurrence of such injuries. Remedial physical training and toughening programs, orthotics, and proper breaking in of footwear might be useful.

▶ [These findings are very similar to what we have found at West Point. The difference is that we begin with a population of women who were highschool athletes and thus were physically active, at least as our society defines physical activity for secondary-school women. The beginning level of physical activity is more intensive at West Point, with aerobic runs beginning at an 8¹/₂-minute-per-mile pace vs. the 10-minute-per-mile pace reported here. However, the injury rates of our population of women when participating in physical activity with men, although not as high as in this study, were significantly higher than the injury rates of the men. It is my judgment that in order to reduce the number of injuries, we must either dramatically change the physical education programs that our women receive in elementary and secondary schools or we must train them separately from men.—J.L.A.] ◄

6–23 **Evaluation of Sports Bras.** Protective brassieres have been recommended for female athletes because of the frequency of sore and tender breasts after exercise and to prevent breast injuries. Gale Gehlsen and Marge Albohm undertook to detect differences in support with selected bras and to assess the effects of binding the breasts over a bra in jogging. Studies were done in 40 female athletes. A camera was used to film joggers. Standard biomechanical procedures were used. Eight sports bras were tested in the biomechanics laboratory as subjects jogged on a treadmill at 6 mph on a flat grade.

Significant differences in linear displacement of the sports bras were found, but there was no significant difference in linear displacement between the size groups. The Bali-Go-Active, Winner, and Play-tops bras allowed the least movement. Vertical displacement could not be related to discomfort, nor could velocity of breast movement. There was, however, a significant effect when the product of mass and velocity was considered, indicating that the mass of the breast in conjunction with the velocity of movement might be related to discomfort during jogging. A 4-in. elastic wrap placed over the bra prevented about 45% of movement.

Some sports bras are better than others for minimizing breast movement and discomfort during strenuous activity. Binding over the bra prevented close to half of breast movement during jogging in this study.

▶ [Given its limitations, this study provides some valuable information concerning the relative effectiveness of the eight sports bras tested in limiting breast displacement and the velocity and acceleration of the displacement. However, the study does not say how long each subject jogged on the treadmill. Also, we do not know whether the bras that best limited breast displacement would be the ones to limit breast pain during and after a marathon run. Although binding over the bra will further limit vertical displacement of the breast, the technique has not been very practical for long-distance running because the wrap is hot and is difficult to keep in place. More research must be done with the sports bra.—J.L.A.] ◄

6–24 **The Female Athlete in Long-Distance Running.** It is the official position of the American College of Sports Medicine that women

(6–23) Physician Sportsmed. 8:89–96, October 1980.
(6–24) Ibid. 8:135–136, January 1980.

should not be denied the opportunity to compete in long-distance running and that they should be allowed to compete over the same distances used by their male counterparts. There is no conclusive evidence to contraindicate long-distance running for the healthy, trained female athlete.

A review of the literature shows that females respond to systematic exercise training in much the same manner as males. Long-distance female runners have significant increases of maximum oxygen uptake and reduced relative body fat content. Also, they are able to tolerate thermal stress and high environmental temperatures and relative humidities as well as the lower partial pressure of oxygen at high altitudes. Although the injury rate in females seems comparable to that in males, the greater pelvic width and joint laxity in women may lead to a higher incidence of injuries in female runners. There is evidence that approximately 33% of competitive female long-distance runners experience at least brief episodes of amenorrhea or oligomenorrhea. This is especially so in women with late onset of menarche, in nulliparous women, and in those who have taken contraceptive hormones. However, there is no evidence that disruption of the menstrual cycle is harmful to the female reproductive system. The role of running in the pathogenesis of menstrual irregularities is unknown.

Thus, because there is no conclusive evidence that long-distance running is harmful to women, they should not be denied the opportunity to compete in such events.

▶ [Again, a call for common sense is heard. There has been no proof that long-distance running is any more harmful or beneficial to a women than a man. Women should be allowed to race the same distances as men. Women as well as men must use some common sense in training, flexibility, and strengthening, and in diet to prepare for these races.—F.G.] ◀

7. Athletic Training

Conditioning, Training, and Injury Prevention

▶ Again, the plea is made for faculty athletic trainers on the high school level. Year after year, article after article, this need has been emphasized. Some slow progress is being made, but not enough for the thousands of high school athletes who are receiving inadequate management of their injuries.

This chapter contains a number of articles concerning the prevention of injuries, which is probably one of the most important duties of the athletic trainer. Training and conditioning programs are included, as well as articles on equipment and athletic shoes and ankle injury prevention, taping, and treatment. ◀

7–1 **An Investigation of Health Care Practices for High School Athletes in Maryland.** Athletics are increasing in popularity for both boys and girls, along with many related problems of proper health care for scholastic athletes. Jerry P. Wrenn (Univ. of Maryland) and David Ambrose (Univ. of Virginia) attempted to determine existing health care practices for high school athletes in Maryland. A questionnaire similar to that used by Redfearn (1975) in his Michigan study was sent to 149 public secondary schools in Maryland. Data were collected in the 1978–1979 academic year. Totals of 45,855 boys and 23,699 girls participated in 19 sports activities at the schools surveyed.

All interscholastic athletes had to have a physical examination by a physician to try out for a team. Only 21% of the schools reporting had a team physician. With few exceptions, physicians attended only football games. The coach generally has primary responsibility for athletic training duties, including initial evaluation of athletic injuries. Only half the schools had a person designated to keep records of injuries. Follow-up care for injuries is by the family physician. A large proportion of school principals expressed a desire for a full-time athletic trainer at their schools. These findings closely parallel those of Redfearn in studying secondary schools in Michigan.

School administrators and parents should attempt to see that all practice sessions and games are attended by persons trained in emergency medical procedures. Where coaches are responsible for dealing with athletic injuries, instruction should be provided as needed. Where possible, competent athletic trainers should be employed. Institutions concerned with professional preparation of teachers should make a particular effort to upgrade and improve their curricular offerings in the area of athletic health care. The knowledge and skills of those directly responsible for the health care of athletes probably

(7–1) Athletic Training 15:85–92, Summer 1980.

should be assessed to determine how competent these persons are for the tasks at hand.

▶ [In previous editions of the YEAR BOOK OF SPORTS MEDICINE, I have made similar comments regarding the need for athletic trainers in high schools. The time has come. The need has been established. The answer is a faculty trainer, an individual certified as an athletic trainer who will teach classes during the school day and serve as an athletic trainer after school hours. It is the most economical and practical solution to the problem. It does work.

The response, "An athletic trainer cannot be afforded," should be answered with, "You cannot afford not to have one." It is unfair to the athlete not to provide him or her with proper prevention and care of injury.—F.G.] ◀

7–2 **Professional Advancement of Athletic Training via Documentation and Publication** is discussed by Sam T. Kegerreis (West Virginia Univ.). The value of undocumented knowledge of various specific sports-related injuries has always been appreciated within the profession of athletic training, and an elite core of individuals has been maintained over the years through transfer of information from established trainers to aspiring young trainers. However, there have been minimal documented data to help the young trainer analyze modern techniques for preventing and treating injuries and rehabilitating athletes after injury. Most sports medical publications are authored by specialists other than athletic trainers. Scholarly productivity has been minimized by the pragmatic nature of athletic training and by demands on the trainer's time by coaching staffs and athletic departments. Athletic training is relatively young as an allied health profession. Another factor is the view that treatment of athletic injuries is an art, not a science.

Professional, public, and political recognition of athletic training is perhaps more important now than ever before. State licensure of athletic trainers is becoming an issue. Unreasonable work loads and dependence on coaching staffs no longer need be accepted by athletic trainers. The emergence of athletic training curricula emphasizes the need for publications by trainers for trainers. In addition, there is a growing public need for education about sport-related injuries. Athletic trainers today have an opportunity via publication to improve their professional status while contributing to the health care of thousands of athletes. They must improve their command of the basic sciences and take the initiative in documenting their successes and failures.

▶ [The author is making a plea to athletic trainers to improve their professional image through scientific publication. The profession of athletic training is young and emerging from a technical to a scientific level. It is my feeling that substantial progress has been made in the past 10 years through education and certification and that the future should continue to bring rapid growth and improvement to this profession.—F.G.] ◀

7–3 **Decision-Making Process in Sports Medicine.** Susan E. (Baltrusaitis) Genuario, William F. Walker (Cincinnati), and Jay A. Bradley (Indianapolis) present a step-by-step method of evaluation to help student trainers at the University of Cincinnati acquire skills needed to evaluate injuries in athletes. Initial evaluation includes specifically

(7–2) Athletic Training 15:47–48, Spring 1980.
(7–3) Ibid., pp. 174–176, Fall 1980.

addressing six points involving talking to and observing the athlete: history, gross deformity, point tenderness, range of motion, swelling, and pain should be noted before deciding on initial mangement. Initial management on the field includes first aid for breathing, circulation, bleeding or shock, as well as routine ice, compression, elevation, and splinting for removal. Whether the athlete returns to competition is determined by follow-up evaluation, which includes reexamination of the six-point evaluation, plus stability tests in the horizontal, vertical, and diagonal planes and functional tests of muscle flexibility, strength, and endurance.

After injury, rehabilitation includes a three-phase program with checkpoints after each stage before the athlete is advanced to the subsequent stage. Initially, the athlete is not participating in sports during the first phase of the program. During phase I, stage I, the objective is to increase range of movement, decrease pain, and control swelling. Therapy to reduce pain-spasm and swelling, support, and passive exercise are used. Stage II aims to increase movement, with continuing therapy and support and active movement of the joint through all pain-free planes. In stage III, disuse atrophy is curtailed, allowing the athlete to return to competition with minimal risk of reinjury. Progressive resistive exercise, with isometrics followed by an isotonic or isokinetic progressive resistance program, is used. Stage IV builds the endurance lost with injury, often generally with a cardiovascular program as well as conditioning of the specific injured musculature. During phase II, the athlete is allowed limited return to play with continuing work of increasing active exercise, strength and endurance, prevention of reinjury, and follow-up evaluation that includes dynamic sport-related assessment. Phase III entails continuation of active exercise, progressive resistive, and endurance programs, as well as preventive padding and strapping while the athlete is fully functioning. Preventive measures addressing nutrition, psychology, taping, wrapping, padding, equipment, conditioning, and health and safety education should be used to protect the athlete and his teammates.

▶ [It is always important to have an evaluation procedure clearly in your mind when determining the extent of an injury. Often, during the excitement of the game, an important test or procedure may be missed. If your procedure is well practiced and the evaluator remains confident and calm in his methods, this is unlikely to occur.

Rehabilitation programs must also follow a regular progression with testing along the way. The athlete is never returned to competition or full practice without a good deal of on-the-field testing of his ability and stage of recovery.—F.G.] ◀

7–4 **Comparison of Effects of Fluid and Electrolyte Replacement Schedules on Work Performance and Circulatory Stress in 30 Members of a High School Football Team.** Twenty-five football-related deaths resulting from heat illness occurred between 1959 and 1965. This led to investigations of the use of water and electrolyte replacement to prevent heat illness during strenuous exercise. W. Donald Myers and Kennon T. Francis (Univ. of Alabama, Birmingham) studied the effects of a commercially available glucose-electro-

(7–4) J. Orthop. Sports Phys. Ther. 1:153–158, Winter 1980.

TABLE 1.—TOTAL WEIGHT, SWEAT, AND URINE LOSS (+SE) IN ATHLETES EXERCISING IN THE HEAT WITH GLUCOSE ELECTROLYTE FLUID ADMINISTERED IN THREE DIFFERENT SCHEDULES

Replacement schedule	Total quantity fluid consumed	Weight loss	Sweat volume	Urine volume
	liters	kg		liters
Control	0.81	3.04 ± 0.19	2.95 ± 0.18	0.08 ± 0.02
120 ml/15 min	0.96	2.72 ± 0.40	2.66 ± 0.40	0.06 ± 0.01
240 ml/15 min	1.92	3.26 ± 0.19	3.21 ± 0.20	0.05 ± 0.00

lyte replacement drink administered in three different schedules on the work performance of 30 high school football players. The drink (Break Time, Johnson & Johnson) contains 23 mEq sodium, 10 mEq potassium, and 23 gm glucose per L. The players consumed the drink ad libitum on the first day of practice (control) and in amounts of 120 ml or 240 ml during 15-minute rest periods on the succeeding 2 days. Environmental conditions were 90–95 degrees F and 60% to 62% relative humidity.

The amount of body weight lost remained essentially constant over the 3 days, regardless of the amount of fluid consumed (Table 1). The prepractice and postpractice physical performance capacities, as measured by predicted oxygen uptake values ($VO_{2 max}$), decreased significantly ($P<.05$) in each group (Table 2). The $VO_{2 max}$ decreased by 31% during the control session, 25% in players following the schedule of 120 ml/15 minutes and 23% in players following the schedule of 240 ml/15 minutes. The physical work capacity measure, as determined by the time required to complete a 300-m. obstacle course, showed contrasting results. During the control session, the time required to complete the course increased from 67.1 seconds (prepractice) to 91.8 seconds (postpractice). However, players following the schedule of 120 ml/15 minutes required 81.7 seconds prepractice to complete the course and only 71.2 seconds after practice. Those following the schedule of 240 ml/15 minutes required 74.0 seconds prepractice and only 53.5 seconds postpractice. The difference between prepractice

TABLE 2.—CHANGES IN MAXIMUM OXYGEN CONSUMPTION IN SUBGROUPS A-1 AND B-1 AND 300-METER OBSTACLE COURSE TIMES IN SUBGROUPS A-2 AND B-2 EXERCISING IN THE HEAT WITH GLUCOSE ELECTROLYTE FLUID ADMINISTERED IN THREE DIFFERENT SCHEDULES

	Replacement schedule	Oxygen consumption groups A-1, B-1	300-Meter obstacle course times groups A-2, B-2
		liter/min	sec
Control	Prepractice	2.85 ± 0.17	69.10 ± 1.93
	Postpractice	1.97 ± 0.10	91.80 ± 5.01
	Δ	−0.71 ± 0.19*	+22.77 ± 5.32[*, a, b]
120 ml/15 min	Prepractice	3.15 ± 0.15	81.67 ± 5.33
	Postpractice	2.37 ± 0.15	71.77 ± 8.10
	Δ	−0.90 ± 0.27*	−18.77 ± 4.63[*, a]
240 ml/15 min	Prepractice	3.07 ± 0.19	74.00 ± 8.61
	Postpractice	2.36 ± 0.23	53.50 ± 4.10
	Δ	−0.77 ± 0.09*	−20.50 ± 5.89[*, b]

*Denotes significance ($P \leq .05$) when practice values were compared to postpractice values. Same superscript letter denotes significance at $P = .50$ level.

and postpractice times was statistically significant (*P*<.05) for each group, as was the difference in times between those following the schedule of 120 ml/15 minutes and those following the one of 240 ml/ 15 minutes (*P*<.05).

The relatively constant body weight loss observed suggests that mandatory consumption of 240 ml of fluids every 15 minutes may be necessary for football players to maintain adequate hydration under conditions similar to those present during this study. The improvement in physical performance is probably attributable to the psychologic, rather than the physiologic, state of the players.

▶ [There is little need to buy expensive commercial fluids under the climate conditions specified—water is as effective as any other replacement fluid. It is not unlikely that all of the fluid emptied from the stomach with a dose of 240 ml/15 minutes; the usual limit of gastric emptying is about 600 ml/hour in an active person. The time of day of competition was 2 to 6 P.M., about the worse possible time, because radiant heating is then at a maximum. In view of the sad toll of deaths from football in this part of the United States, one must ask why the organizers did not have the wisdom to postpone activity until after sundown.—R.J.S.] ◀

7–5 **Primary Prevention of Heat Stroke in Canadian Long-Distance Runs** is outlined by Richard L. Hughson (Univ. of Waterloo). Heat stroke is the most common medical problem in participants in long-distance runs. Although exertional heat stroke can occur in varying climatic conditions, the risk increases with environmental temperature and humidity. Primary prevention appears to be the best approach. Education is the basis for prevention.

In the past, organizers of races have based starting times on convenience, and the commercial influence of sponsors often has outweighed common sense. Many novice and some experienced runners are ignorant of the dangers of competing in very hot weather. If competitive considerations overcome common sense, heat injury may result. Novices may dissociate themselves from the discomfort of effort and force themselves beyond their capabilities. Most cases of exertional heat stroke are preventable.

Races should not be run in July and August, and they should be scheduled to start in the early morning or evening. A course with

---

WARNINGS TO BE GIVEN TO PARTICIPANTS IN LONG-DISTANCE
RUNS, RATED ACCORDING TO AIR TEMPERATURE

Green: Go, but remember to monitor yourself.
Yellow: Caution, be very aware of possible heat injury. Monitor yourself closely for the early warning symptoms of heat injury and be prepared to slow your usual running pace.
Red: Extreme caution: do not enter the race if you are uncertain of your ability. The only way that you will finish is by running much slower than normal.

Air temperature (°C); warning

Months	Green	Yellow	Red
April-June	< 12	12-23	> 23
July-September	< 18	18-27	> 27
Others	< 10	10-20	> 20

(7–5) Can. Med. Assoc. J. 122:1115–119, May 24, 1980.

some shade should be selected. Adequate fluids should be provided every 2–3 km. All race officials should know the warning signs of heat stroke and its management. Warnings should be given to the participants before the race begins, according to the guidelines presented in the table. Medical facilities should be available at the race site and staffed with personnel capable of instituting immediate cooling and full-scale resuscitation. Persons trained in first aid should be stationed around the course. Competitors should know that training in the heat can reduce the risk of heat injury, as can the consumption of 500 ml of water just before the run and 250 ml at every water station. They should know the early symptoms of heat injury. Racers should run with a partner, and each should agree to be responsible for the other's well-being during the run.

▶ [In all sports, *prevention* is the best management of heat stroke. Hopefully, coaches and athletes all understand that drinking water before and during a practice or contest is not harmful. It is probably one of the most beneficial things an athlete can do to help his performance on a hot, muggy day. Coaches should encourage their athletes to drink water, because thirst is a poor indicator of the need for fluid replacement. The American College of Sports Medicine has an excellent position statement: The Prevention of Heat Injuries During Distance Running.

It has been my practice to use the temperature-humidity index (THI) as a guide to follow. When the THI rises above 70, we provide extra water breaks during the practice. Above a THI of 75, we give as much water as the athlete desires, and we reduce our practice time on the field. Above 79, we would not wear equipment and we would have only a light workout in shorts. Above 84, practice is cancelled; we did this once in the past 15 years. By holding the practice very early or late in the day, we can avoid many dangerous THI situations.—F.G.] ◀

7–6 **Referred Visceral Pain in Athletics** is discussed by Christine Elaine Boyd (Univ. of Virginia). All athletes in contact sports are vulnerable to abdominal trauma, and the use of protective gear is not feasible in a majority of sports. When abdominal injury occurs, immediate recognition and treatment are necessary if disastrous sequelae are to be avoided. Abdominal injuries can present rather misleading symptomatology. The viscera are relatively insensitive to painful stimuli, and referred pain often results in confusion and a delay in appropriate diagnosis.

Visceral pain will be noted in the somatic region with which a final common path is shared. Free blood in contact with the peritoneum results in peritonitis, which also presents referred pain corresponding to the site of the incoming afferent impulses. Cardiac pain is felt at the base of the neck and the left jaw, as well as the left shoulder and arm over the ulnar nerve distribution. Irritation of the parietal pleura after lung damage may give rise to pain along the dermatomes corresponding to C8–T8. Diaphragmatic pain typically is referred to the shoulder region. Esophageal injury results in pain in the sternal region of the thorax at a level corresponding to the site of the lesion. Splenic afferent impulses result in sharp cutaneous pain projected to the left shoulder and about one third of the way down the arm. Pancreatic involvement may cause both anterior and posterior pain.

(7–6) Athletic Training 15:20–25, Spring 1980.

Liver and gallbladder pain is referred to the epigastrium and just to the right of it. Pain of gastric origin is most often felt in the epigastrium, usually in the midline or in the left quadrant. Backache or sharp pain in the back may result from intestinal lesions. Kidney pain may be felt high in the costovertebral angle posteriorly, and pain may radiate around the flank into the lower abdominal quadrant. Similar pain results from ureteral involvement. Pain from bladder involvement may be felt in the lower part of the trunk and upper part of the thigh anteriorly.

Visceral injuries can result in the referral of pain to superficial areas of the body considerably removed from the actual site of the lesion. This phenomenon may be the only presenting feature of an internal injury. Trainers can recognize potentially life-threatening situations if they are aware of referred visceral pain.

▶ [Anyone involved with immediate evaluation of athletic injuries must be aware that referred pain is often a symptom of visceral injury. It has been my experience that contusions of the kidneys and testes are fairly common and should be checked by a physician. Injuries to the spleen are, fortunately, not so common, but they do require immediate referral to a physician or hospital. Sports in which an athlete could be hit with an object such as a hockey stick or kicked below the rib cage are associated with higher incidences of splenic injuries. The recognition of referred pain may mean the difference between life and death.—F.G.] ◀

7–7 **Strength Imbalance and Knee Injury.** The prevention of sports-related injuries is often secondary to treatment and rehabilitation. John B. Cage (Texas City, Texas) describes a method for testing the quadriceps and hamstrings for strength imbalances so that any deficiencies found can be corrected before they result in injury.

The testing is performed on an Orthotron machine. The Orthotron has two hydraulic gauges to measure flexion torque and extension torque, respectively. Before testing, the athlete stretches the muscles to be tested to prevent strain. Once the athlete has become accustomed to the machine, testing begins. Both hydraulic valves are set at $2^1/_2$. The athlete performs 3 sets of 3 repetitions with one leg, with a 30-second interval between each set. The procedure is then repeated with the other leg. The readings for the hamstrings should be at least 50% of the maximum torque exerted by the quadriceps. If a significant imbalance is found in one leg compared with the other, an exercise program to correct the imbalance should be started. An athlete having an overall strength deficiency should be enrolled in a weight-training program to develop both legs. If an Orthotron is not available, comparative testing can be performed with conventional weights. This is done by recording the maximal weight lifted with a full knee extension and with a hamstring curl and comparing the findings as one would the recordings on the Orthotron.

Although most high school athletes increase in strength every year, all should be reevaluated annually to determine possible changes in muscle balance.

▶ [Injury prevention is an extremely important aspect of sports medicine. The athletic

(7–7) Physician Sportsmed. 8:140, January 1980.

trainer is in an ideal position to evaluate potential problems and to design exercise programs to eliminate them. Many injuries could be prevented if athletes performed flexibility and strengthening exercises designed to reduce a specific weakness. The screening of athletes to detect these weaknesses can be time-consuming. However, the time is well spent and the results are well worth the effort. The treatment time for one serious injury is considerably longer than any screening program.—.G.] ◄

7–8 **The Development of Specific Function Tests as a Measure of Performance** is discussed by B. Nettleton and C. A. Briggs (Univ. of Melbourne). The most obvious feedback to coaches is the outcome of games, but this will not provide information on areas where coaching should be improved. Previous means of assessing player performance on the field are extremely time-consuming, leading to the use of various simple indirect measures that correlate with on-field performance. A series of "functional fitness tests" has been developed to identify typical responses made by players during a series of games and to standardize the response. Useful tests must include the chief elements of the game in a simple setting that can be readily incorporated into coaching sessions and repeated at intervals. Clear, quick conclusions must be available.

Zelenka devised a test consisting of a sprint with a sharp change in direction, jumping over and then crawling under a hurdle, dribbling a ball around a series of flags, and passing it over 25 m at a target space 2 m wide. Two circuits are completed with a recovery period of 45–60 seconds. This test was administered to 9 soccer players, and a modified version of the test was administered to players of different ability levels. Heart rate responses indicated that the test reproduces the stresses of the game. The modified test includes a short "power agility" run and an information-processing task that simulates the task of the player running with the ball in a game. The modified test discriminated between different levels of competitive league players. The total time needed to complete the test correlated significantly with performance on the field of play, and also with maximal oxygen uptake of the players.

This specific function test can be used to differentiate among various levels of soccer ability. Data may be obtainable from performance on various parts of the test that indicate strengths and weaknesses of individual players. Sections of the test may be usable for discriminating between players whose roles on the field differ.

► [Coaches are often seeking ways to determine how an athlete will perform in a game. A number of parameters are discussed and presented by the authors as a means of determining the ability of soccer players. Similar tests can and have been devised in other sports. Coaches do rely somewhat on these test results; however, in general, less objective means are usually followed to select a starting team. Most coaches still rely on experience and their judgment to evaluate a player's performance.—F.G.] ◄

7–9 **Effect of Dry Land Training on Aerobic Capacity of College Hockey Players.** The Soviets have developed scientific training programs to enhance and maintain superior levels of aerobic capacity, and well-conditioned athletes have been a characteristic of their

(7–8) J. Sports Med. 20:47–54, March 1980.
(7–9) Ibid. 19:271–276, September 1979.

hockey program. They have had considerable success in using dry land training programs to enhance aerobic capacity both before and during the hockey season. Hockey is a very intense sport that relies heavily on both aerobic and anaerobic energy systems. Wallace W. Hutchinson, Gerald M. Maas, and Alan J. Murdoch (Iowa State Univ., Ames) examined the effects of a preseason dry land training program on aerobic capacity in 11 men aged 18–20 years who were members of a collegiate hockey team. The subjects all had participated on high school or juvenile teams, and they were highly skilled. Maximal aerobic capacity was determined by the open circuit method during continuous graded treadmill exercise, before and after a 6-week dry land training period, and 15 weeks later, at the end of the hockey season.

Subjects trained 3 days a week for $1^1/2$ hours for 2 weeks, using flexibility and strength calisthenics exercises and weight-training exercises. They also ran 2 miles, increased progressively to 5 miles. Training then was extended to 6 days a week for about $1^1/2$ hours, and subjects ran 5 miles 3 times a week. Running steps was substituted for weight training 3 days a week. Training resulted in significant changes in maximal oxygen uptake at both posttraining evaluations.

A dry land training program led to an 11% increase in maximal oxygen uptake in hockey players. The frequency and regularity of physical training are very important in maintaining high levels of aerobic capacity during the competitive season.

▶ [Aerobic capacity is an extremely important parameter of fitness for hockey players. Methods that can improve and maintain aerobic capacity should be used in every pre-season conditioning program and be continued during the season. Too often during the season, coaches feel they do not have the time to provide for conditioning-type exercises. Athletes often are in better physical condition, regarding both strength and aerobic capacity, at the beginning of a season than they are at the end of a 3- or 4-month season. "Ice time" is expensive and precious, and I understand why a coach would not use this valuable time for other than improving skills and team work. An off-ice flexibility, strengthening and cardiovascular program must be utilized in the pre-season and be continued on a modified basis during the season.—F.G.] ◀

7–10 **Muscular Development and Lean Body Weight in Body Builders and Weight Lifters.** Weight lifters often exhibit remarkable muscle hypertrophy, but quantification of this hypertrophy has been limited. Victor L. Katch, Frank I. Katch, Robert Moffatt, and Michael Gittleson (Univ. of Michigan) attempted to quantify excess muscle development and levels of lean body weight in 39 male competitive body builders, Olympic weight lifters, and power weight lifters. Five skin fold sites and 8 bone diameters were measured and recorded in addition to standard anthropometric measures.

The 18 body builders had a mean lean body weight of 74.6 kg with 9.3% fat. Thirteen power weight lifters had a mean lean body weight of 73.3 kg with 9.1% fat, and 8 Olympic weight lifters had a lean body weight of 68.2 kg with 10.8% fat. No group differences were found in frame size, percent fat, lean body weight, skin fold thicknesses, or diameter measurements. The body builders had the largest shoulders, chests, biceps, and forearms. Calculations of excess muscle by the Behnke method showed that body builders had 15.6 kg of excess muscle, power weight lifters had an excess of 14.8 kg, and Olympic weight lifters had an excess of 13.1 kg. Somatographic comparisons indicated only slight differences among these groups, while differences from reference man were substantial. Nearly half the subjects reported performing endurance-aerobic conditioning in addition to lifting.

Persons engaged in weight training develop extreme muscular hypertrophy, resulting in excess muscle weights of about 14.5 kg. Body builders exhibited increased amounts of excess muscle weight, even when expressed relative to body weight. Estimates of excess muscle weight are primarily responsible for classifying subjects as overweight, according to weight-for-height standards from actuarial tables.

▶ [Other interesting data that could be obtained from these three groups would be on muscular power, strength, and endurance, as well as histologic determination of muscle fiber type.—J.S.T.] ◀

7–11 **Comparison of Two Methods of Training on the Development of Muscular Strength and Endurance.** Theoretically Nautilus equipment should provide an optimal training stimulus for developing muscle strength and endurance because of its mechanical design, with maximal resistance provided through the full range of motion. Michael T. Sanders (Univ. of Wisconsin, La Crosse) compared training using Nautilus and traditional equipment in college-age men who trained 3 days a week for 5 weeks in 3-minute bouts of rhythmic isometric exercise involving the forearm extensors and shoulder flexors. A dynograph was used to process the load cell signal. Eleven subjects trained with barbells and 11 with Nautilus equipment. The former group performed the bench press and the behind-the-neck seated press. Very similar exercises were performed using the Chest and Shoulder Press Nautilus machines. The progressive-resistance technique was used in both groups.

Significant improvement in the forearm extensors was found with training. The shoulder flexors showed significantly increased strength, with no significant differences between the training methods. Muscle endurance improved significantly in the forearm extensors with both types of training equipment. The shoulder flexors may fatigue more rapidly initially than the forearm extensors.

Within the limits of this study, training with the traditional barbell method and with Nautilus dynamic equipment using the progressive-resistance technique produced significant gains in muscle strength and gains in absolute muscle endurance. The two types of training appeared to be equally effective in developing muscle strength and endurance in this study.

▶ [It has always been my opinion that the type of equipment used is the least important factor in any strength-building program. The motivation of the individual is by far the

(7–11) J. Orthop. Sports Phys. Ther. 1:210–213, Spring 1980.

most important factor. It has often been stated that the motivated athlete using inexpensive weights will far surpass the less-motivated athlete using the most expensive training equipment available.—F.G.] ◄

7–12 **The Caloric Costs of Rope Skipping and Running.** Although rope skipping may have potential for developing cardiorespiratory fitness, some claims of its benefits for training are exaggerated. Bud Getchell and Pat Cleary (Ball State Univ., Muncie, Ind.) measured the energy cost of and the heart rate response to rope skipping in 7 male and 3 female students who were physically active and compared the results with those for similar intensities of jogging. A special apparatus was devised to allow unimpeded rope skipping while respiratory gases were collected to determine oxygen uptake.

Rope skipping substantially increased the heart rate and required considerable energy output, although the energy requirement was lower than that for jogging at the same heart rate. The energy cost for rope skipping during the last minute of each bout was about 66% of the maximal oxygen uptake capacity (11.9 kcal/min^{-1}), whereas the caloric requirement increased to about 74% of maximal oxygen (13.6 kcal/min^{-1}) when the same subjects ran on the treadmill. When the energy cost was expressed in terms of mets, rope skipping required 9.5 mets (9.5 times the energy required at rest), whereas jogging at the same heart rate required 10.9 mets. Men had a greater caloric requirement than women, which supports the fact that larger persons require more energy to perform the same task. The results were comparable to others reported in the literature.

The findings reported here dispel the claim that 10 minutes of rope skipping daily have as beneficial an effect as 30 minutes a day of jogging. On the basis of energy expenditure comparisons, jogging appears to be better than rope skipping for developing physical fitness because it involves more muscle mass than skipping rope. If a person wants to obtain physiologic training benefits from rope skipping, it appears that heart rate intensity and the length of time skipping have to be at least as great as for jogging.

▶ [There have been several studies of rope skipping recently, some more critical than this article. The energy cost of rope skipping can be quite high, but it depends very largely on how high the subject jumps as the rope is turned. While it is a useful indoor activity, it is more difficult to regulate when a suitable training load is being prescribed.—R.J.S.] ◄

7–13 **The Athlete's Mouthpiece** is discussed by Robert Schwartz and Max M. Novich. Effective movement often depends on the subtle guiding, stabilizing, or neutralizing contributions of assistant movers. The actions of a given muscle group can be complemented or hindered by the actions of another muscle or group of muscles. It has been shown that the relation of the mandible to the maxilla affects the strength of some portions of the related musculature. In addition, premature loss of teeth and the disordered dental function that results affect the vascular and nervous structures of the involved part. Loss

(7–12)   Physician Sportsmed. 8:56–60, February 1980.
(7–13)   Am. J. Sports Med. 8:357–359, Sept.–Oct. 1980.

COMPETITIVE RESULTS WITH AND WITHOUT MOUTHPIECES

Athlete's no.	Pushups		440		100-yard dash		Deltoid testing muscle	
	Without MG[a]	With MG	Without MG	With MG	Without MG	With MG	Without MG	With MG
1	23	23	69.3	68.1	13.9	12.2	0	+
2	15	30	75.9	75.2	16.0	15.3	0	+
3	20	28	70.9	66.0	13.1	12.3	0	+
4	9	25	71.9	67.0	13.3	13.1	0	+
5[b]	21	26	80.7	84	15.5	16	0	+
6[c]	43	39	60.6	59.0	12.3	11.7	0	+
7	38	35	58.4	58.1	12.3	11.7	0	+
8[d]	26	28	74.5	74.2	13.3	12.1	0	+

[a]MG indicates mouthguard.
[b]Athlete 5 had participated in a 20-mile bike race the day before the tests. She complained of exhaustion and did not wish to participate in the tests.
[c]Athletes 6 and 7 did not bite down on the mouthpiece while doing pushups.
[d]This athlete was tested with the shot put as well as the other tests reported in the table. His results with the shot put were measurably better with the mouthpiece compared with results without one.

of teeth also can alter the vertical dimension and change the mandibular position in relation to the maxilla. Mandibular position affects the size of the airway as well as the aerobics of the athlete.

Examination of the mouthguards of junior olympic boxing contestants showed a mandibular position compatible with good muscular strength in only 1 of 12 subjects. All the mouthguards examined failed to accord with principles of good aerobics. Track and field athletes had impressions made and casts of their occlusion fabricated. Mouthguards were made for each athlete, and the youngsters then competed in 100- and 440-yd events, did pushups, and underwent a deltoid resistive test, both with and without the newly designed mouthguards. The results are presented in the table.

A properly designed mouthpiece can both protect and add measurably to athletic performance. Appropriate mouthpieces should be designed for participants in boxing, contact sports, and track and field events.

▶ [For many years, mouthpieces have been used in boxing, football, and other contact sports to prevent tooth injuries and hopefully to act as a shock absorber and minimize the severity of cerebral concussions. Recently, the effect of these devices on athletic performance has been questioned. It has been suggested that devices that provide proper temporomandibular joint positioning can improve athletic performance. To date, I have had no experience with these devices and have not seen enough scientific data to support these claims. Certainly, more study should be done in this area under usual scientific testing guidelines.—F.G.] ◀

7–14 **A Specialized Pad for the Acromioclavicular Joint** is described by Charles E. Wershing (Miami Univ.). A pad for the acromioclavicular joint was initially constructed by Lake for use in running backs with acromioclavicular separation.

TECHNIQUE—The pad is fitted to the person who will wear it in competition. The elastic strapping is fitted first. The athlete must loosen the straps

(7–14) Athletic Training 15:102–104, Summer 1980.

before removing the pad. The Temperstik inlay then is fitted. The inlay covers only that part of the foam "toilet seat" pad that rests on the superior aspect of the injured shoulder. The Orthoplast shield then is fitted with the assembly on the athlete. Excess material is removed while it is still pliable. Applying cold packs will hasten cooling of the Orthoplast. A layer of moleskin is applied along the proximal edge of the Orthoplast for added comfort and protection. The Orthoplast shield is secured with a fast-setting cement, and the raised portion is aligned over the acromioclavicular joint. Each inferior post is covered with moleskin.

The acromioclavicular pad provides maximal protection, comfort, and mobility without sacrificing any of these. It is readily and inexpensively constructed.

▶ [Acromioclavicular joint injuries are extremely difficult to protect in contact sports. Varying success has been achieved with some commercial products such as the "toilet seat" pad or a similar pad with cutouts for the acromioclavicular joints, an air-filled apparatus, or even air bags that are inserted under the shoulder pads. The problem to date has been in keeping the protective pad in the proper place. This specialized pad appears to be a good solution. I have had fairly good results with a modification of this protective pad. The shoulder pad insert I use comes with the acromioclavicular joint cutouts. Another major problem is that the telescoping type of injury cannot be protected with this type of pad. These provide protection from the direct blow only.—F.G.] ◀

7–15 **Nine Mistakes Racers Make: Racing Tests the Systems That Running Strengthens.** Steve Subotnick discusses the hazards faced by the inexperienced racer who has enjoyed running, has never intended to be a serious competitor, but nevertheless has entered an open road race. A runner must train at a given rate to know his or her right pace, and this should be done the week before the event so that the body will grow accustomed to it. Knowing how the body will respond to a race will lend confidence to the runner and reduce the chance of having to drop out. Beginning racers tend to be overanxious and not warm up properly. Stretching and warming up are necessary before any run, particularly a race. Most beginners should use their training flats in a race, rather than racing flats. If the latter are to be used, they should be broken in by being used before the race once or twice a week. The risk of blistering is greater during a race than in training. If blisters or mild irritations are present before the race, tincture of Benzoine and moleskin should be used on the affected areas.

A good night's sleep before a race is important, but rest 2 nights before the race is particularly important; nervousness may make it hard to sleep on the eve of the event. Beginners tend to eat too much of the wrong type of food too close to starting time. No food should be taken within 3 hours of a race, and no eggs or bacon should be taken in the prerace meal. Sugar on cereal should be avoided. Water or diluted electrolyte drink should be taken before the race, and water should be taken at aid stations during the event.

Knowledge of the race course will be helpful. To go faster in a race, the cadence, not the stride length, should be increased. Racers should check their breathing during a race and should know the limits of their bodies. In most races the competitor should be able to talk, but should avoid conversation if the best time is to be achieved.

▶ [The author has some good advice for runners who have not raced competitively. Before entering a competitive race, increase your training program to a level that will prepare you for the distance and speed you expect to run. Wear the proper shoes and clothing. Eat a correct diet for weeks prior to the event and a pregame meal if desired. Be sure to warm up properly. If possible, train on the race course or similar terrain. Do not leave these most important factors to chance.—F.G.] ◀

7–16 **Selection of a Running Shoe: If the Shoe Fits—Run.** Bruce Heckman (Univ. of California, Los Angeles) points out that national consciousness for physical fitness through running has led to the creation of a new athletic shoe. The long-distance running shoe, or flat, was designed to protect the foot from the rigors of long-distance running. The protective design of shoes is patterned from infancy and, if the athletic shoe manufacturer recognizes the mechanics of gait, an appropriate design will result. Standards for a normal foot vary with custom and race. The foot and ankle perform as recipients and mediators of ground forces, and on occasion must provide rigidity or flexibility. Ultimately, they must provide stability. Arches or vaults contribute weight distribution, mechanical efficiency, and a protective space for the transmission of important structures. Gait depends on a balanced relationship of the functioning muscles. If shoes were made from a biomechanical standpoint, increased medial support would extend from the heel counter anteriorly to buttress the talar head and navicular during foot pronation. The outer sole and midsole should provide cushioning and flexibility, while the heel counter should be rigid to stabilize heel action. The upper, or vamp, should be made of nylon for comfort and to reduce abrasive forces. A 0.5-in. heel lift will absorb the shock from initial ground contact, but heel height can vary slightly according to street shoe habits. A box toe keeps the upper composition away from the dorsal aspect of the toes to eliminate blisters. At least 0.25 in. of extra toe length should be allowed.

A balanced foot will be least susceptible to the stresses of running and inappropriate footwear. Wear patterns on the tread of the outsole can suggest gait deviations. The long-distance runner is susceptible to unique stresses from his sport, which may facilitate lower leg injury. The biomechanics of foot pronation and the unfolding trauma may be antecedents of further trauma to the lower leg. The running public must be aware of the possible adverse effects of the sport as well as its benefits.

▶ [There is probably no one make or model of running shoe that is best for everyone. Because of foot shape and individual mechanics of running, what is great for one person may not be good for another. Take the time to try the shoe on and walk in it extensively in the store before you buy it. Take all the time to fit and try a pair of running shoes that you would with a pair of ski boots. Too many runners' closets are full of running shoes that were selected without enough examination. Unfortunately, the only true test comes in use. However, proper fit and the basics of what is needed in a good running shoe must always be considered.—F.G.] ◀

(7–16) J. Orthop. Sports Phys. Ther. 2:65–67, Fall 1980.

7–17   **Achilles Peritendinitis** is discussed by Patrick O'Connor and Robert D. Kersey. Achilles tendinitis is second only to knee injuries among long-distance runners. Anatomical and physiologic elements relating to the vulnerability of the Achilles tendon are the fact that peritendon, rather than synovial, tissue forms the sheath and the extremely poor circulation at the middle third of the tendon. Because of the poor circulation, the Achilles tendon seems an unlikely spot for inflammation, nor can it be vulnerable to tenosynovitis. Peritendinitis, rather than tendinitis, is the pathologic condition. In pure peritendinitis there is definite thickening of the peritendon tissue, which is somewhat adherent to the tendon itself. In peritendinitis with tendinosis the tendon itself is found to have thickened and become soft and yellowish. Causes range from running mechanics to the training intensity and duration to the shoes worn.

To avoid being sidelined by an injury, the runner must understand signs and symptoms and initiate treatment at the onset. Cryotherapy before and after running is appropriate with minor strains. Stretching and warm-up exercises, with the knee in both flexed and extended positions, are important. Heel lifts help ease the strain on Achilles tendons. Shoes should be checked for excessive wear. When appropriate, orthotics can correct poor foot position, alignment, or both. Added support can be gained from longitudinal taping of the tendon; circular strappings should be avoided around an injured Achilles tendon for they may aggravate the condition. In cases of acute peritendinitis, immobilization permits healing without constant stress. Splints permit accessibility for cryotherapy, without sacrificing stability. Anti-inflammatory medication and cryotherapy reduce inflammation and increase blood supply. Return to full training schedules should be gradual. Patients with chronic Achilles peritendinitis are hardest to treat, and surgery to release the tendon from sheath tissue and remove any nodules and calcification may be undertaken. Injection of steroids is usually contraindicated; pain may be relieved, but degenerative changes in collagen fibers can result.

▶ [The authors have outlined a good preventive program to avoid the occurrence of these problems. They have included a good description of Achilles peritendinitis, along with a treatment program and rationale. I have no statistical evidence to support the statement, however, that many patients with reported Achilles tendon ruptures complain of a soreness in this area of at least 2 to 3 weeks' duration prior to the rupture. This pain may be an indicator of a severe problem, and the athlete should not try to practice or compete until pain has been relieved and satisfactory rehabilitation exercises performed.—F.G.] ◀

7–18   **Ankle Injuries: Anatomical and Biochemical Considerations Necessary for Development of Injury Prevention Program.** Greg Kaumeyer and Terry Malone (Rehabilitation Services of Mid-America, Inc., Joliet, Ill.) provide a framework for the development of an ankle injury prevention program. The program should be based on anatomical principles of the ankle relating musculoskeletal structure

(7–17)   Athletic Training 15:159–166, Fall 1980.
(7–18)   J. Orthop. Sports Phys. Ther. 1:171–177, Winter 1980.

to ankle stability, ankle biomechanisms, and the mechanisms of ankle injuries.

An adequate prevention program should encompass the following areas: screening of athletes, exercise program to strengthen the ankle, taping or wrapping the ankle prior to sports participation, and attention to shoe type and size, especially with regard to playing surface to be used. Football players with a talar tilt of 5 degrees or more experience the highest incidence of ankle injuries. For screening purposes, the lateral stability of the ankle can be assessed clinically by forcing the foot into inversion and noting the talar tilt. The strength of the peroneal muscle and the flexibility of the gastrocnemius should be assessed. Those found to be susceptible to ankle injury should be enrolled in an exercise program to maintain high levels of strength and flexibility. Although taping or wrapping the ankle reduces jumping ability slightly, it does help to prevent ankle injury. Shoes should have rigid soles. Ankle injuries occur less frequently when high-top basketball shoes are worn rather than the low-cut type.

▶ [The authors have outlined an excellent program for preventing ankle injuries. Preseason screening, exercise programs, taping and wrapping, and types of shoes to be worn are described. Ankle injuries occur very frequently in athletics. A program such as the one described by the authors may reduce the incidence of these injuries.— F.G.] ◀

7–19 **Three-Dimensional Kinematics of the Taped Ankle Before and After Exercise.** The lateral ligament complex of the ankle may be the most frequently injured single structure in the body. Prophylactic ankle taping has become a popular means of preventing ankle sprains, but some oppose the practice as expensive, time-consuming, and essentially useless. Simon found no objective documentation of the value of ankle taping or wrapping. R. K. Laughman, T. A. Carr, E. Y. Chao, J. W. Youdas, and F. H. Sim (Mayo Clinic) used the electrogoniometer to assess the ability of one taping technique to check the active physiologic motions associated with an inversion ankle sprain, both before and after a standardized exercise routine. Ankle and subtalar joint motions were recorded with a triaxial electrogoniometer as subjects walked across a level walkway and a 10-degree side slope. The subjects, of each sex, were aged 20–45 years. Taping was done using a closed basket weave with heel locks and a half-figure-eight technique.

All motions measured showed an average reduction of about 27% between the normal untaped evaluation and the taped preexercise evaluation. Loosening of the tape was noted with exercise, with an average 12% increase in joint motion. Most changes related to efficacy of taping were significant, exceptions being sagittal plane motion in the early stance phase, and parameters for the up leg on the side slope. Analysis of motion around the tibiotalar axis indicated a significant reduction in terminal stance phase plantar flexion for the taped ankle. The taped ankle was maintained in a dorsiflexed position throughout the entire gait cycle.

(7–19) Am. J. Sports Med. 8:425–431, Nov.–Dec. 1980.

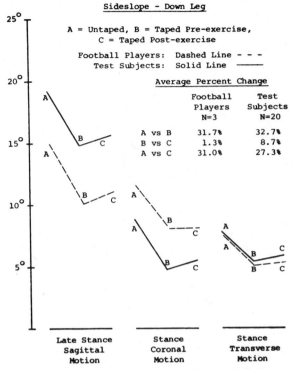

Sideslope - Down Leg

A = Untaped, B = Taped Pre-exercise,
C = Taped Post-exercise

Football Players: Dashed Line - - -
Test Subjects: Solid Line ———

Average Percent Change

	Football Players N=3	Test Subjects N=20
A vs B	31.7%	32.7%
B vs C	1.3%	8.7%
A vs C	31.0%	27.3%

Late Stance Sagittal Motion   Stance Coronal Motion   Stance Transverse Motion

Fig 7–1.—Comparison between data obtained from 3 college football players and 20 test subjects for parameters concerned with an inversion ankle sprain. (Courtesy of Laughman, R. K., et al.: Am. J. Sports Med. 8:425–431, Nov.–Dec. 1980.)

Taping appears to restrict those motions associated with inversion ankle sprain. Its efficacy is more dependent on the tensile strength than on the adhesive properties of the tape. Tape applied correctly to a joint acts as an external ligament that helps restrict excessive joint motion. The observations made in football players are compared with those in test subjects in Figure 7–1, indicating similarity between the two groups. This approach could be used to assess many current training-room practices objectively and to help establish a more scientific foundation for sports medicine.

▶ [The controversy of whether ankles should be taped continues. It has been my practice to tape all recently injured ankles to prevent reinjury or additional damage to an injured ligament. As stated in the 1980 YEAR BOOK, it may take as long as a year before complete ligament strength is restored. Therefore, a recently injured ankle should be taped for the duration of the season. Ankles that are unstable, lax, or chronically sprained should be taped to prevent reinjury. Ankles can be taped to prevent inversion-type sprains with no significant loss of range of motion or torques of ankle movement.—F.G.] ◀

7–20 **Orthoplast Splint: Support Method for a Sprained Ankle.**
Gwen E. Cleaves (Kean College of New Jersey) describes the con-

(7–20) Athletic Training 15:94–95, Summer 1980.

struction and application of the Orthoplast splint, a semirigid support for sprained ankles described by Stover (1979). It is made from Orthoplast shaped in the form of a stirrup, starts from the base of the calf, and extends along both sides of the leg underneath the heel of the foot. The splint permits plantar flexion and dorsiflexion while limiting inversion and eversion. It is relatively easy to make and can be reused.

TECHNIQUE.—A paper pattern first is cut out for the splint. The portion going beneath the heel should be about half the width of the side portions. The Orthoplast is placed in a hydrocollator for about 30 seconds before the splint is cut. While the Orthoplast is still pliable, it is fitted on the athlete's ankle in the position of application. The entire splint should fit snugly against the subject's foot and lower leg. The Orthoplast then is allowed to harden. Moleskin is applied to the parts of the splint lying under the heel and under the base of the calf, and the parts into which the malleoli protrude are padded with the plastic air bubbles used for packaging. A lubricated gauze pad is placed behind the heel and on the instep before the splint is applied. The entire ankle is covered with prewrap. Heel locks are applied with elastic tape to lend stability to the ankle while maintaining a normal range of motion.

▶ [I have experienced good results using this type of splint with first- and second-degree ankle sprains. It allows for easy removal of the splint, and an early treatment regimen can be started. I have read of people being able to participate in athletics with this support. At the university level of competition, I have not found this to be common practice. It is generally too restrictive to allow the necessary ankle mobility required in sports that involve cutting or quick changes in direction. There are similar commercial products on the market that are lined with an inner tube-type plastic bladder. These may be more comfortable, but are not molded to each individual's ankle.—F.G.] ◀

7–21 **Modified Low-Dye Strapping.** Many sports activities cause medial arch strain, plantar fascial strain, and pronation of the foot. Podiatrists have used low-dye strapping to fit orthotics for these arch and foot conditions. Jim Whitesel and Stanley G. Newell (Seattle) have used a modification of this technique, employing moleskin stirrups to support the plantar fascial plane in place of an orthotic. The moleskin stabilizes the head of the first metatarsal by plantar flexing it and holding it in the plantar-grade position, reducing forefoot pronation. The moleskin strapping is stronger than tape, gives the athlete more of an arch, and stands up to the stresses of sports activities.

TECHNIQUE.—The forefoot is cleaned, and tape is applied. Small pieces of moleskin about 1×2 in. are placed below the first and fifth metatarsal heads. A 2-in.-wide adhesive moleskin strip is cut to the size of the foot, and 3×0.5-in. angled pieces are cut from both sides of the midportion. The strip then is placed on the head of the fifth metatarsal and secured along the lateral aspect of the foot. The head of the first metatarsal is depressed, and the rest of the moleskin is secured to it. The longitudinal arch is then strapped with 1-in. adhesive tape by the "X-arch" or "scissors" method. Locking strips are placed around the dorsum of the forefoot, with care being taken not to compress the foot.

Modified low-dye strapping has been used in rehabilitating patients with the posterior tibial syndrome, posterior tibial tendinitis, peripatellar compression pain, Achilles tendon problems, and jumper's knee. James et al. (1978) found this type of conservative treatment to be effective in overuse injuries when combined with rehabilitation exercises.

▶ [I have had good success using this type of taping technique to support the plantar fascial plane of the foot. The heavier the patient, the more supporting material must be used. The moleskin can add a great deal of strength to this taping method with a minimal of added bulk. I have added support to this technique by using a moleskin strip from the metatarsal heads, following the plantar arch to just above the dorsum of the heel.—F.G.] ◀

7–22 **Fitting of Protective Football Equipment** is outlined by Joe Gieck and Frank C. McCue III (Univ. of Virginia). Properly fitted protective equipment is necessary to prevent injuries in football. Many injuries are due to improper fitting rather than inadequate protection from equipment, especially at the secondary school level, where players below the first string may receive inadequate equipment. Improper fit may also increase the severity of injury. The helmet and shoulder pads are the most important items, but other specialized pieces of equipment are also necessary to prevent injury.

The helmet should fit snugly on the head, allowing no excessive twisting in any plane. The frontal crown should be one or two finger-widths above the eyebrow. The posterior aspect should not impinge on the cervical spine with the neck extended. The outside shell should be kept slick.

Both flat shoulder pads, used by limited contact positions, and cantilever pads for constant contact are utilized. The player should be able to extend the arms overhead without impingement on the neck, but also without excessive sliding about the shoulder. The axilla straps should be as tight as is comfortable. Calipers may be used to facilitate proper fitting. A strap has been used successfully to prevent anterior shoulder dislocation. Cervical collars are a common shoulder pad accessory. A donut-fiber pad fitted to the shoulder gives added acromioclavicular protection.

Hip pads, rib pads, knee pads, and thigh pads also are used. Proper pant length and waist size are important. A wider shoe sole appears to prevent the foot and ankle from rolling into inversion and eversion better than the narrow sole. Many pads are available for use on the lower arm, but no hard fiber pad should be worn at the elbow or below. Custom-fitted pads are most important for many individual injuries. Custom-fitted mouthpieces are preferable to stock mouthpieces, although the latter are effective.

▶ [The message here is that no matter how good the equipment is, if it does not fit properly it is not going to protect. Frequently the junior varsity teams receive the leftovers, which may be of good quality but too often are not the correct size. Someone who is knowledgeable (an equipment man, a coach, a trainer) must be responsible for proper fitting of equipment. This fit must be checked periodically, but especially at the end of double sessions. Many times there is significant weight loss at the end of this period. At least once a week, helmets should be checked for loose webbing and screws, preferably the day before a game.—F.G.] ◀

(7–22) Am. J. Sports Med. 8:192–196, May–June 1980.

BUYING AND USING A PFD

Some PFDs are more rugged and durable than others, but they usually cost more too. You should evaluate the trade-offs of cost, intended use, and how often the PFD will have to be replaced when deciding which PFD to buy.

1. Try on the PFD. It should be comfortable and easy to put on and remove. It should be designed to dry quickly.
2. Try it out in the water. Your head and chin should float completely above water level. It is important that children feel comfortable with PFDs in and out of the water so they don't panic. Approved devices will keep a child afloat, but not always in a face-up position.
3. Mark your PFD with your name if you are the only wearer.
4. Do not alter your PFD to fit you. An altered device is no longer Coast Guard approved. If your PFD doesn't fit, buy a new one.
5. PFDs are not intended to be used as fenders or kneeling pads.
6. Inspect your PFD periodically to ensure that it is free of rips or holes, that flotation pads have no leaks, that seams and joints are securely sewn. Kapok fibers may lose their buoyancy after vinyl inserts are split or punctured. When kapok becomes hard or waterlogged, the PFD is no longer serviceable and must be replaced.
7. If the PFD is wet, allow it to dry thoroughly. Don't dry it in front of a radiator or other source of direct heat. Store it in a well-ventilated area.
8. If you must swim while wearing your PFD, use a back stroke or sidestroke.

7-23 **Equipment Update: PFDs Float Into Fashion.** Ray Bloomberg (Seattle) discusses the different types of personal flotation devices (PFDs) available and their proper use. The PFD, used to keep a non-swimmer afloat, includes all types of flotation devices from a life preserver to a survival suit. Type I PFDs have the greatest buoyancy and are designed to turn unconscious persons face-up in the water and keep them there. They are suitable for rough water and situations where rescue may take a long time. They are the easiest type to put on in an emergency. Type II PFDs also can turn a swimmer face-up, but are less effective than the type I device. Type III PFDs are most suitable for use in areas where potential rescuers are nearby. Many look like rain jackets. Type IV PFDs, such as a ring buoy or cushion with straps, are designed to be thrown to a person and grasped until he is rescued; they are suitable only for quick rescue situations and are not recommended for nonswimmers or children. Inflatable PFDs also are available. The Coast Guard has not indicated much support for inflatables; it probably will approve them for limited use, as in offshore sailboats and work boats. A guide to the purchase and use of PFDs is given in the table.

For handicapped persons, PFDs should have greater buoyancy and must take into account the inability of many of these persons to assume a horizontal float or even float with the head above water. Models that can be adjusted for different disabilities are being designed. Proper PFDs will permit handicapped persons to enjoy water recreational activities safely.

▶ [These are a must for all boating enthusiasts. They must never be left stored under a seat, but should be worn at all times. Many boating tragedies could be avoided if these devices were worn.—F.G.] ◀

(7-23) Physician Sportsmed. 8:101-104, July 1980.

PHYSICAL THERAPY AND REHABILITATION OF THE ATHLETE

7-24 **Normal Joint Structures and Their Reactions to Injury.** Dixie L. Hettinga (Wausaw, Wis., Med. Center) discusses the reactions of articular cartilage to injury. Hyaline cartilage is the actual load-carrying surface of the synovial joint. It is only about 1–7 mm thick in healthy joints. Its chief constituents are collagen, protein-polysaccharide, and water. Small numbers of chondrocytes are present, surrounded by a lattice of collagen fibrils enmeshed in ground substance. The matrix of articular cartilage is hyperhydrated. Movement of fluid into and out of articular cartilage appears to be produced by diffusion and osmosis. The collagen fibers as a whole are at right angles to the surface of the subchondral bone to which they are attached. Articular cartilage appears to act primarily as a bearing surface, distributing loads, rather than as a shock absorber. The chief contribution to peak force attenuation is made by the soft tissue structures and bone, rather than the cartilage and synovial fluid.

Microscopic damage may be found when joint stress is insufficient to cause a clinical fracture of the subchondral bone. Trauma to synovial joints can result in subsequent osteoarthritis or degenerative joint disease. The factors in cartilage degeneration are interrelated in Figure 7–2. Early degenerative changes may be asymptomatic until synovitis with effusion develops. Osteophytes can cause extensive deformity of the articular bone ends, pain from stretching of the periosteum, and limited movement (Fig 7–3). Treatment involves heat,

Fig 7–2.—Postulated final pathway of cartilage degeneration. (Courtesy of Hettinga, D. L.: J. Orthop. Sports Phys. Ther. 1:178–185, Winter 1980.)

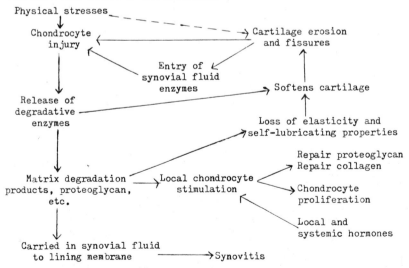

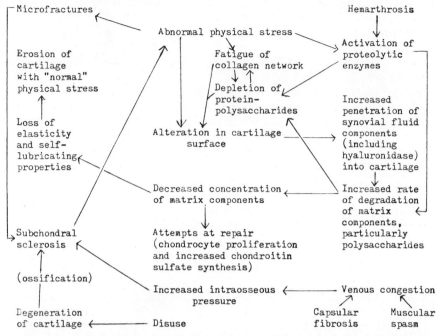

Fig 7–3.—Pathophysiology of osteoarthritis. (Courtesy of Hettinga, D. L.: J. Orthop. Sports Phys. Ther. 1:178–185, Winter 1980.)

and evaluation of daily activities, and active flexion and extension exercises of the joint. After 6–8 weeks, analgesic and anti-inflammatory drugs can be used if necessary, but exercise should still be restricted. Trauma can lead to a form of arthritis through cracking or fibrillation of the intra-articular cartilage with subsequent atrophy, and scarring or weakening of the intra- and extra-articular supporting structures. The ability of the joint to withstand the physiologic trauma caused by motion and weight-bearing is thereby reduced.

▶ [This is the third and final part of an excellent series on joint structures and their reaction to injury. I would strongly recommend the study of this series for all those who are serious about understanding what occurs when a joint is injured.—F.G.] ◀

7–25 **Injuries to the Elbow in Athletics** are discussed by J. Pat Evans (Sports Medicine Clinic of North Texas, Inc., Dallas). The athletic trainer should be able to recognize elbow injuries, since adequate treatment will promote healing and allow a return to function, while inadequate management may result in permanent disability to the athlete. Soft tissue injuries may involve the skin and muscular tissues or the bursae about the elbow. Any forceful stretching of the elbow to gain range of motion only results in subsequent loss of the motion that has been achieved. Injuries to the olecranon bursa are managed with ice, rest, and compression. Acute strain may be pre-

(7–25) Athletic Training 15:78–81, Summer 1980.

vented by adequate training and warm-up and avoidance of sudden excessive overloading by the untrained athlete. The early recognition of overuse and treatment by ice, rest, and gradual active stretching, followed by strengthening exercises, will minimize chronic overuse syndromes. Ultrasound or galvanic stimulation may be helpful in reducing scar tissue formation. In cases of sprain, the athlete must not return prematurely to activities.

Injuries to neural structures about the elbow are most frequent in collision sports, where contusions of the medial arm may bruise the ulnar nerve. Osteochondritis dissecans is seen in the skeletally immature elbow; if abuse continues, a loose body may form. Elbow fractures are not common, even in collision sports, but they may occur in basketball, soccer, and gymnastics. In throwing sports, loose bodies may form, and small osteocartilaginous fractures may develop in the elbow joint. Synovial irritation may require the removal of loose bodies. Spurs and loose bodies can be prevented only by reducing the total amount of throwing done through the years. If the elbow remains asymptomatic during active participation, it may be possible to continue the activity and remove the loose bodies electively at the end of the season.

▶ [When attempting to improve elbow joint range of motion after an injury, I have three words of advice: *CAUTION, CAUTION, CAUTION.* Passive stretching of a contracted elbow must not be done. Increasing triceps strength and active joint extension exercises are the only way to stretch tight elbow flexors. Holding a heavy weight in the hand of a contracted elbow will only increase the stimulus of the flexors to contract.

Overuse syndromes of the elbow can be avoided by using proper technique and sensible exercise programs. Good coaching is a must to teach the proper mechanics of throwing a baseball or javelin or hitting a tennis ball. No matter how much treatment, exercise, and rehabilitation is done, if the athlete uses poor technique and body mechanics the problem will most certainly recur.

The progression of treatment involves: (1) reducing the inflammation; (2) improving flexibility of the wrist, elbow, and shoulder; (3) improving strength of the wrist, elbow, and shoulder; (4) improving throwing or stroking techniques.—F.G.] ◀

7–26 **Effects of Strength Training and Immobilization on Human Muscle Fibers.** The fast twitch (FT) muscle fibers of well-trained weight lifters reportedly are considerably larger than those of endurance-trained athletes, whereas the slow twitch (ST) fibers are the same size in both groups. Compensatory hypertrophy in animals shows a marked increase in the apparent nuclei to fiber ratio. J. D. MacDougall, G. C. B. Elder, D. G. Sale, J. R. Moroz, and J. R. Sutton (McMaster Univ., Hamilton, Ont.) studied the effects of 5–6 months of heavy resistance training and 5–6 weeks of arm immobilization by elbow casts in 7 healthy male volunteers. Cross-sectional fiber areas and nuclei to fiber ratios were calculated for cryostat sections of needle biopsy specimens obtained from the long head of triceps brachii.

Elbow extension strength increased by 98% ($P<.01$) following training and decreased by 41% ($P<.05$) following immobilization. During the control period, the FT fibers were approximately 42% larger than the ST fibers. Comparison of posttraining results with

(7–26) Eur. J. Appl. Physiol. 43:25–34, February 1980.

postimmobilization values showed a 39% increase in FT fiber area and a 31% increase in ST fiber area; when compared with control values, the increases were 17% and 15%, respectively. Immobilization caused a 30% reduction in FT fiber areas and a 25% reduction in ST fiber areas compared with control values. Training produced a 10% increase in the apparent nuclei to fiber ratio, but the increase was not significant. No significant correlations were found between the changes in maximal elbow extension strength and the changes in FT and ST fiber areas.

The results indicate that significant changes occur in FT and ST fibers following resistance training or immobilization, with FT fibers showing the greater increase or decrease. The absence of a significant increase in the nuclei to fiber ratio does not exclude its possibility, because light microscopy is not sufficient to distinguish true nuclei from other possible dark-staining material.

▶ [Of note is the fact that there was little or no correlation between the magnitude of the hypertrophy or atrophy effect and the changes in maximal voluntary contractile strength observed after a training program or period of immobilization.—J.S.T.] ◀

7-27 **Mechanisms of Selected Knee Injuries.** George J. Davies, Lynn A. Wallace, and Terry Malone clarify different mechanisms according to their classification of injury to provide physical therapists a better understanding of knee trauma.

Microtrauma, a series of inflammatory reactions to submaximal loading that eventually produce clinical signs, is caused by normal forces occurring about the knee, by excessive normal forces (overuse syndromes), or by excessive loads produced through abnormal biomechanics. Overuse syndromes can be caused by (1) high repetition, low load or (2) low repetition, high load. Biomechanical abnormalities produce microtrauma because any malalignment causes biomechanical changes, placing abnormal stress on particular tissues. Discrepancies in limb length, insufficient flexibility, unbalanced muscular strengths and power, or improper gait can result in microtrauma. Manifestations of microtrauma are strain, inflammation-tendinitis, effusion, sprain, chondromalacia patellae and Osgood-Schlatter disease.

Macrotrauma results from injury causing immediate clinical signs and symptoms. The resulting sprains or strains are classified as first, second, or third degree (mild, moderate, or severe, respectively); a third-degree injury is complete disruption of the musculotendinous unit or of the noncontractile structures. Straight one-plane instabilities include straight anterior, straight posterior, straight medial (Fig 7-4) and straight lateral instabilities and combined injury. Transverse plane rotatory instabilities include anterior medial, anterior lateral and posterior lateral rotatory instabilities or combinations of the above. Factors affecting the severity of the injury include tension of the tissues on contact, position of the joint, angular velocity of the joint, and the speed, duration, and severity of the impact force. Tis-

(7-27) Phys. Ther. 60:1590-1595, December 1980.

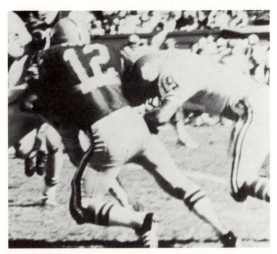

Fig 7–4.—Number 12 (tackler) is sustaining a blow to the lateral aspect of the right leg, stressing the medial structures of the right knee. This produces a contrecoup type of injury. (Courtesy of Davies, G. J., et al.: Phys. Ther. 60:1590–1595, December 1980; reprinted with the permission of the American Physical Therapy Association.)

sues that are taut when force is applied will sustain the most damage.

▶ [The authors have outlined a good description of the mechanisms of knee injuries. They describe mechanisms of injuries involving both microtrauma and macrotrauma of the knee. The injured knee is a major concern of the athletic trainer. Programs have been designed for preseason screening to prevent these injuries, and a number of reconditioning and rehabilitation programs are used to prevent their recurrence.— F.G.] ◄

7–28 **Knee Examination** is outlined by George J. Davies, Terry Malone, and Frank H. Bassett III. Effective management and rehabilitation of the knee begin with a detailed history and a thorough, systematic examination. The uninvolved knee is first examined to obtain a data base for comparison with the involved knee. Forceful procedures are avoided, particularly with an acute knee injury. Usually, the patient has the most awareness of what has occurred. The patient should be allowed to demonstrate actively where possible.

First, the total patient is observed, with special attention to the legs. A gait evaluation then is carried out, and anthropometric measurements are obtained to determine the severity of swelling or muscle atrophy. Leg length measurements are obtained. All joints that could refer pain to the knee and all that could have been injured should be checked. Gentle palpation is used to help locate the injured anatomical structures and sites of irritability. Neurologic testing follows, with assessment of sensation, reflexes, balance, and range of motion. Goniometric measurements are made of passive movements of the hip, knee, ankle, subtalar, and forefoot joints. Resisted movement testing is carried out as part of the neurologic examination.

(7–28) Phys. Ther. 60:1565–1574, December 1980.

Manual muscle testing is done with the muscle in the shortened, mid-range, and stretched positions. Flexibility should be assessed.

Many specific tests exist for further assessment of the anatomical structures involved and of the severity of the injuries sustained. These include tests of ligamentous structures and of rotational instability. Functional tests include such maneuvers as sprinting, running in place, squatting, and running up stairs. The isokinetic dynamometer may add information on strength, power, endurance, and range-of-motion problems. Special-view roentgenograms, arthrography, and arthroscopy may be indicated in various circumstances. Standard knee evaluation forms should be used by clinicians at each facility in order to standardize testing and establish a data base at initial evaluation.

▶ [Examination of the injured knee has developed into a very exact science and should be approached with a great deal of forethought and study. The authors bring out the very important point that forceful procedures are avoided, particularly with the presence of an acute knee injury. I have often wondered how much damage could be done to the acutely injured knee by repeated forceful testing procedures.

The clinical examination of the injured knee is still the most useful diagnostic tool in determining knee dysfunction. A thorough examination must be done before any rehabilitation programs can be instituted.—F.G.] ◀

7–29 **Knee Rehabilitation** is reviewed by Terry Malone, Turner A. Blackburn, and Lynn A. Wallace. The authors' rehabilitation program is based on high repetition and relatively low resistance to minimize stress on the knee. Treatment decisions have been based on empirical data rather than on controlled laboratory studies, and clinical research is needed to verify the procedures. If knee surgery is done, outcome depends on a disciplined exercise program for both athletes and nonathletes. The programs are designed to be used at home. Rehabilitation is begun as soon as possible after injury or operation. The chronically involved knee will benefit from an exercise program to the degree that the problem can be decreased through improved strength or flexibility. Vigorous rehabilitation is indicated after surgery for either acute or chronic problems to rebuild the strength of the involved extremity as well as the entire body.

A quadriceps femoris setting program is instituted after acute injury. Straight-leg raises are done 3 times a day, out of the supporting wrap if possible, and minimum terminal extensions also can be performed to encourage full extension and "squeeze" the knee effusion. In extensor mechanism injuries, resistance for straight-leg-raising exercises is a maximum of 15 lb; most patients should be able to reach 10 lb. Bicycle riding can be encouraged in some instances. Patients with meniscal injuries perform flexion-to-extension exercises to strengthen the quadriceps femoris mechanism. Chronic ligamentous injuries will respond to quadriceps femoris setting, straight-leg raises, and hamstring stretching. Depending on the condition of the joint, flexion-to-extension exercises can be instituted. Posterolateral

(7–29)   Phys. Ther. 60:1602–1609, December 1980.

instabilities are exercised in an arc lacking 10 degrees of full extension. Bicycling is also indicated for these problems.

The time that treatment is begun depends on the patient and on the procedure done. Exercises can be done with the patient in a hinge cast, with resistance kept very low for quadriceps femoris muscle exercises, at 5 lb or below for the first month. The knee must come into extension slowly and under active quadriceps femoris power, and passive extension should be avoided. Subsequently, isokinetic exercise can be used in either a complete or a limited arc. Advanced rehabilitation for athletes stresses the functional and specific aspects of the sport in question. Many patients can benefit from a supportive knee appliance during physical therapy to protect tissue healing, compensate for decreased internal stability, or alter the biomechanics of the knee.

▶ [The authors have stressed the need for an individualized knee rehabilitation program. They have underlined the avoidance of passively stretching the knee into extension. All extension work should be done actively and with slow progression. An entire surgical repair could be compromised by passively stretching the knee into extension. The authors have also stressed the importance of limiting the amount of weight used in straight-leg-raising exercises, because of the stress placed on the hip and low back.

The importance of hamstring stretching is underlined to help prevent compression of the patella against the femur. The need for a wide variety of exercises and structured exercise programs is a very important point brought out in this article.—F.G.] ◀

7–30 **Quadriceps Function and Training After Knee Ligament Surgery.** Quadriceps atrophy is a well-recognized finding after knee injuries. G. Grimby, E. Gustafsson, L. Peterson, and P. Renström (Univ. of Göteborg) report a follow-up study of 30 subjects with a mean age of 26 years. These subjects were operated on for knee ligament injuries, which in all cases but 1 were incurred in sports, usually soccer. The patients had isolated ruptures of the medial collateral ligament or anterior cruciate ligament; some had combination injuries. Sixteen were operated on acutely, whereas 14 had old injuries reconstructed because of knee joint instability. Postoperatively, patients spent 3 weeks in a full leg cast and 3 in a knee cast allowing full weight-bearing. The training program is illustrated in Figure 7–5. Self-training was supervised by a physical therapist, usually once a week, for 2–3 months. The athletes returned to athletic training after a mean time of 14 weeks. The mean time from surgery to the start of training was 14 months. All patients had full knee extension and at least 100 degrees of knee flexion without pain.

Maximal isometric and isokinetic torque for knee extension was measured, and vastus lateralis biopsies were obtained. Maximal torque values were reduced on the side operated on despite the resumption of athletic training. Isokinetic training, weight training, and self-training all led to increased muscle strength; the greatest increase was with isokinetic training. Initially mean fiber areas were somewhat low, especially for type II fibers, and a tendency toward an

(7–30) Med. Sci. Sports Exerc. 12:70–75, Spring 1980.

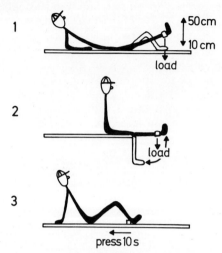

Fig 7–5.—Training program for the self-training group. Training leg is black, nontraining leg is white. All exercises are repeated 25–50 times at each session: **1**, the training leg is raised from 10 to 50 cm with a load of 2–8 kg; **2**, the training leg is fully extended with a load of 2–8 kg; **3**, the training leg is pressed for 10 seconds against a fixed resistance such as a doorstep. (Courtesy of Grimby, G., et al.: Med. Sci. Sports Exerc. 12:70–75, Spring 1980; copyright 1980, the American College of Sports Medicine. Reprinted by permission.)

increase was noted after training. No significant change in adenosine triphosphate, creatine phosphate, or contractile enzyme activities occurred with training.

More systematic follow-up of patients who have had knee injury is needed. Spontaneous activity, including athletic training, often may not suffice to restore muscle function. Additional training should be used for longer periods than conventional physiotherapeutic programs. Isokinetic training can be recommended for well-motivated subjects. With isokinetic training, maximal torque can be achieved through the whole range of motion, in contrast to weight training.

▶ [This study also emphasizes the importance of a structured knee rehabilitation program after knee surgery. Athletes cannot be left to their own devices and ideas to regain proper knee function. The authors state, "The isokinetic training principle can be recommended for well-motivated subjects." It has been my experience that the more motivation athletes have to return to activity, the better they will progress in a rehabilitation program. With the proper instruction and guidance and enough motivation, it is remarkable how well these repaired knees can be rehabilitated.

I will take the liberty to write again that no "one" program is best for all postoperative knees. Each case must be approached individually, and the type of reconstruction must be the basis of the exercise program developed. The speed at which the athlete progresses is also individualized according to pain, swelling, joint motion, and muscle function.—F.G.] ◀

7–31 **Rehabilitation of First- and Second-Degree Sprains of Medial Collateral Ligament.** J. R. Steadman (South Lake Tahoe, Calif.) describes in general terms an active rehabilitation program for grade 1 or 2 sprains of the medial collateral ligament of the knee.

(7–31) Am. J. Sports Med. 7:300–302, Sept.–Oct. 1979.

The presence of cruciate injury should be excluded before therapy is undertaken. Rehabilitation should begin as early as possible with a manual resistive exercise program accompanied by electrical stimulation of the quadriceps; exercise of the uninjured leg can begin immediately. The manual resistive program involves a series of 7 exercises. Initially, the exercises are performed with light resistance and low movement; resistance, speed, and duration are increased as symptoms decrease. The absence of patellofemoral loading with exercise of lower resistance and longer duration is important. If the patient was involved in extensive daily running before the injury occurred, knee exercise for 3–5 minutes seems sensible. As the patient becomes accustomed to manual resistive exercise, a Cybex or other isokinetic machine can be used in rehabilitation. The use of Cybex printouts is valuable in monitoring and evaluating the patient's progress. Variable resistance, the NK table, or a weight shoe can be used if an isokinetic machine is unavailable.

As therapy progresses, the "Tahoe Marathon" exercise is introduced. This consists of 30 knee extensions with about 75% resistance followed by rapid exercise with low resistance until a burning sensation develops in the thigh. The patient then performs an isometric exercise for 1 minute and the cycle is begun again without interruption. Electric stimulation of the muscle during exercise can be provided by faradic, galvanic, or transcutaneous nerve stimulation. Transcutaneous stimulation is preferred because it treats pain simultaneously with muscle stimulation, even though the muscle contractions so induced are not as satisfactory as those induced by stronger units. Stimulation is applied for 5 seconds to achieve tetanic contractions, followed by a rest period of 5 seconds. This regimen is carried out for 1 hour daily, and the entire exercise program is continued for 5–7 days a week. If patellofemoral pain or swelling occurs, appropriate modifications in exercise and electric stimulation should be made.

▶ [One of the many points the author brings out in this article is "The presence of a cruciate injury should be excluded before therapy is begun." The reason for this is that the quadriceps mechanism acts as an antagonist to the support provided by the anterior cruciate ligament. In the presence of anterior cruciate ligament damage, the hamstrings and other knee flexors must be strengthened because they act as synergists to the anterior cruciate ligament. When sufficient knee flexor strength has been developed and enough time has passed for ligament healing to occur, then quadriceps strength can be restored.

The author has also stated the importance of maintaining cardiovascular fitness and has described methods of achieving this despite the knee injury.—F.G.] ◀

7–32 **Patellar Malalignment: Treatment Rationale** is presented by Lonnie Paulos, Ken Rusche, Charles Johnson, and Frank R. Noyes. Patellar malalignment, the most common patellofemoral disorder leading to surgery, may be either permanent or recurrent. Understanding the biomechanics (Fig 7–6) and pathophysiology helps the therapist deal with the surgical procedures and postoperative rehabilitation. The University of Cincinnati Sports Medicine Institute has a four-phase "Patella Protection Program" designed to minimize the

(7–32) Phys. Ther. 60:1624–1632, December 1980.

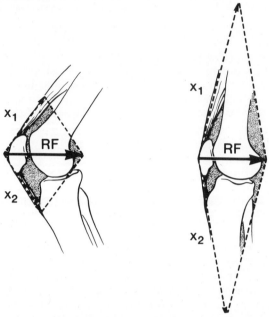

Fig 7–6.—The patellofemoral joint reaction force *(RF)* decreases as the knee moves from flexion to extension. Note how the patella acts as a fulcrum to increase the leverage of the quadriceps femoris muscle. (Courtesy of Paulos, L., et al.: Phys. Ther. 60:1624–1632, December 1980; reprinted with the permission of the American Physical Therapy Association.)

forces across the patellofemoral joint while strengthening the quadriceps. This program is the basis for nonoperative treatment and postoperative rehabilitation. Each phase has specific goals, exercises, and built-in restrictions to guide progression.

Period 1, initial rehabilitation, involves the acutely affected knee. Goals are to relieve pain, decrease atrophic response, and decrease inflammation. Six to ten sets of isometric exercises are repeated ten times daily with 10-second contractions. Flexibility exercises for the total lower extremity are included. Period 2, intermediate rehabilitation, begins when range of motion increases and pain and effusion decrease. The goal is to increase muscular strength without increasing pain or effusion. Terminal extension exercises, using progressive resistance, and lateral step-ups are used. Period 3, advanced rehabilitation, has goals of obtaining maximum strength, alternating endurance activities, and obtaining normal range of motion. This phase is initiated when the patient can do terminal extension exercises with about 10–15 lb of resistance. Isotonic weight equipment is used and the isometric program is discontinued. Extension exercises are limited to 0–30 degrees; resistance increases to about one fourth of body weight. Hamstring exercises are conducted and flexibility exercises continued. Endurance activities such as swimming or cycling are done on alternate days. Period 4, return to activity and maintenance, aims to return the patient slowly to specific activities of choice and to continue strength and endurance training. A 75% level of power and endurance should be obtained before a running program is allowed; 90% should be reached before return to full activity.

The association of chondromalacia with recurrent malalignment is well known, and physical therapists should be aware of the tendency for the condition to progress after surgery. If signs of increasing chondromalacia occur, patellofemoral forces should be decreased at once. Such indications of complication as decreased knee flexion, medial instability, patella infera, recurvatum, rotation of the patella in the femoral groove, rupture of the patellar tendon, infection, peroneal nerve palsy, detachment of the tibial bone block, thrombophlebitis or anterior compartment syndrome must be watched for and reported by the physical therapist.

▶ [The rehabilitation program I use for patients with patella malalignment problems is different. With this type of patient, we never progress to the use of isotonic weight equipment. We never do repetitive-type exercises from 90 degrees of flexion to full extension. Not using this equipment may extend the rehabilitation time. However, we feel it is safer to avoid increasing the patellofemoral joint pressure. A good deal of time is spent with the athlete, explaining the problem and the types of exercise that are allowed.—F.G.] ◀

7–33 **Selective Training of the Vastus Medialis Muscle Using EMG Biofeedback.** Patellofemoral joint problems are a frequent clinical occurrence. The forces produced by the vastus medialis (VM) muscle and the vastus lateralis (VL) affect lateral alignment of the patella, and correct alignment of the extensor mechanism of the knee depends

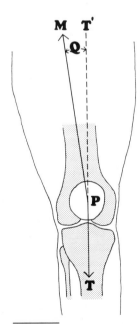

Fig 7–7.—The "Q" angle formed by the resultant vector of the quadriceps femoris muscle *(M)* and by the line of pull of patellar tendon *(T')*: *P*, patella; *T*, vector representing patellar tendon. (Courtesy of LeVeau, B. F., and Rogers, C.: Phys. Ther. 60:1410–1415, November 1980; reprinted with the permission of the American Physical Therapy Association.)

on proper function of the VM. Barney F. LeVeau and Carol Rogers (Univ. of North Carolina, Chapel Hill) attempted to determine whether electromyographic (EMG) biofeedback can be used to train the VM to contract independently of the VL to adjust patellar alignment through muscle control. Determinants of patellar motion are illustrated in Figure 7–7. Poor patellar alignment can result in a hypermobile patella or in chondromalacia.

The VM must be trained to contrast with enough force to balance the force of the VL. Biofeedback training was evaluated in 5 volunteer subjects of each sex, aged 22–29 years. Training sessions were held for 30 minutes 5 days a week for 3 weeks. Electrodes were applied to the areas of greatest muscle bulk of the VM and VL muscles. Subjects were asked to reduce muscle activity in the VL while maintaining a constant percentage of the reference activity level in the VM, over a 2-week period. Then they increased VM activity while maintaining VL activity below a daily determined percentage of the reference level. In this phase, the threshold for VL activity was set at the average percentage for the past 2 days of training, and the VM EMG unit threshold was raised in increments of about 1.25 μl.

The initial procedure had only limited success. The VL muscle activity did decline significantly, but the subjects had some difficulty in maintaining the set muscle activity level for the VM. The later phase of training was more successful. An overall significant difference of 6.5% between the activity levels of the VM and VL was achieved during the 3-week training period. Some subjects apparently benefited from having a pillow placed under the knee. The subjects varied in the ways in which they concentrated to achieve successful results.

If the VM muscle can gain in strength compared with the VL, a conservative treatment procedure might be devised to obtain greater muscle strength in the VM. This may make possible the conservative management of such knee disorders as hypermobile patella, chondromalacia, progressive lateral subluxation, and degenerative arthritis of the patellofemoral joint.

▶ [Selective training of the vastus medialis muscle has been high on the list in many knee rehabilitation programs. Success has not been achieved easily. Many techniques have been attempted, and it appears that the use of biofeedback had some limited success. The vastus lateralis muscle definitely has a biomechanical advantage when extending the knee. This advantage can cause an increase of symptoms in those athletes with chondromalacia and subluxating patellae. In the past few years electric muscle stimulation of the VM has been used with some success in knee rehabilitation programs.—F.G.] ◀

7–34 **Comparison of Electro-Myo Stimulation to Isokinetic Training in Increasing Power of the Knee Extensor Mechanism** is reported by John W. Halbach and Don Straus. The Soviet Union has apparently used Electro-Myo stimulation (EMS) with great success to increase the strength and power of large muscle groups, in less time than is needed with normal weight training. The theory is that, if all the motor units are innervated, the muscle will contract maximally

(7–34) J. Orthop. Sports Phys. Ther. 2:20–24, Summer 1980.

on faradic stimulation. At present, strength and power training in the United States is basically done with isometric, isotonic, and isokinetic exercises over at least 8–10 weeks. Competitive athletes would benefit from a shorter rehabilitation time.

Three subjects using isokinetics and 3 using EMS alone, both with an average age of 27 years, were compared. Fifteen sessions were held over 3 weeks to increase knee extensor power. The faradic setting for EMS was determined by the subject's tolerance. Conventional training was with the Cybex Orthotron.

The isokinetic group had an average total increase of 42% in extensor power over 3 weeks, compared to 22% for the EMS group. Thus, isokinetics appeared to increase power more efficiently than EMS over the same period. The amount of faradic current tolerated increased significantly as training continued, but after treatments at maximal tolerance, there generally was a fall in the amount of current tolerated because of muscle soreness. The isokinetic group had minimal muscle soreness after treatment sessions. Girth measurements could not be related to the outcome of training.

Both isokinetics and EMS increased knee extensor power in this study, but isokinetics were superior to EMS. Pain and burning are the chief limiting factors in the amplitude of faradic current achieved with EMS. Questions remain about the effects of EMS when subjects tolerate over 25 mamp in a treatment session.

▶ [This study indicates that isokinetic exercise is a better method of increasing knee extensor power than electric muscle stimulation. It appears that the subjects were not rehabilitating injured knees. Thus, the question remains: "Is a conventional program of exercise equal to a program of exercise plus electric muscle stimulation for the atrophied quadriceps muscle?" It is possible that if electric muscle stimulation can reduce some of the postoperative or postinjury pain, then more exercise can be done with better and quicker results.—F.G.] ◀

7–35 **Muscle Strength at the Trunk.** Gary L. Smidt, Louis R. Amundsen, and William F. Dostal (Univ. of Iowa) measured trunk flexor and extensor strength during isometric, concentric, and eccentric muscle contraction in 11 normal men aged 21–37. The Iowa Force Table was adapted to test pelvic and lower extremity strength. The men were placed in the side-lying position to minimize the effect of gravity. Muscle strength was expressed as moments of force (the external force times its moment arm) in newton-meter (N-m) units.

The coefficients of correlation between measurements at 20 degrees extension, neutral position, and 20 degrees and 40 degrees flexion was excellent for both extension and flexion. Measurements from isometric contractions were significantly ($P < .05$) more reliable than measurements from dynamic contractions. The extensor-flexor ratio at 20 degree intervals of trunk position ranged from 1.7 to 3.78. A greater N-m was recorded for eccentric (lengthening) contractions than for concentric (shortening) contractions of the same muscle group (Fig 7–8). The N-m recorded during isometric, eccentric, and concentric contractions of trunk extensors was always greater than

(7–35) J. Orthop. Sports Phys. Ther. 1:165–170, Winter 1980.

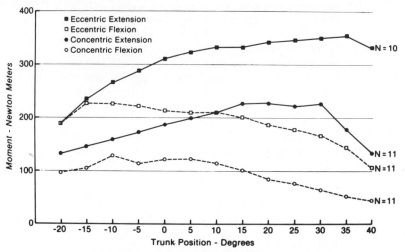

Fig 7–8.—Average moments produced by extensors and flexors through range of trunk motion. (Courtesy of Smidt, G. L., et al.: J. Orthop. Sports Phys. Ther. 1:165–170, Winter 1980.)

that of trunk flexors. Because the effect of table friction on each man was not accounted for, the measurements for concentric contractions were biased downward, whereas those for eccentric contractions were biased upward.

The results have certain clinical implications. Because the flexed position enhanced maximal trunk extensor torque, pelvic tilt exercise is indicated if treatment is intended to improve the efficiency of weak back muscles affected by chronic strain. The results of isometric tests in a 40-degree flexed position indicate that weak back extensors should be exercised when the trunk is flexed. The results provide useful reference data for assessing the significance of trunk muscle weakness in patients with low back dysfunction.

▶ [The best way to rehabilitate patients with chronic low back problems has been a controversial issue among therapists and trainers for many years. At one time, only flexion exercises were ever considered. Then, back extension-type exercise programs came into vogue. It seems that one type of program is not the answer for all back problems. A complete evaluation and workup of each individual problem must be done. Then a proper exercise program can be developed, which may include both types of exercise. Hopefully, the days of the one exercise program for all problems are gone.—F.G.] ◀

7–36 **A Functional Approach in the Rehabilitation of the Ankle and Rear Foot** is described by Russell D. Fiore and John S. Leard. Injuries of the ankle and rear part of the foot still are frequent in sports. The complex of the rear part of the foot involves multiarticular function. The individual joint axes are obliquely oriented to one another and to the cardinal planes of the body, and each of the joints acts in combination with one another to provide a wide variety of motion. Sprains occur when the capsule and ligaments are placed un-

(7–36) Athletic Training 15:231–235, Winter 1980.

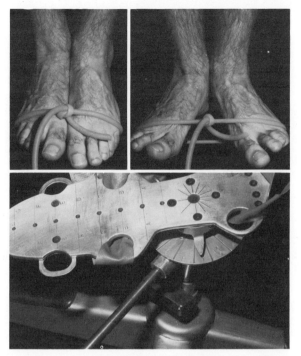

Fig 7–9 (top).—Eversion with rubber tubing. *Left,* tubing in place. *Right,* tubing with feet everted.

Fig 7–10 (bottom).—Close-up view of multiaxial PRE-resistive mechanism.
(Courtesy of Fiore, R. D., and Leard, J. S.: Athletic Training 15:231–235, Winter 1980.)

der excessive stress because the stabilizing muscles are not strong enough or do not act quickly enough to offer protection. Cutting maneuvers in sports such as football and soccer increase inversion sprains. Certain footwear and playing surfaces add traction or rotation and discourage foot release. Incomplete rehabilitation of the ankle after an injury may also increase the risk of injury.

A variety of progressive exercise routines are used in rehabilitation of injuries of the ankle and rear part of the foot. Initial care is designed to limit the extent of injury. Restoration of motion and function follows, with subsequently work to increase strength, agility, and endurance. The gap between the latter phases of rehabilitation can be bridged exercises that may be incorporated into the regimen as soon as possible. Straight plane exercises include heel raises, heel walking, eversion with rubber tubing (Fig 7–9), uniaxial progressive resistance exercise (PRE), manual resistance, and multiaxial PRE (Figs 7–10 and 7–11). Diagonal maneuvers and combinations of diagonal, straight plane, and circumduction maneuvers also are used. Balancing and coordination exercises include unilateral balance, teeter board-uniaxial exercise (Fig 7–12), teeter board-multiaxial exercise (Fig 7–13), and jumping rope. A program using these types of

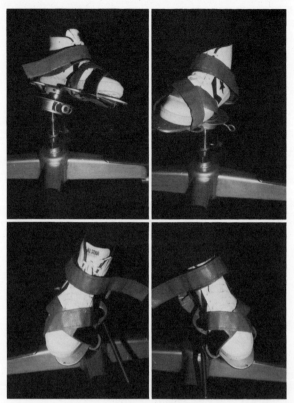

Fig 7–11.—Ranges of movements of multiaxial PRE machine. (Courtesy of Fiore R. D., and Leard, J. S.: Athletic Training 15:231–235, Winter 1980.)

Fig 7–12 (left).—Teeter board, uniaxial (underside view).
Fig 7–13 (right).—Teeter board, multiaxial (underside view).
(Courtesy of Fiore, R. D., and Leard, J. S.: Athletic Training 15:231–235, Winter 1980.)

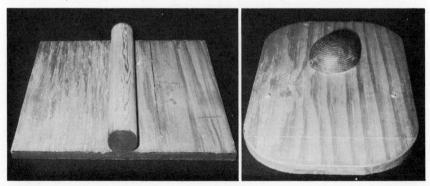

exercises, and which is carefully designed to meet the individual's needs progressively, will insure the best possible functional return and prevent the weakness and imbalance that lead to reinjury.

▶ [As stated in the 1979 YEAR BOOK, strength, flexibility, coordination, and proprioception are all important aspects of ankle rehabilitation. Proper progression in each stage of rehabilitation is important. Final testing of the athlete must be done on the gym floor or on the field, using a series of progressive running and cutting exercises and drills before the athlete is allowed to return to participation.

The multiaxial ankle exerciser is an adjunct to the total ankle rehabilitation program. It is a new device that allows for progressive resistance in straight planes, diagonals, and rotatory patterns.—F.G.] ◀

7–37 **Restoration of Dorsiflexion After Injuries to the Distal Leg and Ankle** is disucssed by Peter G. Kramer (Johnson State College, Johnson, Vt.). Many injuries result in a reduction in ankle motion, most commonly fractures of the distal part of the leg and the ankle. Restricted dorsiflexion often is minimal and is missed on clinical examination, but it must be eliminated to ensure normal function. The relevant bony anatomy is shown in Figures 7–14 and 7–15. Active dorsiflexion is produced by muscles in the anterior compartment of the leg, which are relatively superficial and often are injured with fractures or contusions of the distal part of the leg. The plantar flexors in the posterior compartment often cause restricted dorsiflexion.

Rehabilitation is based on free gliding of the tibia on the talus, return of the plantar flexors to their full amplitude if contractures are present, and the reestablishment of normal mobility of the distal tibiofibular joint. Normal tibiotalar motion is aided by applying traction through the foot parallel to the long axis of the leg to distract the ankle and free the articular surfaces. Tightness of the plantar flexors can be reduced with the use of a modification of Knott's contract-relax technique, or passively by the patient's standing with the

Fig 7–14 (left).—Superior view of the tibial articular surface of the talus.
Fig 7–15 (right).—Frontal view of ankle mortise.
(Courtesy of Kramer, P. G.: J. Orthop. Sports Phys. Ther. 1:159–164, Winter 1980.)

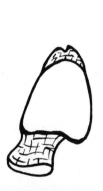
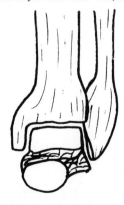

forefoot on a step and allowing the body weight to stretch the muscles. Normal motion in the distal tibiofibular syndesmosis can be restored by stabilizing the tibial malleolus while gliding the distal fibula posteriorly, with the ankle in a few degrees of plantar flexion.

These techniques can be used effectively in most ankle conditions where limited dorsiflexion is present. Any ankle with structural instability or hypermobility must be carefully assessed before starting this type of treatment. Any open reduction or procedure requiring internal fixation must be taken into account. Within these limitations, good results can be expected in a majority of patients with injuries of the leg and ankle.

▶ [I would strongly recommend, as the author does, that full ankle dorsiflexion and flexibility of the posterior ankle musculotendinous unit must be restored after ankle injuries. Tightness of these structures is often a contributing factor in lateral ankle sprains and shin splints. Most ankle reconditioning programs begin with stretching of these structures and range of motion exercises to increase ankle joint dorsiflexion. Special attention must be paid to the flexibility of these structures in joggers and older athletes who participate in racket sports.—F.G.] ◀

7–38 **Ankle Reconditioning With TNS** is described by Al Peppard and Hubert Riegler (SUNY, Brockport). Reconditioning can be started once an ankle sprain has stabilized, usually within 24–48 hours on treatment with rest, immobilization, elevation, and ice. Pain must be reduced to a level permitting comfortable exercise before reconditioning. Cryotherapy is effective when pain is intense and constant. Either cryotherapy or thermotherapy can be tried when pain is dull and mild. If sharp, intermittent pain is present, transcutaneous neural stimulation (TNS) will be effective.

One electrode is placed over the trigger point and the other distal and posterior to the lateral malleolus. If a single-channel TNS unit is used, only the injured ankle is treated. The athlete increases the amplitude at maximal frequency until a comfortably intense sensation is felt, and the pulse width then is gradually increased. The athlete begins exercising after 15 minutes of TNS, keeping the unit in place. Shifting weight from foot to foot and short-step walking are followed by long-step walking, straight-ahead jogging, lazy-S and then sharp-Z running, and short-specific movements. Initial exercise periods may last only 15–20 seconds. Three to 4 bouts are performed during each exercise session, with a 5-minute rest between bouts. Discomfort should be avoided. Exercise sessions are held daily for 2–3 days. If intense pain occurs after exercise, ice is applied; usually the cause is too much exercise.

Many ankles will recover full motion after 2 treatments but will still have intermittent pain. Continued reconditioning, with or without TNS, should reduce the pain within 10–14 days. If there is no response to TNS, cryotherapy or thermotherapy may be tried. Additional pathology must be ruled out.

▶ [The authors have responded to the extremely controversial question of when to begin reconditioning exercises. Their answer is, "Once the injury has stabilized." We should not become involved with a definition of terms regarding this subject, such as,

(7–38) Physician Sportsmed. 8:105–108, June 1980.

"What is *reconditioning*?" "What is the definition of *stabilized*?" The amount or type of reconditioning exercises that should be done is determined by the extent of the injury. Only exercises that will not disrupt tissue repair are permitted in the healing stages of any injury. In reconditioning an ankle injury with no joint or ligament laxity, a TNS unit can be helpful in relieving soreness and discomfort. The less pain experienced, the better the quality and amount of exercise that can be performed. The authors are very careful to explain, "The intensity of exercise should always be guided by the amount of residual pain."—F.G.] ◄

7–39 **Review of Physical Therapy Alternatives for Reducing Muscle Contracture** is presented by Dianne B. Cherry (Cleveland State Univ.). A primary goal of physical therapy is to maintain or regain range of motion in cases of orthopedic or neuromuscular dysfunction, to prevent or reduce myostatic contracture. Manual passive stretching of tight structures may be of limited effectiveness and often is painful. Kinesiologic and neurophysiologic research has provided alternatives. Muscle shortening may be due to intrinsic adaptive changes in response to prolonged positioning, as after orthopedic immobilization, or poor positioning with dynamic imbalance of muscle power, as in poliomyelitis. Contracture also may result from extrinsic influences such as central nervous system (CNS) damage. Any increased motion obtained passively will be lost unless maintained by active motion or by supportive devices.

The weak agonist may be activated or strengthened as an alternative to passive stretch. Such techniques are very useful in orthopedic rehabilitation and also in treating neurologic problems. If the agonist is very weak or inhibited, or both, facilitatory techniques using exteroceptive and proprioceptive stimulation may enhance its function. Vibration may be especially useful where the antagonist is spastic and the agonist is very inhibited. Another approach is inhibition of the tight muscle, which is useful for localized tightness, especially within one muscle group at one joint. Inhibition of muscle tone throughout the body can be achieved through both somatic and autonomic components of the CNS. This approach may be particularly effective where hypertonus or spasticity interferes with normal movement. Advanced muscular dystrophy or peripheral neuropathy may require direct passive lengthening. This is possible through prolonged holding of the desired position at the point of maximum tolerated muscle length, or by manual passive stretching of the tight antagonist. Passive stretching is likely to be most effective where the stretch reflex is inhibited, either by cortical effort at relaxation or in paralytic states.

Further research is needed to determine which procedures are most effective in various types of problems.

► [Much of what the author has presented can be related to the prevention and treatment of athletic injuries. Many teams are using proprioceptive neuromuscular facilitation (PNF) techniques in their stretching and flexibility programs. This is often accomplished through the "buddy system" of stretching. All good rehabilitation programs utilize active strengthening of weak agonists to improve joint range of motion and to restore normal strength and function.—F.G.] ◄

(7–39) Phys. Ther. 60:877–881, July 1980.

7-40 **Cryostretch for Muscle Spasm** is described by Kenneth L. Knight (Indiana State Univ.). Most muscle injuries cause some degree of muscle spasm or tightness. Many mild muscle "pulls" are actually low-grade spasm rather than fiber tears. Cryostretch therapy combines ice application with the hold-relax technique of proprioceptive neuromuscular facilitation, involving static and isometric stretching of the affected muscle. A brief neuromuscular training session is conducted before the first exercise session to help the athlete contract the injured muscle so that the joint moves through as great a range of motion as possible without resistance. The motion is repeated 2 or 3 times.

Each exercise bout consists of a 65-second set of static stretches and isometric contractions, a 20-second rest, and another set of exercises. Three bouts are performed during each treatment session (table), with 2 or 3 sessions each day. The muscle is numbed with a large cold pack or by massage with an ice cone. Initially the extremity or body part is moved until tightness or pain is felt (Fig 7–16). After holding the part in a pain-free position for 20 seconds, the athlete is told to contract the muscle and try to perform the practiced motion, which the therapist will resist. Rapid contraction is avoided; contraction should last about 5 seconds and be as strong as possible. After this, the part again is moved to the point of pain for 10 seconds. The sequence is repeated, ending with a 10-second stretch, and the 65-second set of exercises is repeated after the limb has rested in the anatomical position for 20 seconds.

Combined cryokinetic and cryostretch therapy is instituted when the spasm is partially relieved, often within 2–3 days. Cryokinetic exercises should begin with manually resisted muscle contraction through a full range of motion, and should proceed through graded running and team drills. Full activity must be resumed gradually to avoid reinjury.

▶ [I have found this particular combination of ice massage or ice pack and a contract-

Fig 7–16.—The therapist stretches the injured muscle (here, a hamstring muscle) before isometric contractions are started. (Courtesy of Knight, K. L.: Physician Sportsmed. 8:129, April 1980.)

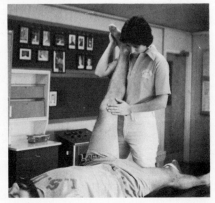

(7–40) Physician Sportsmed. 8:129, April 1980.

CRYOSTRETCH TECHNIQUE

1. Numb with ice (15 to 20 min)
2. Exercise (65 sec)
   20-sec static stretch
   5-sec isometric contraction
   10-sec static stretch
   5-sec isometric contraction
   10-sec static stretch
   5-sec isometric contraction
   10-sec static stretch
3. Rest in anatomical position (20 sec)
4. Repeat exercise (65 sec)
5. Renumb (3 to 5 min)
6. Repeat steps 2 through 5 twice

---

relax type of proprioceptive neuromuscular (PNF) stretch to be most beneficial in treating this type of injury. This same type of contract-relax type of stretching or flexibility exercise can be incorporated into team drills. The technique is easily taught, and athletes are eager to participate in the "buddy system" of stretching. At times, this PNF stretching produces very dramatic results.—F.G.] ◄

7–41 **A Reexamination of Lewis' Cold-Induced Vasodilatation: In the Finger and the Ankle** is reported by K. L. Knight, J. Aquino, S. M. Johannes, and C. D. Urban (Indiana State Univ., Terre Haute). Many sports medicine workers accept cold-induced vasodilatation (CIVD) as an explanation for the success of cryokinetics in the rehabilitation of acute musculoskeletal injuries. Support for this view came from the studies of Lewis of finger temperature on ice-water immersion, which appeared to demonstrate vasodilatation on removal of the cooled finger from the medium. However, Knight and Londeree showed a decrease in blood flow to the ankle during and after cold pack application. The present study used the approach of Lewis. Temperature measurements were made with surface probes in 6 male subjects. Both finger and ankle measurements were recorded in conjunction with ice water immersion.

Finger studies gave results like those reported by Lewis. Temperature decreased to 3 C within 5 minutes and rose to 24.6 C within 4 minutes of removal from ice. By 20 minutes after immersion, the temperature was 33.5 C, and it began decreasing after 10 minutes. The ankle reacted similarly to immersion, but afterward the temperature rose to 15.8 C in the first 10 minutes, and to only 19.2 C at 40 minutes. Differences between the finger and ankle responses after the end of immersion were significant.

These findings cast further doubt on the CIVD theory as an explanation for the success of cryokinetics. If an increase in blood flow to the injured area is critical in increasing the healing rate, as is assumed, treatment with ice application only will fail to promote healing, and may actually retard healing through reducing blood flow for a time, particularly in the ankle. Grant, in promoting cryokinetics for rehabilitation, postulated that early motion and restoration of normal

---

(7–41) Athletic Training 15:248–250, Winter 1980.

function in the injured area is the key to symptomatic improvement and that the use of ice is only an adjunctive measure used to relieve pain and permit early motion. Knight and Londeree obtained data supporting this view. Moore et al. agreed that therapeutic exercise is of prime importance in the success of cryotherapy.

▶ [I have never clearly understood cold-induced vasodilation and why we use ice as a first-aid measure and as a treatment modality. I use ice extensively in both instances for different reasons. As a treatment modality, I use ice to relieve pain and spasm so that more and better exercise can be done. Exercise is the key to increasing circulation and rebuilding flexibility and strength.

I use ice as a first aid measure for all the well-known reasons of increased blood viscosity and control of hemorrhage and on the basis that undamaged tissue adjacent to an injury can be saved from lack of oxygen if this tissue can be put into a temporary state of hibernation and therefore have less need for oxygen.

Cryokinetics is a major portion of most of my treatment programs. It is almost always cold first and then an additional modality. I use the cold until I stop receiving the results I expect to obtain with it.—F.G.] ◀

7–42 **Ice Massage and Transcutaneous Electric Stimulation: Comparison of Treatment for Low Back Pain.** Ice massage of the web between the thumb and index finger has produced greater relief of dental pain than a placebo procedure, indicating that it may be comparable to transcutaneous electric stimulation (TES) and acupuncture and may be mediated by similar neural mechanisms. R. Melzack, M. E. Jeans, J. G. Stratford, and R. C. Monks (McGill Univ.) examined the relative efficacy of ice massage and TES for relieving low back pain in 23 men and 21 women aged 18–73 years who had had pain for a mean of 7.4 years and had failed to respond to conventional treatment. A majority had had diskectomy and/or spinal fusion or

CHANGES IN LOW BACK PAIN WITH ICE MASSAGE AND TRANSCUTANEOUS
ELECTRIC STIMULATION

Study design	Ice massage	TES
Independent samples (N = 22)		
Mean % decrease in PRI	50.4%	48.7%
Range	6.7^-—98^+% *	17.3^+—100^+%
% patients reporting a PRI decrease >33%	68.2%	68.2%
Mean % decrease in PPI	45.5%	41.8%
Range	50^-—100^+%	2^+—100^+%
% patients reporting a PPI decrease >33%	72.7%	59.1%
Mean duration of pain relief	11.7 h	21.8 h
Range	0—96 h	0—2 wks
Crossover (N = 38)		
Mean % decrease in PRI	44.5%	42.8%
Range	76^-—100^+%	0—100^+%
% patients reporting a PRI decrease >33%	69.1%	67.5%
Mean % decrease in PPI	50%	32.5%
Range	50^-—100^+%	16^-—100^+%
% patients reporting a PPI decrease >33%	73.9%	53.4%
Mean duration of pain relief	10.9 h	22.6 h
Range	0—96 h	0—2 wks

*A minus sign represents a pain increase.

(7–42) Pain 9:209, October 1980.

showed radiologic evidence of degenerative disk disease. Ice massage and TES were administered in random order, and pain relief was assessed by the McGill Pain Questionairre. Ice massage was administered with an ice cube and gauze pad at the sites used for TES: the midline at L3 and S1 and the lateral malleolus of the side with the most marked pain.

The results are presented in the table. Both ice massage and TES produced substantial reductions in pain, but there were no significant differences between the treatments in independent samples, and mean reductions in pain scores were comparable on crossover analysis. Both treatments were equally effective with high and low initial pain levels. Thirteen of 29 patients preferred TES, while 9 preferred ice massage, and 5 requested other treatment. Fourteen of 30 patients who had follow-up had continued treatment. Several had purchased or rented TES devices and used them daily or when needed. Five patients still practiced ice massage.

Brief, intense cold appears to have analgesic effects comparable to those produced by TES and acupuncture. Probably intense cold activates brain stem mechanisms that exert descending inhibitory influences on pain signals. Ice massage is clearly effective in relieving low back pain. Both ice massage and TES should be tried in a clinic setting, but ice massage is a more convenient means of treatment at home. It usually is moderately painful, however, and another person must administer it. Patients who after a time find TES less effective than before may try ice massage.

▶ [As I stated above, for acute injuries I usually use ice with other modalities. It may be ice and electric muscle stimulation, or ice and transcutaneous electric stimulation, or ice and ultrasound, but almost always ice and exercise. It is safe, available, inexpensive, and easy to use in a home program. Why not try it? The ultimate test is what you use on yourself when an injury occurs.—F.G.] ◀

7–43 **Considerations in Ultrasound Therapy and Equipment Performance.** The Bureau of Radiologic Health of the Food and Drug Administration has issued, under the authority of The Radiation Control for Health and Safety Act of 1968, a regulatory performance standard for ultrasound therapy equipment manufactured on or after February 17, 1979. Harold F. Stewart, Jesse L. Abzug, and Gerald R. Harris (Food and Drug Administration, Rockville) discuss various topics relevant to the use of ultrasound in physical therapy including the physics of ultrasound, equipment calibration, ultrasonic output, waveform and field distribution specifications, and harmful biologic effects of ultrasound.

Because field tests showed that most ultrasonic therapy equipment was not calibrated within ±20%, the standard requires manufacturers to specify how often their equipment should be calibrated. The standard also requires that for continuous-wave waveforms, the temporal average ultrasonic power and intensity be indicated on the device. For pulsed waveforms, information on the temporal maximum power and intensity must be stated and information on the generator

(7–43) Phys. Ther. 60:424–428, April 1980.

must include the ratio of the temporal maximum intensity to the temporal average intensity, pulse duration and repetition, and a graphic of the shape of the pulse waveform. All units must be able to shut down automatically. Specific information about the spatial intensity variations within the ultrasonic beam should be displayed.

Ultrasonic therapy can produce potentially harmful levels of radiation; therefore, equipment performance standards were designed to ensure maximum safety and efficacy. It is incumbent on the user to maintain the equipment and be informed of possible health hazards.

▶ [The complete article is recommended reading for persons prescribing or administrating ultrasound therapy.—J.S.T.] ◀

7–44   **Phonophoresis: A Review of the Literature and Technique** is presented by William S. Quillen (U.S. Naval Academy). Phonophoresis is a technique whereby molecules of medication are driven subcutaneously by ultrasound application. It is used infrequently, although reports of its clinical efficacy have appeared for over 25 years. Penetration of medication for up to 6 cm by phonophoresis has been described. The indications are essentially those for therapeutic ultrasound, with the limitations imposed by systemic medication.

TECHNIQUE.—A continuous ultrasound waveform is utilized. The area to be treated is washed, preheated, and covered with a layer of cream or petrolatum base. Bony prominences may be treated by immersion in a water bath at 33 C. The dosage rarely exceeds 2.5 watts/sq cm for 5–6 minutes, unless the total surface area is over 100 sq cm. Separate fields are treated where larger areas are present. Both steady linear and circular stroking methods of application have been advocated. From 3 to 9 treatment sessions have been used, with frequencies twice weekly to daily.

Hydrocortisone is used in the great majority of phonophoresis treatments. Prolonged application of steriods to load-bearing structures can lead to their failure under stress. Aldes, in 1954, reported favorable results with injected hydrocortisone followed by ultrasound therapy in common articular orthopedic conditions such as arthritis and bursitis. The most definitive research on therapeutic ultrasound has been done by Griffin and Touchstone et al., using swine tissue as a human homologue (1963, 1965, 1968, and 1972). They showed that ultrasound can drive molecules of topically applied hydrocortisone into paravertebral muscle and nerve. Clinical trials of ultrasound phonophoresis have been limited. Moll (1979) recently reported significant improvement from steroid-lidocaine ultrasound phonophoresis compared to placebo treatment in patients with chronic back pain unresponsive to other conservative measures.

Phonophoresis offers a safe, painless alternative to subcutaneous injections in the treatment of various inflammatory states. Needle phobia is circumvented by this measure, and the hazards of infection and tissue trauma are minimized. With proper application, phonophoresis can be a valuable tool in treating sports-related injuries.

▶ [Phonophoresis and, more notably, a new form of iontophoresis have recieved a

(7–44)   Athletic Training 15:109–110, Summer 1980.

revival of exposure in the literature and at clinical meetings. Iontophoresis was at one time quite popular, then all but disappeared in many practices. The use of phonophoresis has never really become widespread or popular in the treatment of athletic injuries. My own experience with these modalities has paralleled the use of other modalities. I have had some successes and some failures, with few predetermining factors.— F.G.] ◄

7–45 **Electric Muscle Stimulation During Immobilization.** Immobilization of joints is often necessary to allow stretched or torn ligaments to heal. Despite isometric contraction of the muscles surrounding an immobilized joint, the muscular atrophy that results can markedly delay the athlete's return to activity. Kenneth L. Knight (Indiana State Univ., Terre Haute) describes a technique that combines electrical stimulation of the lower leg muscles with isometric contraction during postsurgical immobilization of the knee. The technique can also be used during cast immobilization of a sprained ankle.

TECHNIQUE.—Holes 3–4 sq cm in size are cut in the cast over the distal portions of the anterior tibialis, the peroneal group, and the triceps surae. An active electrode 2½ cm in length is then introduced through each of the holes to provide stimulation of the muscle. A dispersive electrode 7½ cm long is applied above the cast and held firmly to the leg with a rubber strap (Fig 7–17). (It may be necessary to force the dispersive electrode under the cast to obtain optimal muscle stimulation.) A nontetanic (pulse rate less than 40/minute), nonsurge current is applied at a voltage as high as can be comfortably tolerated. Each muscle is stimulated for 1 minute on the first day. On each succeeding day up to 5 days, the stimulation time is increased by 1 minute. Thereafter, each muscle is stimulated for 5 minutes daily. Ten repetitions of isometric contractions should be performed by each muscle before and after stimulation; this should also be done 5–10 additional times throughout the day. Both legs should be exercised isotonically and isometrically to maintain strength, endurance, and quickness. A bicycle should be ridden vigorously for 30–60 minutes daily to maintain cardiovascular fitness.

The technique has produced good results: a basketball player who

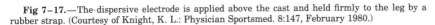

Fig 7–17.—The dispersive electrode is applied above the cast and held firmly to the leg by a rubber strap. (Courtesy of Knight, K. L.: Physician Sportsmed. 8:147, February 1980.)

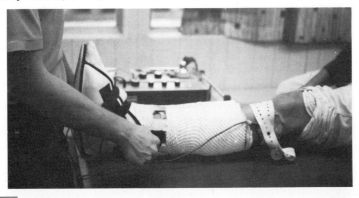

(7–45) Physician Sportsmed. 8:147, February 1980.

had worn a cast for a lateral ankle sprain for 7 weeks was able to play 19 minutes of a game only 2 days after cast removal.

▶ [As I noted in my comment to a previous article in this chapter (7-33), this technique of electric muscle stimulation has been effective in some knee rehabilitation programs. I have had no experience with the use of this technique on casted muscles of the lower leg, but I have had acceptable results with it when stimulating lower leg muscles that are not casted. Any procedure that safely can be used to speed rehabilitation time is worth trying, and this is a good example.—F.G.] ◀

7-46 **Predictors for the Outcome of Treatment With High-Frequency Transcutaneous Electric Nerve Stimulation in Patients With Chronic Pain.** Up to half of patients with chronic pain have reported acceptable pain relief with different kinds of transcutaneous nerve stimulation (TNS), but relief tends to decline in time in some cases. There is much empiricism in the application of various modalities of TNS. F. Johansson, B. G. L. Almay, L. von Knorring (Univ. of Umeå), and L. Terenius (Univ. of Uppsala) evaluated some possible predictors of the outcome of high-frequency TNS in 72 patients with pain for at least 6 months, who had tried several other types of treatment, including surgery, often without gaining adequate relief. None had taken narcotic analgesics. Forty-one patients had neurogenic pain, usually peripheral; 23 had somatogenic pain, and 8 had psychogenic pain. The TNS treatment was carried out with impulses in the range of 80–100 Hz. Positive results consisted of 20% or greater relief on visual analogue scale assessment for more than 30 minutes after stimulation.

Age and sex did not significantly influence the results of treatment, nor was pain intensity a significant predictive factor. Patients with neurogenic pain responded significantly better than those with somatogenic or psychogenic pain. Patients with extremity pain from organic causes benefited significantly more than those with pain in axial structures. Among 22 patients with organic pain, those with a positive response to TNS had somewhat lower mean CSF fraction I endorphin levels, but the difference was not significant.

About half of patients in this study had acceptable pain relief from high-frequency TNS. Patients with neurogenic pain of mostly peripheral origin and those with segmental extremity pain did the best. Patients with lower CSF endorphin levels tended to respond better to TNS. Personality characteristics and psychiatric symptoms may also influence the results of peripheral nerve stimulation for pain relief.

▶ [The problem is deciding which modality to use for best response for relief of pain. The authors have described which type of pain responds best to TNS treatment. As would be expected, those patients with neurogenic pain responded the best. As I mentioned after the article on phonophoresis, there is no one modality that works all the time on every injury. Therefore, we should not expect this to occur with TNS units; TNS units can be effective for the relief of pain with some athletic injuries and not others. It should be tried in the regular treatment regimen, when pain is a major factor of the injury. It should also be tried when pain limits the type of reconditioning exercises that can be performed.—F.G.] ◀

(7–46) Pain 9:55–61, August 1980.

7–47 **Effect of Biofeedback and Static Stretching on Muscle Pain.**
Persons engaging in rigorous muscular activity commonly have muscle pain, during or up to 48 hours after physical activity. Immediate pain is thought to be chiefly due to end products of metabolism and local tissue edema, but the cause of delayed pain or soreness remains unclear. There is considerable evidence that complete relaxation of normal resting muscle can be demonstrated electromyographically and that a normal subject can reduce neuromuscular activity in skeletal muscles through relaxing. George H. McGlynn and Neil Laughlin (Univ. of San Francisco) evaluated biofeedback and static muscle stretching in 48 men aged 18–23 years, in whom muscle soreness was induced through eccentric contraction by means of a dumbbell at a weight 80% of the subject's maximum level. Five 15-minute biofeedback sessions were held from 6 to 54 hours after exercise. Subjects were encouraged to imagine themselves in a warm, confortable situation, to concentrate on specific details of the scene, and to try to

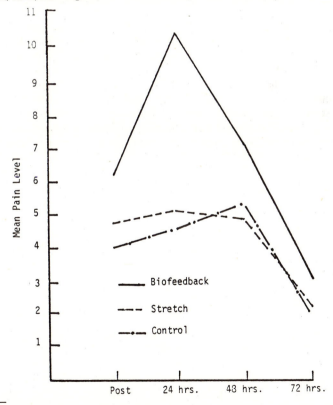

Fig 7–18.—Mean pain levels in the biofeedback, static stretching, and control groups. (Courtesy of McGlynn, G. H., and Laughlin, N.: Athletic Training 15:43–45, Spring 1980.)

relax the muscles in line with the feedback. A static stretch method was used by other subjects at the same intervals.

Pain levels are shown in Figure 7–18. Perceived pain in the biofeedback group was significantly greater than that in the static stretch and control groups. These subjects may have been more conscious of, or sensitive to, pain in the biceps brachii because the biofeedback technique had them focus on this muscle group, and perceived pain is a subjective phenomenon dependent on the focus of each person. In contrast to the other groups, perceived pain in the biofeedback group was considerably greater 24 hours after exercise than immediately after exercise.

Most research on the effects of biofeedback on pain has concerned pain not produced by exercise. The present findings indicate that biofeedback was less effective than both static stretching and rest in reducing exercise-produced pain. Further study is needed of the effects of both biofeedback and static stretching on various types of pain incurred in sports activities.

▶ [As the authors state, "The cause of delayed pain or soreness after exercise remains unclear." Athletic trainers have been advocating stretching and flexibility exercises to relieve exercise-induced delayed muscle soreness. It is sometimes difficult to convince tired athletes that they should do these exercises after practice and in the evening. Once they learn how effective this stretching can be to relieve pain, they soon become advocates of the "postpractice stretch."—F.G.] ◀

7–48   **Electromyographic Biofeedback in Exercise Programs** is discussed by Steven L. Wolf (Emory Univ.). Electronic biofeedback techniques have produced remarkable functional improvements in patients with such conditions as stroke, cerebral palsy, and torticollis, who must relearn control over sensorimotor integration to regain function. Surprisingly few efforts have been made to use biofeedback methods in persons with musculoskeletal dysfunction or those requiring improved muscle strength or athletic skill. Theoretically, such persons should readily process biofeedback signals representing muscle activity or joint position, since neural disruption is not present, and should be able to process them more accurately and rapidly than any verbal cues provided by a coach or clinician assessing motor performance.

Applications of electromyographic (EMG) biofeedback training are listed in the table. The method may be used for relaxation or reduction of muscle tension due to anxiety or muscle splinting or guarding. Biofeedback training is begun soon after knee surgery with an electrode pair over the rectus femoris muscle. The goal is to feed back localized and isolated muscle activity as the patient attempts an isometric quadriceps contraction. More widely spaced electrodes are utilized to recruit more motor unit activity progressively until the entire muscle is activated. Another approach involves control and strength during dynamic movements, with minimization of extraneous muscle activation. Biofeedback units that process 2 EMG channels simulta-

(7–48)   Physician Sportsmed. 8:61–69, November 1980.

APPLICATIONS OF EMG BIOFEEDBACK TRAINING

	PRIMARY STRATEGY	SECONDARY STRATEGY
TRAUMA OR SURGERY		
Weakness following immobilization	Increase EMG activity	Increase range of motion
Muscle reeducation		
Peripheral nerve repair		
Gait training		
Joint contracture	Increase range of motion	Increase EMG activity
Tendon repair		
Soft tissue injury		
Muscle spasm and pain	Relaxation; reduce EMG activity	
IMPROVING ATHLETIC SKILL		
Weakness	Increase EMG activity	
Substitution movements	Decrease extraneous EMG activity	
Target muscle strengthening and sequence timing	Increase EMG activity	

neously are now available. This ratio mode can be used to gain motor control in either clinical or sports-related activities and to enhance motions related to athletic skills.

Little is yet known of how to use EMG biofeedback to develop athletic prowess. Feedback could be used not only to assess the magnitude of muscle activity, but also to ascertain the timing of such activity with respect to other muscles participating in a specific athletic movement. Performance could be altered by gradually changing the demand setting for the magnitude of contraction and the sequencing of muscle activation. More knowledge is needed about the distribution of motor unit types within muscles and the predominant type within each part of a muscle that acts on more than one joint.

▶ [Biofeedback is an–as yet–untouched entity in the search for greater strength, speed, and power. I am not sure why. Even in countries where this type of experimentation has been popular, the use of biofeedback in athletic performance-type situations has not been reported at length. Only one of the author's 25 references concerns biofeedback and athletics.

The preceding article showed disappointing results for the use of biofeedback to relieve delayed exercise-induced pain. Perhaps this technique is only helpful to those with central nervous system disorders. Certainly, more study and experimentation need be done.—F.G.] ◄

Subject Index

Index to Authors

The number after each entry is the reference number of the author's article in the text. The reference number indicates the chapter in which the article appears and its numerical order within the chapter.

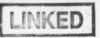

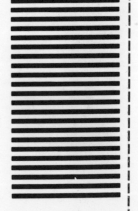